Access Device Standards of Practice
FOR ONCOLOGY NURSING

Edited by
Dawn Camp-Sorrell, RN, MSN, FNP, AOCN®
Laurl Matey, MSN, RN, CHPN

Oncology Nursing Society
Pittsburgh, Pennsylvania

ONS Publications Department
Publisher and Director of Publications: William A. Tony, BA, CQIA
Managing Editor: Lisa M. George, BA
Assistant Managing Editor: Amy Nicoletti, BA, JD
Acquisitions Editor: John Zaphyr, BA, MEd
Copy Editors: Vanessa Kattouf, BA, Andrew Petyak, BA
Graphic Designer: Dany Sjoen
Editorial Assistant: Judy Holmes

First printing, January 2017
Second printing, November 2018

Library of Congress Cataloging-in-Publication Data

Names: Camp-Sorrell, Dawn, editor. | Matey, Laurl, editor. | Oncology Nursing
  Society, issuing body.
Title: Access device standards of practice for oncology nursing / edited by
  Dawn Camp-Sorrell, Laurl Matey.
Description: Pittsburgh, Pennsylvania : Oncology Nursing Society, [2017] |
  Includes bibliographical references and index.
Identifiers: LCCN 2016042284 | ISBN 9781935864905
Subjects: | MESH: Neoplasms–nursing | Vascular Access Devices–standards |
  Infusions, Parenteral–instrumentation | Oncology Nursing–standards |
  Handbooks
Classification: LCC RC266 | NLM WY 49 | DDC 616.99/40231–dc23 LC record available at https://lccn.loc.gov/2016042284

Publisher's Note

This book is published by the Oncology Nursing Society (ONS). ONS neither represents nor guarantees that the practices described herein will, if followed, ensure safe and effective patient care. The recommendations contained in this book reflect ONS's judgment regarding the state of general knowledge and practice in the field as of the date of publication. The recommendations may not be appropriate for use in all circumstances. Those who use this book should make their own determinations regarding specific safe and appropriate patient care practices, taking into account the personnel, equipment, and practices available at the hospital or other facility at which they are located. The editors and publisher cannot be held responsible for any liability incurred as a consequence from the use or application of any of the contents of this book. Figures and tables are used as examples only. They are not meant to be all-inclusive, nor do they represent endorsement of any particular institution by ONS. Mention of specific products and opinions related to those products do not indicate or imply endorsement by ONS. Websites mentioned are provided for information only; the hosts are responsible for their own content and availability. Unless otherwise indicated, dollar amounts reflect U.S. dollars.

ONS publications are originally published in English. Publishers wishing to translate ONS publications must contact ONS about licensing arrangements. ONS publications cannot be translated without obtaining written permission from ONS. (Individual tables and figures that are reprinted or adapted require additional permission from the original source.) Because translations from English may not always be accurate or precise, ONS disclaims any responsibility for inaccuracies in words or meaning that may occur as a result of the translation. Readers relying on precise information should check the original English version.

Printed in the United States of America

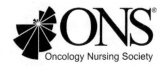

Innovation • Excellence • Advocacy

To our mothers, who brought us together in so many ways.

—Dawn Camp-Sorrell and Laurl Matey

Contributors

Editors

Dawn Camp-Sorrell, RN, MSN, FNP, AOCN®
Oncology Nurse Practitioner
Children's Hospital of Alabama
Birmingham, Alabama
Chapter 4. Nontunneled Central Venous Lines

Laurl Matey, MSN, RN, CHPN
Oncology Clinical Specialist
Oncology Nursing Society
Pittsburgh, Pennsylvania
Chapter 1. Access Device Standards, Recommendations, and Controversies; Chapter 4. Nontunneled Central Venous Lines

Authors

Diane G. Cope, PhD, ARNP-BC, AOCNP®
Oncology Nurse Practitioner
Florida Cancer Specialists and Research Institute
Fort Myers, Florida
Chapter 1. Access Device Standards, Recommendations, and Controversies; Chapter 3. Midline Catheters; Chapter 5. Peripherally Inserted Central Catheters

Carole Marie Elledge, RN, MSN, AOCN®
Clinical Program Specialist
Methodist Hospital
San Antonio, Texas
Chapter 12. Intraventricular Access Devices; Chapter 13. Epidural and Intrathecal Access Devices

Heather Thompson Mackey, RN, MSN, ANP-BC, AOCN®
Nurse Practitioner, Cancer Survivorship
Cone Health Cancer Center
Greensboro, North Carolina
Chapter 2. Short-Term Peripheral Intravenous Catheters; Chapter 6. Tunneled Central Venous Catheters; Chapter 8. Apheresis Catheters; Chapter 15. Pleural Catheters; Chapter 17. Education, Documentation, and Legal Issues for Access Devices

Andrea B. Moran, RN, APRN
Adult Hematology/Oncology Nurse Practitioner
University of Connecticut Health
Farmington, Connecticut
Chapter 10. Subcutaneous (Hypodermoclysis) Infusion Devices; Chapter 16. Ambulatory Infusion Pumps

Miriam Rogers, EdD, MN, RN, AOCN®
Director
CANursing Enrichment
Willow Spring, North Carolina
Chapter 14. Intraperitoneal Catheters

Lisa Schulmeister, RN, MN, ACNS-BC, FAAN
Oncology Nursing Consultant
New Orleans, Louisiana
Chapter 7. Implanted Venous Ports; Chapter 9. Complications of Long-Term Venous Access Devices

Lisa Hartkopf Smith, MS, RN, AOCN®, CNS
Oncology Clinical Nurse Specialist
Riverside Methodist Hospital
Columbus, Ohio
Chapter 11. Arterial Access Devices

Mady Stovall, RN, MSN, ANP-BC
PhD Student
Oregon Health and Science University, School of Nursing
Portland, Oregon
Chapter 13. Epidural and Intrathecal Access Devices

Disclosure

Editors and authors of books and guidelines provided by the Oncology Nursing Society are expected to disclose to the readers any significant financial interest or other relationships with the manufacturer(s) of any commercial products.

A vested interest may be considered to exist if a contributor is affiliated with or has a financial interest in commercial organizations that may have a direct or indirect interest in the subject matter. A "financial interest" may include, but is not limited to, being a shareholder in the organization; being an employee of the commercial organization; serving on an organization's speakers bureau; or receiving research funding from the organization. An "affiliation" may be holding a position on an advisory board or some other role of benefit to the commercial organization. Vested interest statements appear in the front matter for each publication.

Contributors are expected to disclose any unlabeled or investigational use of products discussed in their content. This information is acknowledged solely for the information of the readers.

The contributors provided the following disclosure and vested interest information:

Laurl Matey, MSN, RN, CHPN: American Nurses Association, consultant or advisory role; Grand Canyon University School of Nursing, leadership role

Heather Thompson Mackey, RN, MSN, ANP-BC, AOCN®: Oncology Nursing Society, employment or leadership position

Lisa Hartkopf Smith, MS, RN, AOCN®, CNS: Genentech Gadzyva Program for Nurses, honoraria

Contents

Abbreviations

AANA—American Association of Nurse Anesthetists
ANTT—aseptic no-touch technique
APN—advanced practice nurse
APRN—advanced practice registered nurse
BSI—bloodstream infection
CDC—Centers for Disease Control and Prevention
CHG—chlorhexidine gluconate
CLABSI—central line–associated bloodstream infection
CNS—central nervous system
CRBSI—catheter-related bloodstream infection
CSF—cerebrospinal fluid
CT—computed tomography
CVAD—central venous access device
CVC—central venous catheter
DERS—dose error reduction system
DVT—deep vein thrombosis
EMR—electronic medical record
EtOH—ethanol
HCl—hydrochloric acid
ICU—intensive care unit
IJ—internal jugular
INR—international normalized ratio

INS—Infusion Nurses Society
IP—intraperitoneal
IR—interventional radiology
IV—intravenous
LMWH—low-molecular-weight heparin
MPE—malignant pleural effusion
MRI—magnetic resonance imaging
NCCN—National Comprehensive Cancer Network
NS—0.9% normal saline
ONS—Oncology Nursing Society
OR—operating room
PASV—pressure-activated safety valve
PICC—peripherally inserted central catheter
PIV—peripheral intravenous
RN—registered nurse
SC—subcutaneous
SVC—superior vena cava
TENS—transcutaneous electrical nerve stimulation
tPA—tissue plasminogen activator
TPN—total parenteral nutrition
VAD—venous access device
WHO—World Health Organization

Introduction

For decades, access devices have been used to deliver complex and diverse treatments to patients with cancer. IV therapy is an integral part of modern medicine and nursing, as it is practiced in every healthcare setting, from the hospital to the home. A new generation of access devices is quickly being adapted to provide a safe means to administer therapies into body systems, such as the peritoneal, arterial, epidural, pleural, or intraventricular spaces. The daily use of access devices is central to the care that oncology nurses provide to patients with cancer. With this increased complexity, nurses have an increased responsibility in maintaining access devices and a key role in preventing device-related complications.

Evolving technology continuously leads to newer devices and products used concurrently with access devices. This technology continues to improve existing access devices to decrease the occurrence of the most frequent complications: infection and occlusion. Increased safety features, for both patient and provider, help to decrease accidental exposures or catheter malposition. As new products emerge, nurses must advance their knowledge to provide competent and safe care.

Little empirical evidence and research are available to support evidence-based nursing care related to venous access devices (VADs). Few randomized controlled trials have been conducted to definitively support nursing practices. Practice continues to be dictated by manufacturer recommendations or manufacturer in vitro clinical trials performed for U.S. Food and Drug Administration device or product approval. Government regulations also dictate care from the standpoint of insurance reimbursement, but without clear evidence to support specific practices; in the absence of evidence but in the face of reimbursement losses, practices may be adopted without clear evidence to support them. Expert opinion and institution-specific historical data often are used to develop policies.

Oncology nurses must base practice on evidence-based research when available, but lack of evidence is a professional challenge. Given this challenge, the Oncology Nursing Society (ONS) recognizes that both the unique complexities of patients with cancer and the extensive use of access devices in this population warrants standards and recommendations that meet the specific needs of nurses who specialize in oncology nursing. ONS is well positioned to define the standards of excellence for access device management in the specialty of oncology nursing and has continually updated its access device recommendations since 1989. Terminology used in *Access Device Standards of Practice for Oncology Nursing* is deliberately chosen to distinguish between evidence-based practices and those for which no definitive evidence is available.

Access Device Standards of Practice for Oncology Nursing was developed through a multiphasic process, beginning with an exhaustive analysis of empirical research, meta-analytical summaries, case reports, and review articles. PubMed, Cumulative Index to Nursing and Allied Health Literature, Cochrane Library, Database of Abstracts of Reviews of Effects, National Guideline Clearinghouse, U.S. Preventive Services Task Force, and Turning Research Into Practice databases were queried to ensure complete data inclusion. Although the main focus of these standards is the adult population, research conducted with pediatric populations is included when available and when appropriate to extrapolate findings to adults. Following this synthesis of evidence, clinical experts working in the field of oncology nursing developed each chapter. Several editorial review cycles followed to ensure accuracy and inclusion of all relevant data. Field reviewers, including the Infusion Nurses Society, were invited to provide in-depth analysis and feedback. An open public comment period was offered to ensure a rigorous and transparent review process. Appendix 1 provides evidence demonstrating the strength on which standard statements are made.

The ONS Board of Directors defines the characteristics of a *standard* as "an authoritative document that provides requirements, specifications, and/or characteristics that shall be used consistently across practice settings to ensure that nursing actions, processes, and services are used to achieve desired optimal results" (www.ons.org/practice-resources/standards-reports). Practice statements in this publication are identified as standards, recommendations, or as practice for which no evidence can support a definitive statement in the case of lacking evidence. The following language is used to identify these statements:

- Practice standard: Evidence is sufficient to conclude the acceptance of this practice.
- Practice recommendation: Evidence is less robust; expert opinion, generally accepted practice, and sound nursing judgment warrant consideration of this practice.
- No definitive recommendation can be made: Evidence is lacking to support a definitive practice.

The Standards have been developed from this synthesis of evidence, critical review, and analysis, focusing on those aspects of VAD management for which nursing is accountable and directly associated with VAD care. Historical evidence, when provided, is offered when recent evidence is lacking or to underscore the strength of a standard statement.

Ongoing surveillance of infection and occlusion rates and daily evaluation of access device use will help any institution evaluate policies to determine if revisions in practice are needed. Access device manufacturer websites should be consulted for recommendations on specific brands and device types. With limited research to guide practice, ongoing controversies remain concerning optimal management. Developing the expertise needed to successfully manage access devices is a continual challenge to nursing professionals. The intent of these standards is to provide the foundation for evidence-based practice to guide individual oncology nursing practice.

Access Device Standards of Practice for Oncology Nursing is arranged in chapters for ease of use. Chapter 1 critically reviews controversies in access device care. Standard statements and recommendations made are based on the evidence presented. The remaining chapters detail each venous and specialty device. Patient selection criteria and advantage/disadvantage tables within each chapter can be used to select the best device based on the patient's needs. Chapter 17 explores recommended documentation and key legal ramifications concerning access devices and their management. Examples of competency practicums are provided as appendices.

It is clear that, despite the lack of evidence-based practice for care of access devices, patient quality of life has greatly improved over the past decades with the advances in access device technology. *Access Device Standards of Practice for Oncology Nursing* explores the latest technologies, management procedures, and the controversies that remain.

Dawn Camp-Sorrell, RN, MSN, FNP, AOCN®
Laurl Matey, MSN, RN, CHPN

Chapter 1

Access Device Standards, Recommendations, and Controversies

Diane G. Cope, PhD, ARNP-BC, AOCNP®, and Laurl Matey, MSN, RN, CHPN

- **Practice standard:** Evidence is sufficient to conclude the acceptance of this practice.
- **Practice recommendation:** Evidence is less robust; expert opinion, generally accepted practice, and sound nursing judgment warrant consideration of this practice.
- No definitive recommendation can be made: Evidence is lacking to support a definitive practice.
- Recent evidence: Evidence is used to support standard or recommendation or to demonstrate insufficient evidence to recommend practice.
- Historical evidence: Evidence is provided as a historical reference; may or may not support current standards or recommendation statements.

(See Appendix 1 for a summary of studies related to access devices.)

I. Placement imaging

What is the best evidence regarding imaging studies to ensure proper placement of a central venous access device (CVAD) during or postprocedure?

A. **Practice recommendation:** Consider the use of ultrasound guidance to place central venous catheters (if this technology is available) to reduce the number of cannulation attempts and mechanical complications. Ultrasound guidance should be used only by those fully trained in its technique (Lamperti et al., 2012; O'Grady et al., 2011).

B. No definitive recommendation can be made regarding the use of intracavitary electrocardiography for central venous catheter placement based on the available evidence.

C. Recent evidence

1. Chest imaging, such as x-rays or fluoroscopic images, traditionally has been used to guide and to verify catheter positioning (Roldan & Paniagua, 2015; Zadeh & Shirvani, 2014).

2. Multiple studies and review articles assert that ultrasound-guided insertion by skilled practitioners should be used to decrease the number of cannulation attempts, reduce complications, and guide correct catheter tip placement by those trained and skilled in this technique (Ahn et al., 2012; Bowen, Mone, Nelson, & Scaife, 2014; Brass, Hellmich, Kolodziej, Schick, & Smith, 2015; Gibson & Bodenham, 2013; Lamperti et al., 2012; O'Grady et al., 2011; Teichgräber, Kausche, Nagel, & Gebauer, 2011; Thomopoulos et al., 2014).

3. A retrospective analysis concluded that if a port is placed with ultrasound or fluoroscopy, a postoperative chest x-ray is not needed to confirm placement (Bowen et al., 2014). Additional studies found accurate catheter tip placement with intracavitary electrocardiogram- and fluoroscopy-guided catheter placement. The studies concluded that the requirement of post-procedural chest x-ray to assess catheter tip placement potentially could be eliminated (Thomopoulos et al., 2014; Walker et al., 2015).

4. Multicenter research reveals that an intracavitary electrocardiography is a safe and accurate alternative method of positioning the catheter tip in the pediatric population (Rossetti et al., 2015). Similar findings have been shown in adult patient populations (Walker, Alexandrou, Rickard, Chan, & Webster, 2015; Wang et al., 2015).

5. Ultrasound or electrocardiogram guidance often may be unavailable where CVADs are needed, such as in urgent situations in the emergency department or operating suite. Skillful insertion of CVADs with subsequent radiographic confirmation of tip placement has proven to be safe and

---

Authors' note: This chapter cites "Historical References," which appear in a separate list at the end of this chapter for further information.

effective in ensuring proper tip placement (Gan & Lanigan, 2013; see also Historical References).

II. Dressing types

What is the best evidence regarding type of dressing (transparent versus gauze and tape) for venous access devices (VADs)?

A. No definitive recommendation can be made based on the available evidence.

Until prospective, multisite, randomized studies are conducted using standardized cleansing protocols, frequency of dressing changes, differences in transparent dressing brands, patient characteristics (e.g., patient disease, comorbidities, treatment, age), and outcome variables, determining which type of dressing and maintenance care protocol will result in the least number of complications will remain inconclusive.

B. Recent evidence

1. The Centers for Disease Control and Prevention (CDC) practice guidelines suggest that dressing choice could be a matter of patient preference (O'Grady et al., 2011).

2. A recent Cochrane systematic review of randomized controlled trials evaluated CVAD–related bloodstream infections with available CVAD dressing and securement devices (Ullman et al., 2015). Twenty-two studies involving 7,436 participants were evaluated, analyzing a variety of different interventions and comparisons involving sterile gauze, standard polyurethane, chlorhexidine gluconate (CHG)–impregnated dressings, silver-impregnated dressings, hydrocolloid dressings, second-generation gas-permeable standard polyurethane, and sutureless securement devices. Results indicated that medication-impregnated dressing products, defined as only CHG-impregnated dressings in a patch or a whole dressing, reduced the incidence of CVAD-related bloodstream infection relative to all other dressing types. Most studies were conducted in the intensive care unit, and the authors cautioned that the effectiveness of CHG-impregnated dressings may not be generalizable beyond these settings.

3. In a clinical trial comparing the safety (phlebitis, pain, and leakage) and costs of transparent versus gauze dressings in patients with peripherally inserted central catheters (PICCs), no significant differences in complication rates were found (Chico-Padrón et al., 2011). The authors concluded that increased costs were associated with gauze dressings compared to transparent dressings, as the gauze dressing required frequent replacement.

4. A randomized controlled clinical trial was conducted to compare the effectiveness of gauze and tape dressing and transparent polyurethane film dressing in a sample of 21 catheters (Pedrolo, Danski, & Vayego, 2014). No significant differences were found in catheter-related infections, dressing stability, or exudate absorption. A significant difference in local reaction was found in the gauze and tape group compared to the transparent film dressing group.

C. Historical evidence

1. Past studies, using both retrospective and prospective designs, support and refute the use of gauze and transparent dressings (see Historical References).

   a) Many of these studies had methodologic flaws and insufficient power to detect significant differences in infection rates; therefore, drawing conclusions regarding differences in infection remains inconclusive.

   b) Multiple operational definitions exist of concepts such as catheter-related infections, varying measures of outcomes, different patient populations, cleansing protocols, frequency of dressing changes, catheter dwell times, and types of catheters.

   c) Studies in which prospective designs were used revealed an increase in catheter tip and exit-site infections with transparent occlusive dressings compared to dry gauze dressings; however, the majority of these studies were conducted over 20 years ago.

2. Investigators who conducted studies in which infection rates were higher with transparent dressings concluded that the transparent dressings did not allow for adequate evaporation of perspiration, leading to increased colonization of bacteria at the catheter exit site. Most studies were done with older dressing designs (over 25 years ago, beginning in the 1980s). Current dressing designs are available that may reduce the rate of organism colonization; however, further randomized controlled trials are needed.

3. Newer designs of transparent dressings with semipermeable and highly permeable membranes that allow for increased mois-

ture vapor transmission rates can remove up to eight times more moisture from the exit site than previous types of transparent dressings.

4. Cost: Historical research concluded that the cost of transparent dressings, even when the frequency of dressing changes is considered, remained higher than the cost of dry gauze dressings (see Historical References). More recent data contradict these findings (Chico-Padrón et al., 2011).

5. No dressing versus gauze dressing: One study investigated catheter-related sepsis, comparing no dressing or gauze dressing for newly inserted tunneled catheters in bone marrow transplant recipients (Olson et al., 2004). Findings suggested that no significant difference existed in catheter-related sepsis between the no dressing and gauze dressing groups; however, the gauze dressing group had a significantly shorter time interval to the development of sepsis.

III. Cleansing agents (see Appendix 2)

What is the best evidence regarding type of cleansing procedure for VADs?

A. Before insertion or implantation

1. **Practice standard:** Scrub the skin at the insertion site with 2% CHG and use vigorous friction for 30 seconds. Allow to air-dry for at least 30 seconds (Schiffer et al., 2013).

2. Recent evidence: CHG solution and povidone-iodine use, patient age and gender, presence of malignancy and coexisting diseases, catheter duration, and use of total parenteral nutrition solution or use of blood products were evaluated for the effects on the development of catheter colonization and catheter-related bloodstream infections in patients with CVAD (Atahan et al., 2012). Patients were randomly assigned for insertion site disinfection prior to CVAD insertion, with a povidone-iodine–based or a 1.5% CHG-based solution. A statistically significant reduction in catheter-related bloodstream infection and catheter colonization was only found with the use of CHG in comparison to the povidone-iodine antiseptic solution.

3. Historical evidence: Past studies using various research procedures for the investigation of cleansing agents before catheter insertion and for catheter site care and dressing changes have found diverse results in the reduction of catheter-related infections (see Historical References).

B. Before accessing port

1. **Practice recommendation:** Use > 0.5% CHG as a cleansing agent.

2. Few studies have been conducted to investigate cleansing agents and protocols for skin cleansing prior to implanted port access. Further research is needed (O'Grady et al., 2011; Schiffer et al., 2013).

C. Before access of a needleless connector or hub

1. **Practice standard:** Routinely clean the needleless connector or hub with an appropriate antiseptic prior to use (Flynn, Keogh, & Gavin, 2015; Moureau & Flynn, 2015; Wright et al., 2013).

2. **Practice standard:** Vigorously apply mechanical friction with a cleansing agent before accessing catheter hubs, needleless connectors, or injection ports. Apply mechanical friction for five seconds or more to reduce contamination (Marschall et al., 2014; O'Grady et al., 2011; Shekelle et al., 2013) (see Appendix 2). Needleless connectors have not been well studied, and it is unclear if duration of disinfection can be generalized.

3. Recent evidence

   a) In an experimental study, Hong, Morrow, Sandora, and Priebe (2013) evaluated different scrub times (e.g., swipe, 5 seconds, 15 seconds, 30 seconds) using CHG alcohol compared to alcohol on needleless connectors for residual disinfectant activity. The swipe with alcohol method did not adequately disinfect needleless connectors, especially with *Staphylococcus aureus* or *Pseudomonas aeruginosa* contamination. CHG alcohol and alcohol performed similarly with scrubs that last at least five seconds; however, CHG alcohol resulted in residual disinfectant activity for up to 24 hours.

b) A systematic review was conducted to evaluate literature from 1977 to December 2014 regarding disinfection of needleless connectors to develop recommendations for aseptic access (Moureau & Flynn, 2015). The review included 140 publications pertaining to disinfection and catheter hub and needleless connector contamination, with a combined 34 abstracts and posters. The authors cautioned that the evidence for the effectiveness of the disinfection strategies was low level. Recommendations for practice regarding infection prevention and aseptic access included the following:

(1) Use an appropriate antiseptic agent (e.g., CHG alcohol, povidone-iodine, iodophor, 70% alcohol) on the surfaces of needleless connectors, stopcocks, and other intravascular access ports immediately prior to any connection, infusion, or aspiration.

(2) Passive continuous hub disinfection on needleless connections may be achieved with antimicrobial caps or port protectors with frictional antiseptic wiping between applications and access (Sweet, Cumpston, Briggs, Craig, & Hamadani, 2012).

(3) Hand hygiene, gloving, and aseptic practices should be maintained prior to any contact with IV devices and add-on equipment.

(4) Clinical staff should be educated to disinfect catheter hubs, needleless connectors, and ports prior to and after each access. Moureau and Flynn (2015) concluded that large, randomized controlled trials are needed to establish quality evidence for disinfection practices, including efficacy of antiseptic type, to disinfect needleless connectors.

c) An in vitro study was conducted to evaluate the effect of alcohol disinfection duration on bacterial load on catheter hubs (Simmons, Bryson, & Porter, 2011). Catheter hubs were contaminated with bacterial solution and allowed to dry for 24 hours. Then the hubs were disinfected with alcohol for 3, 10, or 15 seconds. No significant difference was found in the duration of disinfection and reduction in bacterial load.

4. Historical evidence

a) Past studies for the investigation of disinfection practices of catheter protective caps prior to puncture with a needle or access of a needleless connector hub found diverse results in the reduction of catheter-related infections (see Historical References).

b) Several studies have suggested that the use of a novel antiseptic barrier or connector cap significantly decreased the risk of microorganisms (see Historical References). Further research is needed. No conclusion can be drawn to affect practice.

D. Skin cleansing with dressing changes

1. **Practice standard:** Clean skin with a > 0.5% CHG alcohol preparation during dressing changes. If a contraindication or allergy to CHG exists, a tincture of iodine, an iodophor, or 70% alcohol can be used (O'Grady et al., 2011). Large, prospective, randomized clinical trials investigating different cleansing agents and different cleansing duration with controlled dressing types are needed to determine the most appropriate cleansing agent.

2. No definitive recommendation can be made for the use of CHG in infants younger than two months of age (O'Grady et al., 2011).

3. Recent evidence

a) The effects of CHG and povidone-iodine were compared for the prevention of bloodstream infection associated with access of venous ports (Kao et al., 2014). No significant difference was found in preventing the occurrence of port-associated bloodstream infections. The most common pathogens were gram-negative bacteria followed by gram-positive bacteria and fungi. CHG was associated with a significant improvement in time to first bloodstream infection caused by gram-positive bacteria; however, no significant preventive effects of CHG on time to first bloodstream infection caused by gram-negative bacteria or fungi were found.

b) CHG, octenidine, and povidone-iodine were compared for effects in preventing catheter-related infections by cleansing the skin with the designated antisepsis before insertion of the catheter and using the same antisepsis in the following days (Bilir, Yelken, & Erkan, 2013). Catheter-related sepsis was 10.5% in the povidone-iodine and octenidine hydrochlorodine groups, and catheter-related colonization was 26.3% in the povidone-iodine group and 21.5% in the octenidine hydrochlorodine group. There was no catheter-related sepsis or colonization in the CHG group.

c) Alcohol povidone-iodine was compared with a CHG antiseptic solution for the prevention of CVAD-related infections (Girard, Comby, & Jacques, 2012). When users switched from povidone-iodine to CHG, a significant reduction in colonization was noted; however, no significant difference in CVAD-related infection or bacteremia was found. Povidone-iodine was associated with a higher risk of colonization and infection.

E. Before epidural catheter placement
1. No definitive recommendation can be made based on the available evidence. The American Association of Nurse Anesthetists (AANA) supports CHG as the preferred skin preparation agent; however, povidone-iodine is a suitable alternative when CHG is contraindicated. Parachoroxylenol may be used as a cleansing agent, but it is less effective than CHG and povidone-iodine at eliminating microorganisms. Iodine base with alcohol also may be used (AANA, 2015).
2. Recent evidence
    a) A prospective study was conducted to compare the efficacy of 10% povidone-iodine and 2% CHG for skin disinfection prior to the placement of an epidural and CVADs (Kulkarni & Awode, 2013). The sample included a total of 60 patients, with 50 having epidural placement. Study findings suggested no difference in cost, efficacy, or side effects between 2% CHG and 10% povidone-iodine for skin disinfection.
    b) Alcohol-based CHG was compared to povidone-iodine for skin disinfection

prior to a neuraxial blockade procedure (Krobbuaban, Diregpoke, Prasan, Thanomsat, & Kumkeaw, 2011). Results showed that the incidence of positive skin culture was significantly lower in the CHG group compared to the povidone-iodine group.

3. Historical evidence: Past studies for the investigation of cleansing agents prior to epidural placement have found diverse results in the reduction of catheter-related infections (see Historical References).

IV. Flushing agents
What is the best evidence regarding the type of flushing protocol for VADs?
A. No definitive recommendation can be made regarding a specific flushing protocol based on the available evidence (Bradford, Edwards, & Chan, 2015; Conway, McCollom, & Bannon, 2014; Ferroni et al., 2014; Goossens, 2015; Goossens et al., 2013; Gorji, Rezaei, Jafari, & Cherati, 2015; Guiffant, Durussel, Merckx, Flaud, Vigier, & Mousset, 2012; Murray, Precious, & Alikhan, 2013; Odabas et al., 2014). Variability in studies involving heparin and saline flushing frequency, volume, concentration, and varying outcome measures prevent a definitive recommendation for a flushing solution protocol.
B. **Practice standard:** Flush all VADs with 0.9% normal saline (NS) following all blood sampling and medication administration.
C. **Practice recommendation:** Based on hydrodynamic flow studies and evidence of intraluminal fibrin buildup, use of pulsatile (push-pause) flushing techniques should be considered.
D. Recent evidence
    1. Gorji et al. (2015) conducted a randomized, double-blind study to compare the effects of heparin saline solution and NS solution in maintenance of CVAD patency. The sample, which included 84 patients with nontunneled CVADs in an intensive care unit, was randomized to a heparin saline flush (3 ml) or an NS flush (10 ml) following medication administration. No significant difference was found in catheter patency between both solutions.
    2. A systematic review was conducted to evaluate heparin versus 0.9% sodium chloride, with intermittent flushing for the prevention of occlusion in CVADs in adults (López-Briz et al., 2014). The review included six studies with heparin concentrations varying from 10–5,000 IU/ml and follow-up varying from 20–180 days for use

in tunneled and nontunneled CVADs. No conclusive evidence of differences between heparin intermittent flushing and NS for efficacy and safety was found. Further, no differences were noted in rates of thrombosis, infection, bleeding, heparin-induced thrombocytopenia, mortality, or catheter survival.

3. In a randomized trial to evaluate blood withdrawal occlusion, catheter-related bacteremia, and occurrence of functional problems, heparin lock (300 IU/3 ml) was compared to 10 ml NS lock in a sample of 802 patients with cancer who had newly inserted nonvalved implanted venous ports (Goossens et al., 2013). No significant difference was found between heparin lock and NS lock. The authors concluded that NS is an effective solution if combined with a consistent pulsatile flushing technique followed by a positive pressure locking technique.

4. To evaluate maintenance of CVAD patency, Schallom, Prentice, Sona, Micek, and Skrupky (2012) conducted a randomized controlled trial of 341 patients with multilumen CVADs. The study compared 10 ml NS every eight hours with 10 ml NS followed by 3 ml heparin lock flush (10 IU/ml) every eight hours. No significant difference in catheter occlusion was found between heparin and NS lock.

5. A prospective, randomized, one-way, single-blinded post-test with a control group study of 90 noncancer homecare patients with PICCs was conducted to investigate three flushing protocols for the development of patency-related complications and issues, such as sluggishness, occlusion, missed medication doses, catheter replacement, additional nursing visits, and the use of alteplase (Lyons & Phalen, 2014). Results indicated that the saline flush group had

the highest incidence of PICC occlusion requiring alteplase use. The higher concentration of heparin flush group and the saline flush group had similar number episodes of PICC sluggishness, and the lower concentration of heparin flush group had the lowest number of episodes of occlusions and use of alteplase. The three flushing protocols were as follows:

   a) Study group I: Saline flush with 10 ml, followed by administration of IV medication, then by a saline flush with 10 ml
   b) Study group II: Saline flush with 10 ml, followed by administration of IV medication, then by a saline flush with 10 ml, and finally by a heparinized saline solution with concentration of 100 IU/ml (3 ml or 300 IU)
   c) Study group III: Same sequence as study group II but with heparin concentration of 10 IU/ml (5 ml or 50 IU)

6. The efficacy of pulsatile flushing to prevent bacterial colonization of VADs was compared with continuous flushing and no flushing in 576 *Staphylococcus aureus*–contaminated polyurethane short-term venous access catheters (Ferroni et al., 2014). *Staphylococcus aureus* endoluminal contamination was significantly higher with continuous flushing than with pulsatile flushing.

E. Historical evidence: Past studies of flushing protocols have found diverse results in the reduction of catheter-related occlusions and complications (see Historical References).

What is the best evidence regarding flushing protocols in patients with heparin-induced thrombocytopenia?

F. No definitive recommendation can be made based on the available evidence. Consideration should be given to insert devices with distal tip valve design and to use NS flush.

What is the best evidence regarding flushing protocols for short-term arterial pressure lines?

G. No definitive recommendation can be made based on the available evidence. Evidence comparing the use of heparin solution and NS solution for flushing and maintaining the patency of arterial pressure lines is inconclusive. Inconsistency in study variables involving heparin and saline flushing frequency, volume, concentration, and varying outcome measures prevent the establishment of a recommendation for a flushing solution protocol.

H. Recent evidence: A systematic review was conducted to compare NS and heparin in varying dosages in maintaining the patency of arterial intravascular catheters in adult patients without a hematologic disorder (Robertson-Malt, Malt, Farquhar, & Greer, 2014). As a result of the clinical and statistical heterogeneity of the seven included studies, no meta-analysis was completed and no conclusion could be drawn. The authors concluded that further research was needed with well-defined primary and secondary outcomes and the use of various heparin doses.

I. Historical evidence: Past studies for the investigation of flushing protocols of arterial pressure lines have found diverse results in the reduction of catheter-related occlusions and complications (see Historical References).

What is the best evidence regarding the volume and flushing frequency needed for VADs?

J. No definitive recommendation can be made based on the available evidence.
   1. The issues of volume and frequency of flushing continue to be controversial among institutions across the United States. Multisite, randomized prospective studies examining the relationship of these variables with factors such as patency, type of device, patient characteristics, infection, and cost are needed to standardize protocols used in multiple institutions.
   2. Little evidence exists regarding the current state of flushing practice. Mechanisms to reduce complications in VADs have included evaluation of optimizing patency through flush volumes, types of flush preparations (prefilled syringes versus manually filled syringes), and flushing. Volume and frequency variations typically are not evaluated independently of other variables.

V. VAD without blood return
What is the best evidence regarding the use of a VAD without a blood return?

A. No definitive recommendation can be made based on the available evidence. No studies to date have provided a research-based answer as to when to administer medication through a VAD without a blood return. No definitive evidence exists to guide surveillance intervals to determine ongoing accuracy of VAD placement.

B. **Practice standard:** It is expert opinion and generally accepted practice in various clinical settings that prior to administering medications through VADs in which no blood return exists, verification of catheter placement and function should be established through imaging studies (Polovich, Olsen, & LeFebvre, 2014).

C. **Practice standard:** Do not administer antineoplastic agents in the absence of a blood return.

D. Interventions (Polovich et al., 2014)
   1. Attempt to flush with NS using gentle pulsatile (push-pause) technique.
   2. Reposition the patient.
   3. Ask the patient to cough and deep breathe.
   4. Obtain a provider order for declotting procedure, as appropriate.
   5. Obtain a provider order for possible imaging study.

E. **Practice standard:** Remove peripheral and midline catheters and reinsert if no blood return (Gonzalez, 2013; Polovich et al., 2014; Schulmeister, 2011).

F. **Practice standard:** If no other options exist after verification of VAD intactness, position, and patency and confirmation by imaging study of the lack of backflow, obtain a provider order to use a VAD when there is no blood return (Polovich et al., 2014).

What is the best evidence regarding type or frequency of imaging study to perform to evaluate a VAD with no blood return?

G. No definitive recommendation can be made based on the available evidence. No studies to date have provided a research-based answer regarding the best imaging or study to determine safe use of a VAD with no blood return.
   1. Management of a catheter without blood return requires evaluation of the location of the catheter's tip. Imaging is ordered and may include injection of contrast (i.e., venogram) or cross-sectional computed tomography (CT) scan.
   2. Expert opinion suggests that it is better to leave a questionable device in situ and to consult a vascular surgeon or interventional radiologist rather than to immediately remove the device (Gibson & Bodenham, 2013).
   3. A chest x-ray will visualize catheter tip positioning and is best for evaluating malposition, migration, kinking, and pinch-off syndrome.
   4. An ultrasound will visualize the vein where the catheter is located and the tip location and is superior in evaluating for clots in the catheter tip. If the VAD is completely occluded, an ultrasound is beneficial in evaluating the VAD.
   5. CT imaging will visualize catheter intactness or the portal body and is useful in detecting malposition of the catheter or port.
   6. A cathetergram (dye study) will visualize the intactness of the catheter and the flow

from the distal tip to evaluate for backflow. It is useful in detecting obstruction, catheter fracture, the fluid pathway, and backflow along the catheter.

VI. Catheter occlusion

What is the best evidence regarding the treatment of a VAD occlusion due to suspected thrombosis?

A. Additional large multicenter trials are needed with direct comparisons of fibrinolytic agents, drug concentrations, the effect on mineral precipitants or lipids, the type of device, and dwelling times in order to establish optimal treatment for catheter occlusion.

B. **Practice standard:** Use 2 mg alteplase (tissue plasminogen activator [tPA]) to restore patency and maintain catheter function (Schiffer et al., 2013).

C. Recent evidence: The successful use of tPA for restoration of catheter patency has been confirmed in numerous studies, among various patient populations and settings, and in catheters placed for various indications (Ernst, Chen, Lipkin, Tayama, & Amin, 2014; Ponce, Mendes, Silva, & Oliveira, 2015; Ragsdale, Oliver, Thompson, & Evans, 2014; Tebbi et al., 2011).

D. Historical evidence: The use of alteplase for catheter occlusion has been found to be safe and effective (see Historical References).

What is the best evidence regarding use of tPA locks or infusions as maintenance therapy for occlusion prevention for VADs?

E. No definitive recommendation can be made regarding use of tPA locks, infusions, or overnight dwells.

F. Recent evidence
1. Most studies evaluating tPA for locking catheters, specific dwells, or continuous infusions (during hemodialysis) have been conducted in the dialysis population, utilizing arteriovenous fistulas. Low-dose tPA directly infused continuously into the fistula during dialysis has been shown to decrease clot burden in a small sample of patients (van der Merwe, Luscombe, & Kiaii, 2015).
2. A twice-weekly recombinant tPA/heparin lock protocol used in each lumen of hemodialysis catheters demonstrated a mean overall cost and efficacy similar to that of a three times per week heparin lock protocol (Manns et al., 2014).
3. The efficacy of an alteplase 30-minute dwell protocol versus an alteplase push protocol (< 30 minutes) in hemodialysis patients with central VADs proved no statistical difference in the resultant blood flow rates

from either group (Vercaigne, Zacharias, & Bernstein, 2012).

G. Historical evidence
1. Although dosing and administration recommendations outlined in drug package inserts for alteplase do not include protocols for overnight drug dwells, research in a homecare population used a three-dose protocol comparing partially and completely occluded devices. Alteplase was administered in partially and fully occluded CVADs up to three repeated doses as needed, with the third instillation dwelling overnight. Approximately 66.7% of all catheters were successfully cleared using this protocol (Moureau, Mlodzik, Pharm, & Pool, 5005).
2. Various protocols for VADs have been recommended, including allowing alteplase to dwell overnight depending on institutional practice and policy (see Historical References).

VII. Catheter occlusion prophylaxis

What is the best evidence regarding effective anticoagulant prophylaxis for the prevention of catheter-related thrombosis?

A. **Practice standard:** Do not use prophylactic, low-dose warfarin or low-molecular-weight heparin as prevention for thrombosis related to VADs in patients with cancer. This, along with the use of oral anticoagulants, is not recommended (D'Ambrosio, Aglietta, & Grignani, 2014; Kahn et al., 2012; Schiffer et al., 2013)

B. Recent evidence
1. A systematic review found that heparin (low molecular or unfractionated) or vitamin K antagonists compared to no therapy did reduce the incidence of symptomatic deep vein thrombosis in patients with cancer who also had a VAD. Heparin was associated with a higher risk of thrombocytopenia and asymptomatic deep vein thrombosis when compared to vitamin K antagonists; benefits must outweigh harms (Akl et al., 2014).
2. Studies investigating the use of low-molecular-weight heparin and vitamin K antagonists for the prevention of catheter-related thrombosis have shown a significant reduction in the rate of catheter-related thrombosis (Lavau-Denes et al., 2013; see also Historical References).

C. Historical evidence: Past randomized trials investigating low-molecular-weight heparin have not found efficacy in prevention of catheter-related thrombosis (see Historical References).

D. No definitive recommendation can be made regarding the use of heparin-bonded catheters for prolonging patency.
   1. Recent evidence: Shah and Shah (2014) conducted a systematic review of heparin-bonded and central venous catheter patency in children. Two studies were included in the review. Results found no difference in catheter-related thrombosis with the use of heparin-bonded catheters compared to non–heparin-bonded catheters.
   2. Historical evidence: Additional historical studies investigating heparin-bonded catheters and flushing protocols for prevention of catheter-related thrombosis have found conflicting results (see Historical References).

VIII. Infection and infection control
   What is the best evidence regarding effective prophylaxis for the prevention of catheter-related infections?
   A. The presence of bacterial biofilms or deposits on the surfaces of VAD catheters is of clinical importance. However, their presence has the potential to serve as a nidus (focus) for infection and bacteremia (Miglietta et al., 2015; Mirijello et al., 2015; Pérez-Granda, Guembe, Cruces, Barrio, & Bouza, 2016; Zhang, Gowardman, Morrison, Runnegar, & Rickard, 2016; see also Historical References). Several recommendations exist to prevent catheter-related infections.
   B. **Practice standard:** Do not routinely replace peripheral IV catheters unless clinically indicated (Helm, Klausner, Klemperer, Flint, & Huang, 2015; Rickard et al., 2012; Webster, Osborne, Rickard, & New, 2015). Recent studies in various settings have shown no difference in rates of phlebitis, occlusion, infiltration, infection, or mortality when peripheral catheters are changed as clinically indicated versus every 72–96 hours (Paşalioğlu & Kaya, 2014).
   C. **Practice standard:** Do not routinely replace central venous catheters (O'Grady et al., 2011; Schiffer et al., 2013).
   D. **Practice standard:** For short-term, nontunneled VADs, use a catheter coated with chlorhexidine and silver sulfadiazine or minocycline and rifampin prior to insertion to decrease the risk of catheter-related infections, especially in high-risk bone marrow transplant recipients and patients with leukemia (Lai et al., 2013; O'Grady et al., 2011; Schiffer et al., 2013).
   E. **Practice standard:** Due to the increased risk for fungal infections and antimicrobial resistance, antimicrobial ointment should not be used at the insertion site (Schiffer et al., 2013).

F. **Practice standard:** Use povidone-iodine antiseptic ointment or bacitracin/gramicidin/polymyxin-B ointment at the exit site of hemodialysis catheters after insertion and at the end of each dialysis session (O'Grady et al., 2011).
G. **Practice standard:** Use a CHG-impregnated sponge dressing for all catheters, including specialty catheters in patients older than two months of age, unless sensitive to CHG (Karpanen et al., 2016; Kerwat et al., 2015; Safdar et al., 2014; Timsit et al., 2012; Ullman et al., 2015; Wibaux et al., 2015).
   1. Following CHG skin preparation, it is recommended to use a CHG-impregnated sponge dressing for any long-term infusion (defined as exceeding 4–6 hours) or if the port remains accessed for intermittent long-term infusions.
   2. Recent evidence
      a) Research demonstrated benefit from the use of CHG-impregnated sponge dressings in preventing catheter colonization and bloodstream infection in patients with VADs. The authors recommended routine use in patients at high risk for catheter-related bloodstream infections in VADs or short-term arterial catheters (Safdar et al., 2014). Additional research suggested that the use of CHG-impregnated sponge dressings significantly reduced the rate of central venous and epidural catheter–related infections (Kerwat et al., 2015; Wibaux et al., 2015).
      b) CHG antimicrobial dressing was compared to gauze and tape dressing in a sample of 85 patients with nontunneled CVADs (Pedrolo et al., 2014). No statistically significant differences were found in bloodstream infections, local reactions, and dressing adherence between the dressings.
   3. Historical evidence: Past reviews suggested utility in the use of CHG-impregnated dressings (see Historical References).
H. **Practice standard:** Monitor all device exit sites visually or by palpation through an intact dressing on a regular basis, depending on the clinical situation of individual patients (O'Grady et al., 2011).
I. **Practice standard:** Use maximum sterile barrier precautions for insertion of all access devices except peripheral venous catheters. Sterile gloves are not necessarily required for insertion of

peripheral catheters if an aseptic no-touch technique is used (Institute for Healthcare Improvement, 2015; Schiffer et al., 2013).

J. **Practice standard:** Use clean or sterile gloves when changing the dressing on VADs (O'Grady et al., 2011).

    1. Historical evidence: One retrospective descriptive study investigated infection rate in 62 patients. An aseptic technique was used for accessing and deaccessing implantable ports. Nonsterile gloves were worn. Results indicated only two of the six infections that occurred could be attributed to the aseptic nonsterile glove technique for accessing and deaccessing implantable ports (Camp-Sorrell, 2009).

    2. The Wound, Ostomy and Continence Nurses Society (2011) and the Association for Professionals in Infection Control and Epidemiology updated their guidelines to reflect the most recent evidence regarding clean versus sterile dressing technique for chronic wounds. They concluded that no definitive evidence exists that sterile technique is superior to clean technique or that it improves outcomes. They also noted a lack of agreement among expert opinion as to what constitutes sterile versus nonsterile technique.

    3. The National Institute for Health and Care Excellence guidelines (2012) state that aseptic technique must be used for all VAD catheter care and when accessing the system.

K. **Practice standard:** Maintain aseptic technique for the care of intravascular catheters (O'Grady et al., 2011).

L. **Practice standard:** Avoid the use of the femoral vein for VAD insertion (O'Grady et al., 2011; Schiffer et al., 2013).

M. **Practice recommendation:** Although evidence does not exist to support sterile maintenance procedures for specialty access devices (e.g., access to cerebrospinal fluid), expert opinion and sound nursing judgment supports the use of sterile technique when accessing or maintaining these devices, as life-threatening infection could occur.

N. No definitive recommendation can be made regarding a preferred vein for insertion of a tunneled VAD (O'Grady et al., 2011; Schiffer et al., 2013). Ge et al. (2012) found that subclavian and internal jugular central venous access routes had similar risks for catheter-related complications in long-term catheterization in patients with cancer. Additional results suggested that subclavian central venous access was preferable to femoral sites in short-term catheterization, and femoral and internal jugular central venous access had similar risks in short-term hemodialysis catheterization, except for higher risks of mechanical complications in internal jugular central venous access.

O. No definitive recommendation can be made regarding coating a catheter with platinum/silver, as studies have shown conflicting results; recommendation for or against the use of these catheters cannot be made (O'Grady et al., 2011).

P. No definitive recommendation can be made regarding the routine use of antibiotic lock techniques for the prevention of catheter-associated infections because of the potential of an increased risk of microbial antibiotic resistance (van de Wetering, van Woensel, & Lawrie, 2013).

Q. **Practice standard:** Consider the use of antibiotic lock therapy if patient is diagnosed with catheter-related infection or is at high risk of infection; however, the frequency, length of dwell time, and whether or not to discard or flush antibiotic dwell has not been determined. Sensitivities of the organism dictate antibiotic use (Chesshyre, Goff, Bowen, & Carapetis, 2015; Fernández-Hidalgo & Almirante, 2014; Justo & Bookstaver, 2014; Mirijello et al., 2015; Raad & Chaftari, 2014; van de Wetering et al., 2013; Zhang et al., 2016).

R. **Practice standard:** Use of a combined antibiotic and heparin flushing or locking solution may increase microbial antibiotic resistance; therefore, it should be reserved for patients at high risk or where baseline VAD infection rates are high (> 15%) (CDC, 2016; Justo & Bookstaver, 2014; Raad & Chaftari, 2014; van de Wetering et al., 2013).

    1. Recent evidence

       a) The value of using an antibiotic lock technique in the port reservoir to prevent catheter-related sepsis is controversial. After investigation of numerous compounds, patient population heterogeneity, and limitations in sample size or study design, a recommendation for or against use cannot be made (O'Grady et al., 2011; Schiffer et al., 2013; Schoot, van Dalen, van Ommen, & van de Wetering, 2013).

       b) A retrospective study was conducted to investigate the efficacy of 70% adjunctive ethanol-lock therapy in combination with systemic antimicrobial treatment for central line–associated bloodstream infections (CLABSIs) and catheter salvage (Kubiak et al., 2014). Findings suggested a trend toward CVAD salvage with the addition of 70% ethanol-lock therapy. The authors concluded that ethanol-lock was a well-tolerated, potentially effective therapy that warranted further large, randomized controlled trials.

    c) Flushing or locking long-term VADs with a combined antibiotic and heparin solution appears to reduce gram-positive catheter-related sepsis in people at risk for neutropenia from chemotherapy or bone marrow disease (van de Wetering et al., 2013).

  2. Historical evidence: Past reviews suggested some utility in the prevention of VAD removal associated with catheter-related sepsis with the use of antibiotic lock technique (see Historical References).

S. **Practice recommendation:** Change needleless connector after each use, with catheter change, or more frequently if damaged or signs of blood or precipitate. Use strict aseptic technique at all times (Flynn et al., 2015; Martinez et al., 2015; Moureau & Flynn, 2015; Sherertz, Karchmer, Palavecino, & Bischoff, 2011; Tabak, Jarvis, Sun, Crosby, & Johannes, 2014; Wright et al., 2013).

T. **Practice recommendation:** Consider the use of connectors with design features such as those with a visible fluid path to assess efficacy of flush technique and a solid, flat, and smooth access surface that easily is disinfected.

U. No definitive recommendation can be made to support time intervals for changing needleless connectors. Additional evidence-based research is needed. Studies support vigorous cleaning of needleless connectors but do not provide clear evidence for changing protocols or whether one type of connector is superior to another. Data support development of biofilm within connectors. The presence of blood in connectors contributes to biofilm foundation. Given that the standard of practice is to verify blood return prior to determining use, it follows that residual blood will remain within the connector, contributing to biofilm development and ultimately increasing risk for bloodstream infection (Martinez et al., 2015; Sherertz et al., 2011).

  1. Recent evidence: Martinez et al. (2015) used a nonrandomized, prospective sample of neutropenic hematology patients with long-term tunneled Hickman®-type catheters to study the effect of a bundle of interventions to reduce bloodstream infections.

During a five-month period, a study group was compared to a control group from the previous six months prior to implementation of the bundle, which consisted of the use of a neutral pressure mechanical valve connector, more frequent changes of the connector (twice weekly and after each blood sample for a new fever episode), and a more efficient 2% CHG solution to clean the connectors. Researchers concluded that the bundle quickly resulted in a significant reduction in bloodstream infections and catheter-related bloodstream infection rates.

2. During a 21-month period, Sherertz et al. (2011) evaluated for the presence of pathogens from samples drawn from three different needleless connector designs. Researchers found pathogens in samples from the Clearlink® connectors to meet CDC criteria for bloodstream infections; however, these patients were asymptomatic. Researchers concluded that pathogens may reside in the needleless connectors alone, causing false positive results.

3. In a retrospective analysis of 150 patients with Hickman catheters, results implied that needleless connector care using an aseptic no-touch technique coupled with hand hygiene, when compared to sterile technique, was not associated with an increase in catheter-associated bloodstream infections. The authors cautioned that the sample size was small (Flynn et al., 2015).

4. A systematic review of 140 studies and 34 abstracts on needleless connector disinfection, hub disinfection, and measure of education and compliance in use of strict aseptic technique concluded that the greatest risk for contamination for the catheter after insertion is the needleless connector. Disinfection compliance was found to be generally as low as 10%. Researchers cautioned that the optimal timing and tech-

nique for connector maintenance is not yet identified; vigorous scrubbing and use of passive alcohol disinfection caps positively affect catheter infection rates. Researchers stressed the importance of strict aseptic compliance (Moureau & Flynn, 2015).

5. Sandora et al. (2014) evaluated the association between needleless connector change frequency and CLABSI rates using an in vitro experimental model of pediatric stem cell transplant connector use. Three data collection periods included a baseline sampling, during which the connector was changed every 96 hours regardless of the infusate to which it was exposed. The connector was changed every 24 hours with blood or lipid infusions. The third sampling mirrored the first study group. Researchers concluded that changing the connectors in a simulated pediatric population increased CLABSI rates but that national recommendations regarding connector change frequency require clarification.

6. Tabak et al. (2014) reviewed studies reporting CLABSI in patients using a newer design of a positive-displacement needleless connector compared to negative- or neutral-displacement needleless connector design. Four out of seven studies occurred in the intensive care setting. Results demonstrated that newer design, positive-displacement connectors (a connection with visible fluid path to assess efficacy of flush technique; a solid, flat, smooth access surface that is easily disinfected; an open fluid pathway that facilitates high flow and avoids hemolysis; a tight septum seal; and a single-part activation of the fluid path) was associated with lower CLABSI risk.

V. No definitive recommendation can be made regarding preferential use of one type of VAD over any other to decrease the risk of bloodstream infection. This risk is unknown, with no recently published evidence (Schiffer et al., 2013).

1. Historical evidence: One previous study found higher rates of bloodstream infections with short-term noncuffed CVADs and non-medication-coated CVADs compared to IV catheters and midline catheters, while short-term arterial catheters and PICCs had bloodstream infection rates similar to CVADs (Maki, Kluger, & Crnich, 2006).

2. Ports usually are inserted in patients with solid tumors receiving less aggressive regimens; therefore, the patients do not have

as prolonged nadirs as those with hematologic cancers or those who are undergoing stem cell transplant. However, tunneled catheters, usually multilumen, are placed in patients with hematologic cancers who receive aggressive regimens that result in prolonged nadirs.

3. Further research is needed that includes the type of device, therapy, maintenance protocols, and diagnosis, comorbidities, age, and manual dexterity.

IX. Removal of VADs in the presence of bacteremia
What is the best evidence regarding VAD removal for infection?

A. No definitive recommendation can be made based on the available evidence. Deciding when to remove VADs in the presence of catheter-related bacteremia is controversial and dependent on individual patient status. Immunosuppressed and thrombocytopenic patients are placed at higher risk for infections and bleeding if the existing catheter is removed and a new one is placed.

B. Recent evidence

1. In a prospective observational study, Lorente et al. (2014) evaluated central venous management of suspected catheter-related infection and its influence on patient mortality. Findings showed no significant difference in mortality in patients with confirmed catheter-related bloodstream infections related to catheter removal at the moment of suspicion versus removal of the catheter at any later point. The authors concluded that immediate removal of CVADs with suspected infection may not be necessary in all patients.

2. Catheter removal may be considered when VAD-related septicemia is confirmed; tunnel infection exists; signs and symptoms of septicemia persist despite antibiotics; or the causative organism is fungi, bacilli, or pseudomonas (Schiffer et al., 2013; see also Historical References).

3. In 2008, the Centers for Medicare and Medicaid Services implemented a payment system, which stipulated that preventable conditions, including vascular catheter–associated infections, would not be reimbursed to Medicare- and Medicaid-certified hospitals unless conditions were present on admission. Measures to prevent catheter-related infections in hospitalized patients are critical. Medicare has not given guidelines regarding prevention of infections (Centers for Medicare and Medicaid Services, 2008).

C. No definitive recommendation can be made on when to insert a new VAD after removal of a VAD for infection.

X. Blood sampling from VADs

What is the best evidence regarding obtaining blood cultures from VADs?

A. **Practice standard:** When fever or suspicion of an infected VAD is present, obtain blood cultures from the CVAD and from another peripheral site (Schiffer et al., 2013).

B. **Practice standard:** Accessing and obtaining blood cultures from an implantable port with clinical signs of an infection is recommended before the initiation of antibiotic therapy (Schiffer et al., 2013).

C. No definitive recommendation can be made regarding the frequency of blood culture sampling, blood discard volumes, methods of collection, or use of discarded blood for culture samples.

   1. No specific professional or regulatory recommendations exist regarding the frequency in obtaining, discarding, or reusing blood drawn from CVADs for culture.

   2. Blood culture collections of 10–20 cc for adults and 1–3 cc for children for each blood culture set; drawing one set through the vascular device and one set from a separate venipuncture is supported (O'Grady et al., 2011; Septimus, 2015).

D. Recent evidence

   1. A study of 62 pediatric patients with cancer with CVADs and blood culture orders had blood drawn aseptically, with the normally discarded first 5 ml of blood injected into the second specimen culture bottle. In all cases where both culture bottles from a single source were positive for pathogens, the normally discarded specimen contained the same pathogen as the usual care specimen. In four cases, the normally discarded specimen demonstrated earlier time to positivity compared to the usual care specimen, allowing for earlier identification and treatment (Winokur et al., 2014).

   2. A study compared individual blood cultures taken from each catheter lumen versus a pooled blood culture bottle containing samples from all catheter lumens to diagnose catheter-related bloodstream infection. The study demonstrated that the sampling of multiple lumens from a central line and incubating them in the same culture bottle is as effective as individual culture bottles in the diagnosis of either colonization or of catheter-related bloodstream infec-

tion. The researchers concluded that sampling multiple lumens using one culture bottle is a better choice than sampling only one lumen when sending three different culture bottles (Herrera-Guerra, Garza-González, Martínez-Resendez, Llaca-Díaz, & Camacho-Ortiz, 2015).

What is the best evidence regarding blood sampling techniques to use when drawing from VADs?

E. **Practice standard:** Blood-sparing techniques should be considered as best practice when drawing blood samples (Berg, Ahee, & Berg, 2011; McEvoy & Shander, 2013; Parco, Visconti, & Vascotto, 2014; World Health Organization [WHO], 2010).

F. **Practice standard:** Organize work to minimize the number of accesses of a device; if possible, time blood sampling to coincide with other indications for accessing a device, such as the administration of another medication (e.g., antibiotic) (WHO, 2010).

What is the best evidence regarding blood sampling from VADs for coagulation studies?

G. No definitive recommendation can be made regarding coagulation test sampling technique and blood discard volume from heparinized VADs. Further research is needed in investigating blood sampling, amount of discard, type of blood specimen, and blood collection methods in different types of VADs.

H. Recent evidence

   1. A 2015 systematic review of the literature concluded that the only reliable method for obtaining coagulation test results from CVADs is to flush then waste or discard prior to obtaining a sample; however, this has been studied only in PICCs. The review noted significant variability in sampling technique and in discard volume practices (Dalton, Aucoin, & Meyer, 2015).

   2. Blood specimens drawn from PICCs using a 10 ml saline flush, followed by a 6 ml blood waste, then by blood collection for evaluation of partial thromboplastin time and prothrombin time/international normalized ratio (INR) were compared to specimens drawn from peripheral venipunctures. After specimens were collected from the PICCs, the lines were flushed with another 10 ml NS and 2 ml of heparinized saline. Although the sample size was small, high correlation was found between all of the values obtained from both types of samples, except for the INR samples (Humphries, Baldwin, Clark, Tenuta, & Brumley, 2012). These findings

support earlier findings, although CVAD type was not specified in the study (see Historical References).

3. In a prospective comparison study, coagulation tests consisting of prothrombin time, activated partial thromboplastin time, and INR were obtained from a peripheral venipuncture and a VAD after discarding 6 ml, 9 ml, and 12 ml of blood (Zu-Kei Lin, Fowler, Dise, & Bustami, 2009). Results indicated a high correlation between peripheral venipuncture and all VAD blood samples. No differences were found between the three VAD samples, indicating that 6 ml was an adequate discard volume.

I. Historical evidence
1. Past research has reported mixed conclusions. INR specimens from heparinized CVADs and activated partial thromboplastin time specimens obtained from PICCs have shown no significant difference compared to samples obtained from peripheral venipuncture (see Historical References); however, past research found that coagulation testing from heparinized tunneled VADs was significantly different compared to peripheral samples.
2. One study found similar laboratory results with the push-pull method and the discard method of obtaining blood samples from CVADs; however, previous research suggested not reinfusing the discard blood collection because of the presence of clots and because the push-pull method can increase the risk of hemolysis with the agitation of blood (see Historical References).

XI. Power injection of contrast media
A. **Practice standard:** Power-injectable VADs are safe when used by skilled personnel using appropriate administration technique.
B. Power-injectable VADs have become increasingly popular to use in oncology clinical practice.

C. Recent evidence
1. Studies investigating the safety and efficacy of power-injectable VADs are limited.
2. In a small retrospective study, implantable venous power ports placed in the femoral vein were evaluated for indication, technical success, and complications (Goltz, Janssen, Petritsch, & Kickuth, 2014). Findings suggested that femoral placement is safe and that ports perform with high technical success when used.
3. The benefit of power-injectable ports was evaluated for safety, use for contrast media injections, and tip location (Teichgräber, Nagel, Kausche, & Enzweiler, 2012). Results indicated that the power-injectable port complication rate was similar to standard port systems.
D. Historical evidence: Past studies have focused on different catheter types and sizes and the power injection of contrast media (see Historical References).
E. Although studies evaluating power ports, tunneled catheters, or PICCs and the use of power injections are limited, numerous radiographic suites will use only VADs specifically designed for power injection of contrast material.

XII. Controversial issues related to nursing practice
A. Suturing of PICCs by RNs
1. No definitive recommendation can be made based on the available evidence.
2. Suturing of PICCs by RNs is defined by each state board of nursing's scope of practice. Several states permit trained RNs to stabilize a PICC with sutures. No research has been conducted investigating RN suturing of PICCs. Opinions on training requirements for insertion of PICCs vary from state to state and from institution to institution, and a lack of uniformity exists regarding certification criteria for inserting these catheters. Training received in one state is not necessarily transferable to another. Further research is needed to investigate the RN scope of practice in suturing PICCs.
3. As universal IV securement devices are used more frequently, suturing PICCs for stabilization is becoming less common.
B. Removal of tunneled catheters by RNs
1. No definitive recommendation can be made based on the available evidence.
2. Several, but not all, state boards of nursing allow trained RNs to remove tunneled catheters.

3. Further research is needed to investigate the RN scope of practice in removing tunneled catheters.

C. Role of assistive personnel in the care of VADs
1. No definitive recommendation can be made based on the available evidence.
2. It is unclear whether assistive nursing personnel or other department personnel (e.g., radiology) may perform procedures such as accessing or flushing VADs or obtaining blood samples. Training requirements may vary depending on state or institution.
3. Nurses in supervisory positions should review their state nurse practice act and establish appropriate policies and procedures for the care of VADs by assistive personnel within their institutions.
4. Further research is needed to investigate the role of assistive personnel in caring for VADs.

References

Ahn, S.J., Kim, H.-C., Chung, J.W., An, S.B., Yin, Y.H., Jae, H.J., … Park, J.H. (2012). Ultrasound and fluoroscopy-guided placement of central venous ports via internal jugular vein: Retrospective analysis of 1254 port implantations at a single center. *Korean Journal of Radiology, 13*, 314–323. doi:10.3348/kjr.2012.13.3.314

Akl, E.A., Ramly, E.P., Kahale, L.A., Yosuico, V.E.D., Barba, M., Sperati, F., … Schünemann, H. (2014). Anticoagulation for people with cancer and central venous catheters. *Cochrane Database of Systematic Reviews, 2014*(10). doi:10.1002/14651858.CD006468.pub5

American Association of Nurse Anesthetists. (2015). Infection prevention and control guidelines for anesthesia care. Retrieved from http://www.aana.com/resources2/professionalpractice/Pages/Infection-Prevention-and-Control-Guidelines-for-Anesthesia-Care.aspx

Atahan, K., Cokmez, A., Bekoglu, M., Durak, E., Tavusbay, C., & Tarcan, E. (2012). The effect of antiseptic solution in central venous catheter care. *Bratislava Medical Journal, 113*, 548–551. doi:10.4149/bll_2012_123

Berg, J.E., Ahee, P., & Berg, J.D. (2011). Variation in phlebotomy techniques in emergency medicine and the incidence of haemolysed samples. *Annals of Clinical Biochemistry, 48*, 562–565. doi:10.1258/acb.2011.011099

Bilir, A., Yelken, B., & Erkan, A. (2013). Chlorhexidine, octenidine or povidone iodine for catheter related infections: A randomized controlled trial. *Journal of Research in Medical Sciences, 18*, 510–512.

Bowen, M.E., Mone, M.C., Nelson, E.W., & Scaife, C.L. (2014). Image-guided placement of long-term central venous catheters reduces complications and cost. *American Journal of Surgery, 208*, 937–941. doi:10.1016/j.amjsurg.2014.08.005

Bradford, N.K., Edwards, R.M., & Chan, R.J. (2015). Heparin versus 0.9% sodium chloride intermittent flushing for the prevention of occlusion in long term central venous catheters in infants and children. *Cochrane Database of Systematic Reviews, 2015*(11). doi:10.1002/14651858.CD010996.pub2

Brass, P., Hellmich, M., Kolodziej, L., Schick, G., & Smith, A.F. (2015). Ultrasound guidance versus anatomical landmarks for internal jugular vein catheterization. *Cochrane Database of Systematic Reviews, 2015*(1). doi:10.1002/14651858.CD006962.pub2

Camp-Sorrell, D. (2009). Accessing and deaccessing ports: Where is the evidence? *Clinical Journal of Oncology Nursing, 13*, 587–590. doi:10.1188/09.CJON.587-590

Centers for Disease Control and Prevention. (2016). Vital signs: Preventing antibiotic-resistant infections in hospitals–United States, 2014. Retrieved from http://www.cdc.gov/mmwr/volumes/65/wr/mm6509e1.htm

Centers for Medicare and Medicaid Services. (2008). Medicare takes new steps to help make your hospital stay safer. Retrieved from https://www.cms.gov/Newsroom/MediaReleaseDatabase/Fact-sheets/2008-Fact-sheets-items/2008-08-045.html

Chesshyre, E., Goff, Z., Bowen, A., & Carapetis, J. (2015). The prevention, diagnosis and management of central venous line infections in children. *Journal of Infection, 71*(Suppl. 1), S59–S75. doi:10.1016/j.jinf.2015.04.029

Chico-Padrón, R.M., Carrión-García, L., Della-Vedove-Rosales, L., González-Vargas, C.S., Marrero-Perera, M., Medina-Chico, S., … Jiménez-Sosa, A. (2011). Comparative safety and costs of transparent versus gauze wound dressings in intravenous catheterization. *Journal of Nursing Care Quality, 26*, 371–376. doi:10.1097/ncq.0b013e318210741b

Conway, M.A., McCollom, C., & Bannon, C. (2014). Central venous catheter flushing recommendations: A systematic evidence-based practice review. *Journal of Pediatric Oncology Nursing, 31*, 185–190. doi:10.1177/1043454214532028

Dalton, K.A., Aucoin, J., & Meyer, B. (2015). Obtaining coagulation blood samples from central venous access devices: A review of the literature. *Clinical Journal of Oncology Nursing, 19*, 418–423. doi:10.1188/15.CJON.19-04AP

D'Ambrosio, L., Aglietta, M., & Grignani, G. (2014). Anticoagulation for central venous catheters in patients with cancer. *New England Journal of Medicine, 371*, 1362–1363. doi:10.1056/NEJMc1408861

Ernst, F.R., Chen, E., Lipkin, C., Tayama, D., & Amin, A.N. (2014). Comparison of hospital length of stay, costs, and readmissions of alteplase versus catheter replacement among patients with occluded central venous catheters. *Journal of Hospital Medicine, 9*, 490–496. doi:10.1002/jhm.2208

Fernández-Hidalgo, N., & Almirante, B. (2014). Antibiotic-lock therapy: A clinical viewpoint. *Expert Review of Anti-Infective Therapy, 12*, 117–129. doi:10.1586/14787210.2014.863148

Ferroni, A., Gaudin, F., Guiffant, G., Flaud, P., Durussel, J.J., Descamps, P., … Merckx, J. (2014). Pulsative flushing as a strategy to prevent bacterial colonization of vascular access devices. *Medical Devices: Evidence and Research, 7*, 379–383. doi:10.2147/MDER.S71217

Flynn, J.M., Keogh, S.J., & Gavin, N.C. (2015). Sterile v aseptic non-touch technique for needle-less connector care on central venous access devices in a bone marrow transplant population: A comparative study. *European Journal of Oncology Nursing, 19*, 694–700. doi:10.1016/j.ejon.2015.05.003

Gan, J., & Lanigan, C. (2013). Alternative methods to improve probability of CVC catheter placement. *British Journal of Anaesthesia, 111*, 123–124. doi:10.1093/bja/aet180

Ge, X., Cavallazzi, R., Li, C., Pan, S.M., Wang, Y.W., & Wang, F.-L. (2012). Central venous access sites for the prevention of venous thrombosis, stenosis and infection. *Cochrane Database of Systematic Reviews, 2012*(3). doi:10.1002/14651858.CD004084.pub3

Gibson, F., & Bodenham, A. (2013). Misplaced central venous catheters: Applied anatomy and practical management. *British Journal of Anaesthesia, 110*, 333–346. doi:10.1093/bja/aes497

Girard, R., Comby, C., & Jacques, D. (2012). Alcoholic povidone-iodine or chlorhexidine-based antiseptic for the prevention of central venous catheter-related infections: In-use comparison. *Journal of Infection and Public Health, 5*, 35–42. doi:10.1016/j.jiph.2011.10.007

Goltz, J.P., Janssen, H., Petritsch, B., & Kickuth, R. (2014). Femoral placement of totally implantable venous power ports as an alternative implantation site for patients with central vein occlusions. *Supportive Care in Cancer, 22,* 383–387. doi:10.1007/s00520-013-1984-3

Gonzalez, T. (2013). Chemotherapy extravasations: Prevention, identification, management, and documentation. *Clinical Journal of Oncology Nursing, 17,* 61–66. doi:10.1188/13.CJON.61-66

Goossens, G.A. (2015). Flushing and locking of venous catheters: Available evidence and evidence deficit. *Nursing Research and Practice, 2015,* 985686. doi:10.1155/2015/985686

Goossens, G.A., Jérôme, M., Janssens, C., Peetermans, W.E., Fieuws, S., Moons, P., ... Stas, M. (2013). Comparing normal saline versus diluted heparin to lock non-valved totally implantable venous access devices in cancer patients: A randomized, non-inferiority, open trial. *Annals of Oncology, 24,* 1892–1899. doi:10.1093/annonc/mdt114

Gorji, M.A.H., Rezaei, F., Jafari, H., & Cherati, J.Y. (2015). Comparison of the effects of heparin and 0.9% sodium chloride solutions in maintenance of patency of central venous catheters. *Anesthesiology and Pain Medicine, 5,* e22595. doi:10.5812/aapm.22595

Guiffant, G., Durussel, J.J., Merckx, J., Flaud, P., Vigier, J.P., & Mousset, P. (2012). Flushing of intravascular access devices (IVADs): Efficacy of pulsed and continuous infusions. *Journal of Vascular Access, 13,* 75–78.

Helm, R.E., Klausner, J.D., Klemperer, J.D., Flint, L.M., & Huang, E. (2015). Accepted but unacceptable: Peripheral IV catheter failure. *Journal of Infusion Nursing, 38,* 189–203. doi:10.1097/NAN.0000000000000100

Herrera-Guerra, A.S., Garza-González, E., Martínez-Resendez, M.F., Llaca-Díaz, J.M., & Camacho-Ortiz, A. (2015). Individual versus pooled multiple-lumen blood cultures for the diagnosis of intravascular catheter-related infections. *American Journal of Infection Control, 43,* 715–718. doi:10.1016/j.ajic.2015.02.028

Hong, H., Morrow, D.F., Sandora, T.J., & Priebe, G.P. (2013). Disinfection of needleless connectors with chlorhexidine-alcohol provides long-lasting residual disinfectant activity [Online exclusive]. *American Journal of Infection Control, 41,* e77–e79. doi:10.1016/j.ajic.2012.10.018

Humphries, L., Baldwin, K., Clark, K.L., Tenuta, V., & Brumley, K. (2012). A comparison of coagulation study results between heparinized peripherally inserted central catheters and venipunctures. *Clinical Nurse Specialist, 26,* 310–316. doi:10.1097/NUR.0b013e31826e3efb

Institute for Healthcare Improvement. (2015). Evidence-based care bundles. Retrieved from http://www.ihi.org/Topics/Bundles/Pages/default.aspx

Justo, J.A., & Bookstaver, P.B. (2014). Antibiotic lock therapy: Review of technique and logistical challenges. *Journal of Infection and Drug Resistance, 7,* 343–363. doi:10.2147/IDR.S51388

Kahn, S.R., Lim, W., Dunn, A.S., Cushman, M., Dentali, F., Akl, E.A., ... Muraad, M.H. (2012). Prevention of VTE in nonsurgical patients: Antithrombotic therapy and prevention of thrombosis, 9th edition: American College of Chest Physicians evidence-based clinical practice guidelines. *Chest, 141*(Suppl. 2), e195S–e226S. doi:10.1378/chest.11-2296

Kao, H.-F., Chen, I.-C., Hsu, C., Chang, S.-Y., Chien, S.-F., Chen, Y.-C., ... Yeh, K.-H. (2014). Chlorhexidine for the prevention of bloodstream infection associated with totally implantable venous ports in patients with solid cancers. *Supportive Care in Cancer, 22,* 1189–1197. doi:10.1007/s00520-013-2071-5

Karpanen, T.J., Casey, A.L., Whitehouse, T., Nightingale, P., Das, I., & Elliott, T.S.J. (2016). Clinical evaluation of a chlorhexidine intravascular catheter gel dressing on short-term central venous catheters. *American Journal of Infection Control, 44,* 54–60. doi:10.1016/j.ajic.2015.08.022

Kerwat, K., Eberhart, L., Kerwat, M., Hörth, D., Wulf, H., Steinfeldt, T., & Wiesmann, T. (2015). Chlorhexidine gluconate dressings reduce bacterial colonization rates in epidural and peripheral

regional catheters. *BioMed Research International, 2015,* 149785. doi:10.1155/2015/149785

Krobbuaban, B., Diregpoke, S., Prasan, S., Thanomsat, M., & Kumkeaw, S. (2011). Alcohol-based chlorhexidine vs. povidone iodine in reducing skin colonization prior to regional anesthesia procedures. *Journal of the Medical Association of Thailand, 94,* 807–812.

Kubiak, D.W., Gilmore, E.T., Buckley, M.W., Lynch, R., Marty, F.M., & Koo, S. (2014). Adjunctive management of central line–associated bloodstream infections with 70% ethanol-lock therapy. *Journal of Antimicrobial Chemotherapy, 69,* 1665–1668. doi:10.1093/jac/dku017

Kulkarni, A.P., & Awode, R.M. (2013). A prospective randomized trial to compare the efficacy of povidone-iodine 10% and chlorhexidine 2% for skin disinfection. *Indian Journal of Anaesthesia, 57,* 270–275. doi:10.4103/0019-5049.115619

Lai, N.M., Chaiyakunapruk, N., Lai, N.A., O'Riordan, E., Pau, W.S.C., & Saint, S. (2013). Catheter impregnation, coating or bonding for reducing central venous catheter-related infections in adults. *Cochrane Database of Systematic Reviews, 2013*(6). doi:10.1002/14651858.CD007878.pub2

Lamperti, M., Bodenham, A.R., Pittiruti, M., Blaivas, M., Augoustides, J.G., Elbarbary, M., ... Verghese, S.T. (2012). International evidence-based recommendations on ultrasound-guided vascular access. *Intensive Care Medicine, 38,* 1105–1117. doi:10.1007/s00134-012-2597-x

Lavau-Denes, S., Lacroix, P., Maubon, A., Preux, P.M., Genet, D., Vénat-Bouvet, L., ... Tubiana-Mathieu, N. (2013). Prophylaxis of catheter-related deep vein thrombosis in cancer patients with low-dose warfarin, low molecular weight heparin, or control: A randomized, controlled, phase III study. *Cancer Chemotherapy and Pharmacology, 72,* 65–73. doi:10.1007/s00280-013-2169-y

López-Briz, E., Garcia, V.R., Cabello, J.B., Bort-Marti, S., Sanchis, R.S., & Burls, A. (2014). Heparin versus 0.9% sodium chloride intermittent flushing for prevention of occlusion in central venous catheters in adults. *Cochrane Database of Systematic Reviews, 2014*(10). doi:10.1002/14651858.CD008462.pub2

Lorente, L., Martín, M.M., Vidal, P., Rebollo, S., Ostabal, M.I., & Solé-Violán, J. (2014). Should central venous catheter be systematically removed in patients with suspected catheter related infection? *Critical Care, 18,* 564. doi:10.1186/s13054-014-0564-3

Lyons, M.G., & Phalen, A.G. (2014). A randomized controlled comparison of flushing protocols in home care patients with peripherally inserted central catheters. *Journal of Infusion Nursing, 37,* 270–281. doi:10.1097/NAN.0000000000000050

Maki, D.G., Kluger, D.M., & Crnich, C.J. (2006). The risk of bloodstream infection in adults with different intravascular devices: A systematic review of 200 published prospective studies. *Mayo Clinic Proceedings, 81,* 1159–1171. doi:10.4065/81.9.1159

Manns, B.J., Scott-Douglas, N., Tonelli, M., Ravani, P., LeBlanc, M., Dorval, M., ... Hemmelgarn, B.R. (2014). An economic evaluation of rt-PA locking solution in dialysis catheters. *Journal of the American Society of Nephrology, 25,* 2887–2895. doi:10.1681/ASN.2013050463

Marschall, J., Mermel, L.A., Fakih, M., Hadaway, L., Kallen, A., O'Grady, N.P., ... Yokoe, D.S. (2014). Strategies to prevent central line–associated bloodstream infections in acute care hospitals: 2014 update. *Infection Control and Hospital Epidemiology, 35,* 753–771. doi:10.1086/676533

Martinez, J.M., Leite, L., França, D., Capela, R., Viterbo, L., Varajão, N., ... Mariz, J. (2015). Bundle approach to reduce bloodstream infections in neutropenic hematologic patients with a long-term central venous catheter. *Acta Médica Portuguesa, 28,* 474–479. doi:10.20344/amp.6002

McEvoy, M.T., & Shander, A. (2013). Anemia, bleeding, and blood transfusion in the intensive care unit: Causes, risks, costs, and new strategies. *American Journal of Critical Care, 22,* eS1–eS13. doi:10.4037/ajcc2013729

Miglietta, F., Letizia Faneschi, M., Braione, A., Palumbo, C., Rizzo, A., Lobreglio, G., & Pizzolante, M. (2015). Central venous catheter-related fungemia caused by Rhodotorula gutinis. *Medical Mycology Journal, 56,* E17–E19. doi:10.3314/mmj.56.E17

Mirijello, A., Impagnatiello, M., Zaccone, V., Ventura, G., Pompa, L., Addolorato, G., & Landolfi, R. (2015). Catheter-related bloodstream infections by opportunistic pathogens in immunocompromised hosts. *European Review for Medical and Pharmacological Sciences, 19,* 2440–2445.

Moureau, N.L., & Flynn, J. (2015). Disinfection of needleless connector hubs: Clinical evidence systematic review. *Nursing Research and Practice, 2015,* 796762. doi:10.1155/2015/796762

Moureau, N., Mlodzik, L., Pharm, D., & Pool, S.M. (2005). The use of alteplase for treatment of occluded central venous catheters in home care. *Journal of the Association for Vascular Access, 10,* 123–129. doi:10.2309/java.10-3-7

Murray, J., Precious, E., & Alikhan, R. (2013). Catheter-related thrombosis in cancer patients. *British Journal of Haematology, 162,* 748–757. doi:10.1111/bjh.12474

National Institute for Health and Care Excellence. (2012). Healthcare-associated infections: Prevention and control in primary and community care. Retrieved from https://www.nice.org.uk/guidance/cg139/chapter/Patient-centred-care

Odabas, H., Ozdemir, N.Y., Ziraman, I., Aksoy, S., Abali, H., Oksuzoglu, B., ... Zengin, N. (2014). Effect of port-care frequency on venous port catheter-related complications in cancer patients. *International Journal of Clinical Oncology, 19,* 761–766. doi:10.1007/s10147-013-0609-7

O'Grady, N.P., Alexander, M., Burns, L.A., Dellinger, E.P., Garland, J., Heard, S.O., ... Healthcare Infection Control Practices Advisory Committee. (2011). Guidelines for the prevention of intravascular catheter-related infections. *Clinical Infectious Diseases, 52,* E162–E193. doi:10.1093/cid/cir257

Olson, K., Rennie, R.P., Hanson, J., Ryan, M., Gilpin, J., Falsetti, M., ... Gaudet, S. (2004). Evaluation of a no-dressing intervention for tunneled central venous catheter exit sites. *Journal of Infusion Nursing, 27,* 37–44. doi:10.1097/00129804-200401000-00006

Parco, S., Visconti, P., & Vascotto, F. (2014). Hematology point of care testing and laboratory errors: An example of multidisciplinary management at a children's hospital in northeast Italy. *Journal of Multidisciplinary Healthcare, 7,* 45–50. doi:10.2147/JMDH.S53904

Paşalioğlu, K.B., & Kaya, H. (2014). Catheter indwell time and phlebitis development during peripheral intravenous catheter administration. *Pakistan Journal of Medical Sciences, 30,* 725–730. doi:10.12669/pjms.304.5067

Pedrolo, E., Danski, M.T.R., Mingorance, P., De Lazzari, L.S.M., & Johann, D.A. (2011). Clinical controlled trial on central venous catheter dressings. *Acta Paulista de Enfermagem, 24,* 278–283. doi:10.1590/S0103-21002011000200019

Pedrolo, E., Danski, M.T.R., & Vayego, S.A. (2014). Chlorhexidine and gauze and tape dressings for central venous catheters: A randomized trial. *Revista Latino-Americana de Enfermagem, 22,* 764–771. doi:10.1590/0104-1169.3443.2478

Pérez-Granda, M.J., Guembe, M., Cruces, R., Barrio, J.M., & Bouza, E. (2016). Assessment of central venous catheter colonization using surveillance culture of withdrawn connectors and insertion site skin. *Critical Care, 20,* 32. doi:10.1186/s13054-016-1201-0

Polovich, M., Olsen, M., & LeFebvre, K.B. (Eds.). (2014). *Chemotherapy and biotherapy guidelines and recommendations for practice* (4th ed.). Pittsburgh, PA: Oncology Nursing Society.

Ponce, D., Mendes, M., Silva, T., & Oliveira, R. (2015). Occluded tunneled venous catheter in hemodialysis patients: Risk factors and efficacy of alteplase. *Artificial Organs, 39,* 741–747. doi:10.1111/aor.12462

Raad, I.I., & Chaftari, A.-M. (2014). Advances in prevention and management of central line–associated bloodstream infections in patients with cancer. *Clinical Infectious Diseases, 59*(Suppl. 5), S340–S343. doi:10.1093/cid/ciu670

Ragsdale, C.E., Oliver, M.R., Thompson, A.J., & Evans, M.C. (2014). Alteplase infusion versus dwell for clearance of partially occluded central venous catheters in critically ill pediatric patients. *Pediatric Critical Care Medicine 15,* e253–e260. doi:10.1097/PCC.0000000000000125

Rickard, C.M., Webster, J., Wallis, M.C., Marsh, N., McGrail, M.R., French, V., ... Whitby, M. (2012). Routine versus clinically indicated replacement of peripheral intravenous catheters: A randomised controlled equivalence trial. *Lancet, 380,* 1066–1074. doi:10.1016/S0140-6736(12)61082-4

Robertson-Malt, S., Malt, G.N., Farquhar, V., & Greer, W. (2014). Heparin versus normal saline for patency of arterial lines. *Cochrane Database of Systematic Reviews, 2014*(5). doi:10.1002/14651858.CD007364.pub2

Roldan, C.J., & Paniagua, L. (2015). Central venous catheter intravascular malpositioning: Causes, prevention, diagnosis, and correction. *Western Journal of Emergency Medicine, 16,* 658–664. doi:10.5811/westjem.2015.7.26248

Rossetti, F., Pittiruti, M., Lamperti, M., Graziano, U., Celentano, D., & Capozzoli, G. (2015). The intracavitary ECG method for positioning the tip of central venous access devices in pediatric patients: Results of an Italian multicenter study [Online exclusive]. *Journal of Vascular Access, 16,* e137–e143. doi:10.5301/jva.5000281

Safdar, N., O'Horo, J.C., Ghufran, A., Bearden, A., Didier, M.E., Chateau, D., & Maki, D.G. (2014). Chlorhexidine-impregnated dressing for prevention of catheter-related bloodstream infection: A meta-analysis. *Critical Care Medicine, 42,* 1703–1713. doi:10.1097/CCM.0000000000000319

Sandora, T.J., Graham, D.A., Conway, M., Dodson, B., Potter-Bynoe, G., & Margossian, S.P. (2014). Impact of needleless connector change frequency on central line–associated bloodstream infection rate. *American Journal of Infection Control, 42,* 485–489. doi:10.1016/j.ajic.2014.01.022

Schallom, M.E., Prentice, D., Sona, C., Micek, S.T., & Skrupky, L.P. (2012). Heparin or 0.9% sodium chloride to maintain central venous catheter patency: A randomized trial. *Critical Care Medicine, 40,* 1820–1826. doi:10.1097/CCM.0b013e31824e11b4

Schiffer, C.A., Mangu, P.B., Wade, J.C., Camp-Sorrell, D., Cope, D.G., El-Rayes, B.F., ... Levine, M. (2013). Central venous catheter care for the patient with cancer: American Society of Clinical Oncology clinical practice guideline. *Journal of Clinical Oncology, 31,* 1357–1370. doi:10.1200/JCO.2012.45.5733

Schoot, R.A., van Dalen, E.C., van Ommen, C.H., & van de Wetering, M.D. (2013). Antibiotic and other lock treatments for tunneled central venous catheter-related infections in children with cancer. *Cochrane Database of Systematic Reviews, 2013*(6). doi:10.1002/14651858.CD008975.pub2

Schulmeister, L. (2011). Extravasation management: Clinical update. *Seminars in Oncology Nursing 27,* 82–90. doi:10.1016/j.soncn.2010.11.010

Septimus, E. (2015). Clinician guide for collecting cultures. Retrieved from http://www.cdc.gov/getsmart/healthcare/implementation/clinicianguide.html

Shah, P.S., & Shah, N. (2014). Heparin-bonded catheters for prolonging the patency of central venous catheters in children. *Cochrane Database of Systematic Reviews, 2014*(2). doi:10.1002/14651858.CD005983.pub3

Shekelle, P.G., Wachter, R.M., Pronovost, P.J., Schoelles, K., McDonald, K.M., Dy, S.M., ... Winters, B.D. (2013, March). *Making health care safer II: An updated critical analysis of the evidence for patient safety practices* (Comparative Effectiveness Review No. 211, prepared by the Southern California-RAND Evidence-based Practice Center under Contract No. 290-2007-10062-I, AHRQ Publication No.

13-E001-EF). Retrieved from http://www.ahrq.gov/research/findings/evidence-based-reports/ptsafetyuptp.html

Sherertz, R.J., Karchmer, T.B., Palavecino, E., & Bischoff, W. (2011). Blood drawn through valved catheter hub connectors carries a significant risk of contamination. *European Journal of Clinical Microbiology and Infectious Diseases, 30,* 1571–1577. doi:10.1007/s10096-011-1262-6

Simmons, S., Bryson, C., & Porter, S. (2011). "Scrub the hub": Cleaning duration and reduction in bacterial load on central venous catheters. *Critical Care Nursing Quarterly, 34,* 31–35. doi:10.1097/CNQ.0b013e3182048073

Sweet, M.A., Cumpston, A., Briggs, F., Craig, M., & Hamadani, M. (2012). Impact of alcohol-impregnated port protectors and needleless neutral pressure connectors on central line–associated bloodstream infections and contamination of blood cultures in an inpatient oncology unit. *American Journal of Infection Control, 40,* 931–934. doi:10.1016/j.ajic.2012.01.025

Tabak, Y.P., Jarvis, W.R., Sun, X., Crosby, C.T., & Johannes, R.S. (2014). Meta-analysis on central line–associated bloodstream infections associated with a needleless intravenous connector with a new engineering design. *American Journal of Infection Control, 42,* 1278–1284. doi:10.1016/j.ajic.2014.08.018

Tebbi, C., Costanzi, J., Shulman, R., Dreisbach, L., Jacobs, B.R., Blaney, M., ... Begelman, S.M. (2011). A phase III, open-label, single-arm study of tenecteplase for restoration of function in dysfunctional central venous catheters. *Journal of Vascular Interventional Radiology, 22,* 1117–1123. doi:10.1016/j.jvir.2011.02.034

Teichgräber, U.K.M., Kausche, S., Nagel, S.N., & Gebauer, B. (2011). Outcome analysis in 3,160 implantations of radiologically guided placements of totally implantable central venous port systems. *European Radiology, 21,* 1224–1232. doi:10.1007/s00330-010-2045-7

Teichgräber, U.K.M., Nagel, S.N., Kausche, S., & Enzweiler, C. (2012). Clinical benefit of power-injectable port systems: A prospective observational study. *European Journal of Radiology, 81,* 528–533. doi:10.1016/j.ejrad.2011.01.038

Thomopoulos, T., Meyer, J., Staszewicz, W., Bagetakos, I., Scheffler, M., Lomessy, A., ... Morel, P. (2014). Routine chest x-ray is not mandatory after fluoroscopy-guided totally implantable venous access device insertion. *Annals of Vascular Surgery, 28,* 345–350. doi:10.1016/j.avsg.2013.08.003

Timsit, J.F., Mimoz, O., Mourvillier, B., Souweine, B., Garrouste-Orgeas, M., Alfandari, S., ... Lucet, J.C. (2012). Randomized controlled trial of chlorhexidine dressing and highly adhesive dressing for preventing catheter-related infections in critically ill adults. *American Journal of Respiratory and Critical Care Medicine, 186,* 1272–1278. doi:10.1164/rccm.201206-1038OC

Ullman, A.J., Cooke, M.L., Mitchell, M., Lin, F., New, K., Long, D.A., ... & Rickard, C.M. (2015). Dressings and securement devices for central venous catheters (CVC). *Cochrane Database of Systematic Reviews, 2015*(9). doi:10.1002/14651858.CD010367.pub2

van de Wetering, M.D., van Woensel, J.B.M., & Lawrie, T.A. (2013). Prophylactic antibiotics for preventing gram positive infections associated with long-term central venous catheters in oncology patients. *Cochrane Database of Systematic Reviews, 2013*(11). doi:10.1002/14651858.CD003295.pub3

van der Merwe, E., Luscombe, R., & Kiaii, M. (2015). The use of tissue plasminogen activator as continuous infusion into an arteriovenous hemodialysis access in the hemodialysis unit: A case series. *Canadian Journal of Kidney Health and Disease, 30,* 2. doi:10.1186/s40697-015-0035-z

Vercaigne, L.M., Zacharias, J., & Bernstein, K.N. (2012). Alteplase for blood flow restoration in hemodialysis catheters: A multicenter, randomized, prospective study comparing "dwell" versus "push" administration. *Clinical Nephrology, 78,* 287–296. doi:10.5414/CN107351

Walker, G., Alexandrou, E., Rickard, C.M., Chan, R.J., & Webster, J. (2015). Effectiveness of electrocardiographic guidance in CVAD tip placement. *British Journal of Nursing, 24*(Suppl. 14), S4, S6, S8–S12. doi:10.12968/bjon.2015.24.Sup14.S4

Wang, G., Guo, L., Jiang, B., Huang, M., Zhang, J., & Qin, Y. (2015). Factors influencing intracavitary electrocardiographic P-wave changes during central venous catheter placement. *PLOS ONE, 10,* e0124846. doi:10.1371/journal.pone.0124846

Webster, J., Osborne, S., Rickard, C.M., & New, K. (2015). Clinically-indicated replacement versus routine replacement of peripheral venous catheters. *Cochrane Database of Systematic Reviews, 2015*(8). doi:10.1002/14651858.cd007798.pub4

Wibaux, A., Thota, P., Mastej, J., Prince, D.L., Carty, N., & Johnson, P. (2015). Antimicrobial activity of a novel vascular access film dressing containing chlorhexidine gluconate. *PLOS ONE, 10,* e0143035. doi:10.1371/journal.pone.0143035

Winokur, E.J., Pai, D., Rutledge, D.N., Vogel, K., Al-Majid, S., Marshall, C., & Sheikewitz, P. (2014). Blood culture accuracy: Discards from central venous catheters in pediatric oncology patients in the emergency department. *Journal of Emergency Nursing, 40,* 323–329. doi:10.1016/j.jen.2013.04.007

World Health Organization. (2010). *WHO guidelines on drawing blood: Best practices in phlebotomy.* Retrieved from http://www.ncbi.nlm.nih.gov/books/NBK138665

Wound, Ostomy and Continence Nurses Society. (2011). Clean vs. sterile dressing techniques for management of chronic wounds: A fact sheet. Retrieved from http://www.wocn.org/news/76597/Clean-vs.-Sterile-Dressing-Techniques-for-Management-of-Chronic-Wounds-A-Fact-Sheet.htm

Wright, M.-O., Tropp, J., Schora, D.M., Dillon-Grant, M., Peterson, K., ... Peterson, L.R. (2013). Continuous passive disinfection of catheter hubs prevents contamination and bloodstream infection. *American Journal of Infection Control, 15,* 33–38. doi:10.1016/j.ajic.2012.05.030

Zadeh, M.K., & Shirvani, A. (2014). The role of routine chest radiography for detecting complications after central venous catheter insertion. *Saudi Journal of Kidney Diseases and Transplantation, 25,* 1011–1016. doi:10.4103/1319-2442.139895

Zhang, L., Gowardman, J., Morrison, M., Runnegar, N., & Rickard, C.M. (2016). Microbial biofilms associated with intravascular catheter-related bloodstream infections in adult intensive care patients. *European Journal of Clinical Microbiology and Infectious Diseases, 35,* 201–205. doi:10.1007/s10096-015-2530-7

Zu-Kei Lin, R., Fowler, S., Dise, C.A., & Bustami, R. (2009). Venous access devices: Obtaining coagulation tests in adult inpatients with cancer. *Clinical Journal of Oncology Nursing, 13,* 347–349. doi:10.1188/09.CJON.347-349

Historical References

Aslam, S. (2008). Effect of antibacterials on biofilms. *American Journal of Infection Control, 36,* S175.e9–S175.e11. doi:10.1016/j.ajic.2008.10.002

Aufwerber, E.W.A., Ringertz, S., & Ransjö, U. (1991). Routine semi-quantitative cultures and central venous catheter-related bacteremia. *Acta Pathologica, Microbiologica, et Immunologica Scandinavica, 99,* 627–630. doi:10.1111/j.1699-0463.1991.tb01237.x

Banton, J. (2006). Techniques to prevent central venous catheter infections: Products, research, and recommendations. *Nutrition in Clinical Practice, 21,* 56–61. doi:10.1177/011542650602100156

Barton, S.J., Chase, T., Latham, B., & Rayens, M.K. (2004). Comparing two methods to obtain blood specimens from pediatric central venous catheters. *Journal of Pediatric Oncology Nursing, 21,* 320–326.

Bestul, M.B., & VandenBussche, H.L. (2005). Antibiotic lock technique: Review of the literature. *Pharmacotherapy, 25,* 211–227. doi:10.1592/phco.25.2.211.56947

Biffi, R., Orsi, F., Pozzi, S., Pace, U., Bonomo, G., Monfardini, L., … Goldhirsch, A. (2009). Best choice of central venous insertion site for the prevention of catheter-related complications in adult patients who need cancer therapy: A randomized trial. *Annals of Oncology, 20,* 935–940. doi:10.1093/annonc/mdn701

Birnbach, D.J., Meadows, W., Stein, D.J., Murray, O., Thys, D.M., & Sordillo, E.M. (2003). Comparison of povidone iodine and Dura-Prep, an iodophor-in-isopropyl alcohol solution, for skin disinfection prior to epidural catheter insertion in parturients. *Anesthesiology, 98,* 164–169. doi:10.1097/00000542-200301000-00026

Bishop, L., Dougherty, L., Bodenham, A., Mansi, J., Crowe, P., Kibbler, C., … Treleaven, J. (2007). Guidelines on the insertion and management of central venous access devices in adults. *International Journal of Laboratory Hematology, 29,* 261–278. doi:10.1111/j.1751-553X.2007.00931.x

Blaney, M., Shen, V., Kerner, J.A., Jacobs, B.R., Gray, S., Armfield, J., & Semba, C.P. (2006). Alteplase for the treatment of central venous catheter occlusion in children: Results of a prospective, open-label, single-arm study (the Cathflo Activase Pediatric Study). *Journal of Vascular and Interventional Radiology, 17,* 1745–1751. doi:10.1097/01.RVI.0000241542.71063.83

Bonawitz, S.C., Hammell, E.J., & Kirkpatrick, J.R. (1991). Prevention of central venous catheter sepsis: A prospective randomized trial. *American Surgeon, 57,* 618–623.

Boraks, P., Seale, J., Price, J., Bass, G., Ethell, M., Keeling, D., … Marcus, R. (1998). Prevention of central venous catheter associated thrombosis using minidose warfarin in patients with haematological malignancies. *British Journal of Haematology, 101,* 483–486. doi:10.1046/j.1365-2141.1998.00732.x

Bowers, L., Speroni, K.G., Jones, L., & Atherton, M. (2008). Comparison of occlusion rates by flushing solutions for peripherally inserted central catheters with positive pressure Luer-activated devices. *Journal of Infusion Nursing, 31,* 22–27. doi:10.1097/01.NAN.0000308542.90615.c2

Boyd, A., Dunne, A., Townsend, K., & Pai, A.B. (2006). Sampling for international normalized ratios in patients on hemodialysis with central venous catheters. *Nephrology Nursing Journal, 33,* 408–411.

Btaiche, I.F., Kovacevich, D.S., Khalidi, N., & Papke, L.F. (2011). The effects of needleless connectors on catheter-related thrombotic occlusions. *Journal of Infusion Nursing, 34,* 89–96. doi:10.1097/NAN.0b013e31820b3ea9

Buchman, A.L., Spapperi, J., & Leopold, P. (2009). A new central venous catheter cap: Decreased microbial growth and risk for catheter-related bloodstream infection. *Journal of Vascular Access, 10,* 11–21.

Carr, K.M., & Rabinowitz, I. (2000). Physician compliance with warfarin prophylaxis for central venous catheters in patients with solid tumors. *Journal of Clinical Oncology, 18,* 3665–3667.

Carratalá, J., Niubó, J., Fernández-Sevilla, A., Juvé, E., Castellsagué, X., Berlanga, J., … Gudiol, F. (1999). Randomized, double-blind trial of an antibiotic-lock technique for prevention of Gram-positive central venous catheter-related infection in neutropenic patients with cancer. *Antimicrobial Agents and Chemotherapy, 43,* 2200–2204.

Cesaro, S., Tridello, G., Cavaliere, M., Magagna, L., Gavin, P., Cusinato, R., … Carli, M. (2009). Prospective, randomized trial of two different modalities of flushing central venous catheters in pediatric patients with cancer. *Journal of Clinical Oncology, 27,* 2059–2065. doi:10.1200/JCO.2008.19.4860

Chaiyakunapruk, N., Veenstra, D.L., Lipsky, B.A., & Saint, S. (2002). Chlorhexidine compared with povidone-iodine solution for vascular catheter–site care: A meta-analysis. *Annals of Internal Medicine, 136,* 792–801. doi:10.7326/0003-4819-136-11-200206040-00007

Chatzinikolaou, I., Hanna, H., Darouiche, R., Samonis, G., Tarrand, J., & Raad, I.I. (2006). Prospective study of the value of quantitative culture of organisms from blood collected through central venous catheters in differentiating between contamination and blood stream infection. *Journal of Clinical Microbiology, 44,* 1834–1835. doi:10.1128/JCM.44.5.1834-1835.2006

Conly, J.M., Grieves, K., & Peters, B. (1989). A prospective, randomized study comparing transparent and dry gauze dressings for central venous catheters. *Journal of Infectious Diseases, 159,* 310–319. doi:10.1093/infdis/159.2.310

Cook, D., Randolph, A., Kernerman, P., Cupido, C., King, D., Soukup, C., & Brun-Buisson, C. (1997). Central venous catheter replacement strategies: A systematic review of the literature. *Critical Care Medicine, 25,* 1417–1424. doi:10.1097/00003246-199708000-00033

Cosca, P.A., Smith, S., Chatfield, S., Meleason, A., Muir, C.A., Nerantzis, S., … Williams, S. (1998). Reinfusion of discard blood from venous access devices. *Oncology Nursing Forum, 25,* 1073–1076.

Coyle, D., Bloomgarden, D., Beres, R., Patel, S., Sane, S., & Hurst, E. (2004). Power injection of contrast media via peripherally inserted central catheters for CT. *Journal of Vascular Interventional Radiology, 15,* 809–814. doi:10.1097/01.RVI.0000128812.20864.EC

Cummings-Winfield, C., & Mushani-Kanji, T. (2008). Restoring patency to central venous access devices. *Clinical Journal of Oncology Nursing, 12,* 925–934. doi:10.1188/08.CJON.925-934

Darouiche, R.O., Raad, I.I., Heard, S.O., Thornby, J.I., Wenker, O.C., Gabrielli, A., … Mayhall, G. (1999). A comparison of two antimicrobial-impregnated central venous catheters. *New England Journal of Medicine, 340,* 1–8. doi:10.1056/NEJM199901073400101

Debreceni, G., Meggyesi, R., & Mestyán, G. (2007). Efficacy of spray disinfection with a 2-propanol and benzalkonium chloride containing solution before epidural catheter insertion—A prospective, randomized, clinical trial. *British Journal of Anaesthesia, 98,* 131–135. doi:10.1093/bja/ael288

De Cicco, M., Matovic, M., Balestreri, L., Steffan, A., Pacenzia, R., Malafronte, M., …Veronesi, A. (2009). Early and short-term acenocumarine or dalteparin for the prevention of central vein catheter-related thrombosis in cancer patients: A randomized controlled study based on serial venographies. *Annals of Oncology, 20,* 1936–1942. doi:10.1093/annonc/mdp235

Del Cotillo, M., Grané, N., Llavoré, M., & Quintana, S. (2008). Heparinized solution vs. saline solution in the maintenance of arterial catheters: A double blind randomized clinical trial. *Intensive Care Medicine, 34,* 339–343. doi:10.1007/s00134-007-0886-6

Dickerson, N., Horton, P., Smith, S., & Rose, R.C. (1989). Clinically significant central venous catheter infections in a community hospital: Association with type of dressing. *Journal of Infectious Diseases, 160,* 720–722. doi:10.1093/infdis/160.4.720

Do, A.N., Ray, B.J., Banerjee, S.N., Illian, A.F., Barnett, B.J., Pham, M.H., … Jarvis, W.R. (1999). Bloodstream infection associated with needleless device use and the importance of infection-control practices in the home health care setting. *Journal of Infectious Diseases, 179,* 442–448. doi:10.1086/314592

Douard, M.C., Arlet, G., Longuet, P., Troje, C., Rouveau, M., Ponscarme, D., & Eurin, B. (1999). Diagnosis of venous access port–related infections. *Clinical Infectious Diseases, 29,* 1197–1202. doi:10.1086/313444

D'souza, N., Gupta, B., Sawhney, C., & Chaturvedi, A. (2010). Misdirected central venous catheter. *Journal of Emergencies, Trauma, and Shock, 3,* 209–210. doi:10.4103/0974-2700.62100

Esteve, F., Pujol, M., Limón, E., Saballs, M., Argerich, M.J., Verdaguer, R., … Gudiol, F. (2007). Bloodstream infection related to catheter connections: A prospective trial of two connection systems. *Journal of Hospital Infection, 67,* 30–34. doi:10.1016/j.jhin.2007.05.021

Field, K., McFarlane, C., Cheng, A.C., Hughes, A.J., Jacobs, E., Styles, K., … Athan, E. (2007). Incidence of catheter-related bloodstream infection among patients with a needleless, mechanical valve–based intravenous connector in an Australian hematology-oncology unit. *Infection Control and Hospital Epidemiology, 28,* 610–613. doi:10.1086/516660

Fraenkel, D., Rickard, C.B., Thomas, P.B., Faoagali, J., George, N., & Ware, R. (2006). A prospective, randomized trial of rifampicin-minocycline-coated and silver-platinum-carbon-impregnated central venous catheters. *Critical Care Medicine, 34,* 668–675. doi:10.1097/01.CCM.0000201404.05523.34

Frey, A.M. (2003). Drawing blood samples from vascular access devices: Evidence-based practice. *Journal of Infusion Nursing, 26,* 285–293. doi:10.1097/00129804-200309000-00004

Garland, J.S., Alex, C.P., Mueller, C.D., Otten, D., Shivpuri, C., Harris, M.C., … Maki, D.G. (2001). A randomized trial comparing povidone-iodine to a chlorhexidine gluconate-impregnated dressing for prevention of central venous catheter infections in neonates. *Pediatrics, 107,* 1431–1436. doi:10.1542/peds.107.6.1431

Gillies, D., Carr, D., Frost, J., O'Riordan, E., Gunning, R., & O'Brien, I. (2003). Gauze and tape and transparent polyurethane dressings for central venous catheters. *Cochrane Database of Systematic Reviews, 2003*(3). doi:10.1002/14651858.CD003827

Goetz, A.M., Wagener, M.M., Miller, J.M., & Muder, R.R. (1998). Risk of infection due to central venous catheters: Effect of site of placement and catheter type. *Infection Control and Hospital Epidemiology, 19,* 842–845. doi:10.1086/647742

Hall, K.F., Bennetts, T.M., Whitta, R.K., Welman, L., & Rawlins, P. (2006). Effect of heparin in arterial line flushing solutions on platelet count: A randomized double-blind study. *Critical Care and Resuscitation, 8,* 294–296.

Harter, C., Salwender, H.J., Bach, A., Egerer, G., Goldschmidt, H., & Ho, A.D. (2002). Catheter-related infection and thrombosis of the internal jugular vein in hematologic-oncologic patients undergoing chemotherapy: A prospective comparison of silver-coated and uncoated catheters. *Cancer, 94,* 245–251. doi:10.1002/cncr.10199

Heard, S.O., Wagle, M., Vijayakumar, E., McLean, S., Brueggemann, A., Napolitano, L.M., … Doern, G.V. (1998). Influence of triple-lumen central venous catheters coated with chlorhexidine and silver sulfadiazine on the incidence of catheter-related bacteremia. *Archives of Internal Medicine, 158,* 81–87. doi:10.1001/archinte.158.1.81

Heath, J., & Jones, S. (2001). Utilization of an elastomeric continuous infusion device to maintain catheter patency. *Journal of Intravenous Nursing, 24,* 102–106.

Herts, B.R., O'Malley, C.M., Wirth, S.L., Lieber, M.L., & Pohlman, B. (2001). Power injection of contrast media using central venous catheters: Feasibility, safety, and efficacy. *American Journal of Roentgenology, 176,* 447–453. doi:10.2214/ajr.176.2.1760447

Hibbard, J.S., Mulberry, G.K., & Brady, A.R. (2002). A clinical study comparing the skin antisepsis and safety of ChloraPrep, 70% isopropyl alcohol, and 2% aqueous chlorhexidine. *Journal of Infusion Nursing, 25,* 244–249. doi:10.1097/00129804-200207000-00007

Hinds, P.S., Quargnenti, A., Gattuso, J., Kumar Srivastova, D., Tong, X., Penn, L., … Head, D. (2002). Comparing the results of coagulation tests on blood drawn by venipuncture and through heparinized tunneled venous access devices in pediatric patients with cancer [Online exclusive]. *Oncology Nursing Forum, 29,* E26–E34. doi:10.1188/02.ONF.E26-E34

Ho, K.M., & Litton, E. (2006). Use of chlorhexidine-impregnated dressing to prevent vascular and epidural catheter colonization and infection: A meta-analysis. *Journal of Antimicrobial Chemotherapy, 58,* 281–287. doi:10.1093/jac/dkl234

Hoffmann, K.K., Weber, D.J., Samsa, G.P., & Rutala, W.A. (1992). Transparent polyurethane film as an intravenous catheter dressing: A meta-analysis of the infection risks. *JAMA, 267,* 2072–2076. doi:10.1001/jama.1992.03480150078041

Holmes, K.R. (1998). Comparison of push-pull versus discard method from central venous catheters for blood testing. *Journal of Intravenous Nursing, 21,* 282–285.

Homer, L.D., & Holmes, K.R. (1998). Risks associated with 72- and 96-hour peripheral intravenous catheter dwell times. *Journal of Intravenous Nursing, 21,* 301–305.

Horne, M.K., III, McCloskey, D.J., Calis, K., Wesley, R., Childs, R., & Kasten-Sportes, C. (2006). Use of heparin versus lepirudin flushes to prevent withdrawal occlusion of central venous access devices. *Pharmacotherapy, 26,* 1262–1267. doi:10.1592/phco.26.9.1262

Jaeger, K., Osthaus, A., Heine, J., Ruschulte, H., Kuhlmann, C., Weissbrodt, H., … Karthaus, M. (2001). Efficacy of a benzalkonium chloride-impregnated central venous catheter to prevent catheter-associated infection in cancer patients. *Chemotherapy, 47,* 50–55.

Jaeger, K., Zenz, S., Jüttner, B., Ruschulte, H., Kuse, E., Heine, J., … Karthaus, M. (2005). Reduction of catheter-related infections in neutropenic patients: A prospective controlled randomized trial using a chlorhexidine and silver sulfadiazine–impregnated central venous catheter. *Annals of Hematology, 84,* 258–262. doi:10.1007/s00277-004-0972-6

Jones, P.M. (1987). Indwelling central venous catheter-related infections and two different procedures of catheter care. *Cancer Nursing, 10,* 123–130. doi:10.1097/00002820-198706000-00001

Kaler, W., & Chinn, R. (2007). Successful disinfection of needleless access ports: A matter of time and friction. *Journal of the Association for Vascular Access, 12,* 140–142. doi:10.2309/java.12-3-9

Kalfon, P., de Vaumas, C., Samba, D., Boulet, E., Lefrant, J.-Y., Eyraud, D., … Riou, B. (2007). Comparison of silver-impregnated with standard multi-lumen central venous catheters in critically ill patients. *Critical Care Medicine, 35,* 1032–1039. doi:10.1097/01.CCM.0000259378.53166.1B

Kallen, A.J., Patel, P.R., & O'Grady, N.P. (2010). Preventing catheter-related bloodstream infections outside the intensive care unit: Expanding prevention to new settings. *Clinical Infectious Diseases, 5,* 335–341. doi:10.1086/653942

Karthaus, M., Kretzschmar, A., Kröning, H., Biakhov, M., Irwin, D., Marschner, N., … Reichardt, P. (2006). Dalteparin for prevention of catheter-related complications in cancer patients with central venous catheters: Final results of a double-blind, placebo-controlled phase III trial. *Annals of Oncology, 17,* 289–296. doi:10.1093/annonc/mdj059

Kasuda, H., Fukuda, H., Togashi, H., Hotta, K., Hirai, Y., & Hayashi, M. (2002). Skin disinfection before epidural catheterization: Comparative study of povidone-iodine versus chlorhexidine ethanol. *Dermatology, 204*(Suppl. 1), 42–46. doi:10.1159/000057724

Kefeli, U., Dane, F., Yumuk, P.F., Karamanoglu, A., Iyikesici, S., Basaran, G., & Turhal, N.S. (2009). Prolonged interval in prophylactic heparin flushing for maintenance of subcutaneous implanted port care in patients with cancer. *European Journal of Cancer Care, 18,* 191–194. doi:10.1111/j.1365-2354.2008.00973.x

Kelly, C., Dumenko, L., McGregor, S.E., & McIutchion, M.E. (1992). A change in flushing protocols of central venous catheters. *Oncology Nursing Forum, 19,* 599–605.

Khare, M.D., Bukhari, S.S., Swann, A., Spiers, P., McLaren, I., & Myers, J. (2007). Reduction of catheter-related colonisation by the use of a silver zeolite-impregnated central vascular catheter in adult critical care. *Journal of Infection, 54,* 146–150. doi:10.1016/j.jinf.2006.03.002

Kinirons, B., Mimoz, O., Lafendi, L., Naas, T., Meunier, J., & Nordmann, P. (2001). Chlorhexidine versus povidone iodine in preventing colonization of continuous epidural catheters in children: A randomized, controlled trial. *Anesthesiology, 94,* 239–244. doi:10.1097/00000542-200102000-00012

Kuo, Y.S., Schwartz, B., Santiago, J., Anderson, P.S., Fields, A.L., & Goldberg, G.L. (2005). How often should a Port-A-Cath be flushed? *Cancer Investigation, 23,* 582–585. doi:10.1080/07357900500276923

Laura, R., Degl'Innocenti, M., Mocali, M., Alberani, F., Boschi, S., Giraudi, A., … Peron, G. (2000). Comparison of two different time interval protocols for central venous catheter dressing in bone marrow transplant patients: Results of a randomized, multicenter study. The Italian Nurse Bone Marrow Transplant Group (GITMO). *Haematologica, 85*, 275–279.

Levy, I., Katz, J., Solter, E., Samra, Z., Vidne, B., Birk, E., ... Dagan, O. (2005). Chlorhexidine-impregnated dressing for prevention of colonization of central venous catheters in infants and children: A randomized controlled study. *Pediatric Infectious Disease Journal, 24*, 676–679. doi:10.1097/01.inf.0000172934.98865.14

Liu, C.Y., Jain, V., Shields, A.F., & Heilbrun, L.K. (2004). Efficacy and safety of reteplase for central venous catheter occlusion in patients with cancer. *Journal of Vascular and Interventional Radiology, 15*, 39–44. doi:10.1097/01.RVI.0000106385.63463.EC

Longuet, P., Douard, M.C., Arlet, G., Molina, J.M., Benoit, C., & Leport, C. (2001). Venous access port–related bacteremia in patients with acquired immunodeficiency syndrome or cancer: The reservoir as a diagnostic and therapeutic tool. *Clinical Infectious Diseases, 32*, 1776–1783. doi:10.1086/320746

Madeo, M., Martin, C., & Nobbs, A. (1997). A randomized study comparing IV 3000 (transparent polyurethane dressing) to a dry gauze dressing for peripheral intravenous catheter sites. *Journal of Intravenous Nursing, 20*, 253–256.

Magagnoli, M., Masci, G., Castagna, L., Pedicini, V., Poretti, D., Morenghi, E., ... Santoro, A. (2006). Prophylaxis of central venous catheter-related thrombosis with minidose warfarin in patients treated with high-dose chemotherapy and peripheral-blood stem-cell transplantation: Retrospective analysis of 228 cancer patients. *American Journal of Hematology, 81*, 1–4. doi:10.1002/ajh.20512

Mann, T.J., Orlikowski, C.E., Gurrin, L.C., & Keil, A.D. (2001). The effect of the biopatch, a chlorhexidine impregnated dressing, on bacterial colonization of epidural catheter exit sites. *Anaesthesia and Intensive Care, 29*, 600–603.

Martinez, E., Mensa, J., Rovira, M., Martínez, J.A., Marcos, A., Almela, M., & Carreras, E. (1999). Central venous catheter exchange by guidewire for treatment of catheter-related bacteraemia in patients undergoing BMT or intensive chemotherapy. *Bone Marrow Transplantation, 23*, 41–44. doi:10.1038/sj.bmt.1701538

McDonald, L.C., Banerjee, S.N., & Jarvis, W.R. (1998). Line-associated bloodstream infections in pediatric intensive-care-unit patients associated with a needleless device and intermittent intravenous therapy. *Infection Control and Hospital Epidemiology, 19*, 772–777.

Menyhay, S.Z., & Maki, D.G. (2006). Disinfection of needleless catheter connectors and access ports with alcohol may not prevent microbial entry: The promise of a novel antiseptic-barrier cap. *Infection Control and Hospital Epidemiology, 27*, 23–27. doi:10.1086/500280

Menyhay, S.Z., & Maki, D.G. (2008). Preventing central venous catheter-associated bloodstream infections: Development of an antiseptic barrier cap for needleless connectors. *American Journal of Infection Control, 36*, S174.e1–S174.e5. doi:10.1016/j.ajic.2008.10.006

Mermel, L.A. (2007). Prevention of central venous catheter-related infections: What works other than impregnated or coated catheters? *Journal of Hospital Infection, 65*(Suppl. 2), 30–33. doi:10.1016/S0195-6701(07)60011-5

Mermel, L.A., Allon, M., Bouza, E., Craven, D.E., Flynn, P., O'Grady, N.P., ... Warren, D.K. (2009). Clinical practice guidelines for the diagnosis and management of intravascular catheter-related infection: 2009 update by the Infectious Diseases Society of America. *Clinical Infectious Diseases, 49*, 1–45. doi:10.1086/599376

Middleton, R. (2006). Suturing as an advanced skill for registered nurses in the emergency department. *Australian Journal of Rural Health, 15*, 258–262. doi:10.1111/j.1440-1584.2006.00826.x

Minassian, V.A., Sood, A.K., Lowe, P., Sorosky, J.I., Al-Jurf, A.S., & Buller, R.E. (2000). Long-term central venous access in gynecologic cancer patients. *Journal of the American College of Surgeons, 191*, 403–409. doi:10.1016/S1072-7515(00)00690-6

Moll, S., Kenyon, P., Bertoli, L., De Maio, J., Homesley, H., & Deitcher, S.R. (2006). Phase II trial of alfimeprase, a novel-acting fibrin degradation agent, for occluded central venous access devices. *Journal of Clinical Oncology, 24*, 3056–3060. doi:10.1200/JCO.2006.05.8438

Moss, H.A., Tebbs, S.E., Faroqui, M.H., Herbst, T., Isaac, J.L., Brown, J., & Elliott, T.S.J. (2000). A central venous catheter coated with benzalkonium chloride for the prevention of catheter-related microbial colonization. *European Journal of Anaesthesiology, 17*, 680–687. doi:10.1097/00003643-200011000-00005

Ng, R., Li, X., Tu, T., & Semba, C.P. (2004). Alteplase for treatment of occluded peripherally inserted central catheters: Safety and efficacy in 240 patients. *Journal of Vascular and Interventional Radiology, 15*, 45–49. doi:10.1097/01.RVI.000099538.29957.F7

Niers, T.M., Di Nisio, M., Klerk, C.P.W., Baarslag, H.J., Büller, H.R., & Biemond, B.J. (2007). Prevention of catheter-related venous thrombosis with nadroparin in patients receiving chemotherapy for hematologic malignancies: A randomized, placebo-controlled study. *Journal of Thrombosis and Haemostasis, 5*, 1878–1882. doi:10.1111/j.1538-7836.2007.02660.x

Nikoletti, S., Leslie, G., Gandossi, S., Coombs, G., & Wilson, R. (1999). A prospective, randomized, controlled trial comparing transparent polyurethane and hydrocolloid dressings for central venous catheters. *American Journal of Infection Control, 27*, 488–496. doi:10.1016/S0196-6553(99)70026-X

Opilla, M. (2008). Epidemiology of bloodstream infection associated with parenteral nutrition. *American Journal of Infection Control, 36*, S173.e5–S173.e8. doi:10.1016/j.ajic.2008.10.007

Osma, S., Kahveci, S.F., Kaya, F.N., Akalin, H., Özakin, C., Yilmaz, E., & Kutlay, O. (2006). Efficacy of antiseptic-impregnated catheters on catheter colonization and catheter-related bloodstream infections in patients in an intensive care unit. *Journal of Hospital Infection, 62*, 156–162. doi:10.1016/j.jhin.2005.06.030

Owens, L. (2002). Reteplase for clearance of occluded venous catheters. *American Journal of Health-System Pharmacy, 59*, 1638–1640.

Paice, J.A., DuPen, A., & Schwertz, D. (1999). Catheter port cleansing techniques and the entry of povidone-iodine into the epidural space. *Oncology Nursing Forum, 26*, 603–605.

Petrosino, B., Becker, H., & Christian, B. (1988). Infection rates in central venous catheter dressings. *Oncology Nursing Forum, 15*, 709–717.

Ponec, D., Irwin, D., Haire, W.D., Hill, P.A., Li, X., & McCluskey, E.R. (2001). Recombinant tissue plasminogen activator (alteplase) for restoration of flow in occluded central venous access devices: A double-blind placebo-controlled trial—The Cardiovascular Thrombolytic to Open Occluded Lines (COOL) efficacy trial. *Journal of Vascular Interventional Radiology, 12*, 951–955. doi:10.1016/S1051-0443(07)61575-9

Raad, I.I., & Bodey, G.P. (1992). Infectious complications of indwelling vascular catheters. *Clinical Infectious Diseases, 15*, 197–210. doi:10.1093/clinids/15.2.197

Raad, I.I., Hanna, H., & Maki, D. (2007). Intravascular catheter-related infections: Advances in diagnosis, prevention, and management. *Lancet Infectious Diseases, 7*, 645–657. doi:10.1016/S1473-3099(07)70235-9

Ramritu, P., Halton, K., Collignon, P., Cook, D., Fraenkel, D., Battistutta, D., ... Graves, N. (2008). A systematic review comparing the relative effectiveness of antimicrobial-coated catheters in intensive care units. *American Journal of Infection Control, 36*, 104–117. doi:10.1016/j.ajic.2007.02.012

Rondina, M.T., Markewitz, B., Kling, S.J., Nohavec, R., & Rodgers, G.M. (2007). The accuracy of activated partial thromboplastin times when drawn through a peripherally inserted central catheter. *American Journal of Hematology, 82*, 738–739. doi:10.1002/ajh.20900

Rubin, L.G., Shih, S., Shende, A., Karayalcin, G., & Lanzkowsky, P. (1999). Cure of implantable venous port-associated bloodstream infections in pediatric hematology-oncology patients without catheter removal. *Clinical Infectious Diseases, 29,* 102–105. doi:10.1086/520135

Ruschulte, H., Franke, M., Gastmeier, P., Zenz, S., Mahr, K.H., Buchholz, S., … Piepenbrock, S. (2009). Prevention of central venous catheter related infections with chlorhexidine gluconate impregnated wound dressings: A randomized controlled trial. *Annals of Hematology, 88,* 267–272. doi:10.1007/s00277-008-0568-7

Safdar, N., & Maki, D.G. (2005). Risk of catheter-related bloodstream infection with peripherally inserted central venous catheters used in hospitalized patients. *Chest, 128,* 489–495. doi:10.1378/chest.128.2.489

Salgado, C.D., Chinnes, L., Paczesny, T.H., & Cantey, J.R. (2007). Increased rate of catheter-related bloodstream infection associated with use of a needleless mechanical valve device at a long-term acute care hospital. *Infection Control and Hospital Epidemiology, 28,* 684–688. doi:10.1086/516800

Sanelli, P.C., Deshmukh, M., Ougorets, I., Caiati, R., & Heier, L.A. (2004). Safety and feasibility of using a central venous catheter for rapid contrast injection rates. *American Journal of Roentgenology, 183,* 1829–1834. doi:10.2214/ajr.183.6.01831829

Schilling, S., Doellman, D., Hutchinson, N., & Jacobs, B.R. (2006). The impact of needleless connector device design on central venous catheter occlusion in children: A prospective, controlled trial. *Journal of Parenteral and Enteral Nutrition, 30,* 85–90. doi:10.1177/014860710603000285

Seymour, V.M., Dhallu, T.S., Moss, H.A., Tebbs, S.E., & Elliott, T.S.J. (2000). A prospective clinical study to investigate the microbial contamination of a needleless connector. *Journal of Hospital Infection, 45,* 165–168. doi:10.1053/jhin.2000.0726

Shivnan, J.C., McGuire, D., Freedman, S., Sharkazy, E., Bosserman, G., Larson, E., & Grouleff, P. (1991). A comparison of transparent adherent and dry sterile gauze dressings for long-term central catheters in patients undergoing bone marrow transplant. *Oncology Nursing Forum, 18,* 1349–1356.

Smith, P.B., Benjamin, D.K., Jr., Cotten, C.M., Schultz, E., Guo, R., Nowell, L., … Thornburg, C.D. (2008). Is an increased dwell time of a peripherally inserted catheter associated with an increased risk of bloodstream infection in infants? *Infection Control and Hospital Epidemiology, 29,* 749–753. doi:10.1086/589905

Stephens, L.C., Haire, W.D., Tarantolo, S., Reed, E., Schmit-Pokorny, K., Kessinger, A., & Klein, R. (1997). Normal saline versus heparin flush for maintaining central venous catheter patency during apheresis collection of peripheral blood stem cells (PBSC). *Transfusion Science, 18,* 187–193. doi:10.1016/S0955-3886(97)00008-8

Terrill, K.R., Lemons, R.S., & Goldsby, R.E. (2003). Safety, dose and timing of reteplase in treating occluded central venous catheters in children with cancer. *Journal of Pediatric Hematology and Oncology, 25,* 864–867. doi:10.1097/00043426-200311000-00008

Timsit, J.-F., Schwebel, C., Bouadma, L., Geffroy, A., Garrouste-Orgeas, M., Pease, S., … Lucet, J.-C. (2009). Chlorhexidine-impregnated sponges and less frequent dressing changes for prevention of catheter-related infections in critically ill adults: A randomized controlled trial. *JAMA, 301,* 1231–1241. doi:10.1001/jama.2009.376

Toscano, C.M., Bell, M., Zukerman, C., Shelton, W., Novicki, T.J., Nichols, W.G., … Jarvis, W.R. (2009). Gram-negative bloodstream infections in hematopoietic stem cell transplant patients: The roles of needleless device use, bathing practices, and catheter care. *American Journal of Infection Control, 37,* 327–334. doi:10.1016/j.ajic.2008.01.012

Treston-Aurand, J., Olmsted, R.N., Allen-Bridson, K., & Craig, C.P. (1997). Impact of dressing materials on central venous catheter infection rates. *Journal of Intravenous Nursing, 20,* 201–206.

Tripepi-Bova, K.A., Woods, K.D., & Loach, M.C. (1997). A comparison of transparent polyurethane and dry gauze dressings for peripheral i.v. catheter sites: Rates of phlebitis, infiltration, and dislodgment by patients. *American Journal of Critical Care, 6,* 377–381.

Tuten, S.H., & Gueldner, S.H. (1991). Efficacy of sodium chloride versus dilute heparin for maintenance of peripheral intermittent intravenous devices. *Applied Nursing Research, 4,* 63–71. doi:10.1016/S0897-1897(05)80057-6

Veenstra, D.L., Saint, S., Saha, S., Lumley, T., & Sullivan, S.D. (1999). Efficacy of antiseptic-impregnated central venous catheters in preventing catheter-related bloodstream infection: A meta-analysis. *JAMA, 284,* 261–267. doi:10.1001/jama.281.3.261

Verso, M., Agnelli, G., Bertoglio, S., Di Somma, F.C., Paoletti, F., Ageno, W., … Mosca, S. (2005). Enoxaparin for the prevention of venous thromboembolism associated with central vein catheter: A double-blind, placebo-controlled, randomized study in cancer patients. *Journal of Clinical Oncology, 23,* 4057–4062. doi:10.1200/JCO.2005.06.084

Verso, M., Agnelli, G., Kamphuisen, P.W., Ageno, W., Bazzan, M., Lazzaro, A., … Bertoglio, S. (2008). Risk factors for upper limb deep vein thrombosis associated with the use of central vein catheter in cancer patients. *Internal and Emergency Medicine, 3,* 117–122. doi:10.1007/s11739-008-0125-3

Vescia, S., Baumgärtner, A.K., Jacobs, V.R., Kiechle-Bahat, M., Rody, A., Loibl, S., & Harbeck, N. (2008). Management of venous port systems in oncology: A review of current evidence. *Annals of Oncology, 19,* 9–15. doi:10.1093/annonc/mdm272

Whitta, R.K., Hall, K.F., Bennetts, T.M., Welman, L., & Rawlins, P. (2006). Comparison of normal or heparinised saline flushing on function of arterial lines. *Critical Care and Resuscitation, 8,* 205–208.

Williamson, E.E., & McKinney, J.M. (2001). Assessing the adequacy of peripherally inserted central catheters for power injection of intravenous contrast agents for CT. *Journal of Computer Assisted Tomography, 25,* 932–937. doi:10.1097/00004728-200111000-00016

Worthington, T., & Elliott, T.S.J. (2005). Diagnosis of central venous catheter related infection in adult patients. *Journal of Infection, 51,* 267–280. doi:10.1016/j.jinf.2005.06.007

Yoshida, J., Ishimaru, T., Fujimoto, M., Hirata, N., Matsubara, N., & Koyanagi, N. (2008). Risk factors for central venous catheter-related bloodstream infection: A 1073-patient study. *Journal of Infection and Chemotherapy, 14,* 399–403. doi:10.1007/s10156-008-0637-9

Yücel, N., Lefering, R., Maegele, M., Max, M., Rossaint, R., Koch, A., … Neugebauer, E.A.M. (2004). Reduced colonization and infection with miconazole-rifampicin modified central venous catheters: A randomized controlled clinical trial. *Journal of Antimicrobial Chemotherapy, 54,* 1109–1115. doi:10.1093/jac/dkh483

Chapter 2

Short-Term Peripheral Intravenous Catheters

Heather Thompson Mackey, RN, MSN, ANP-BC, AOCN®

I. History (Dychter, Gold, Carson, & Haller, 2012)
   A. The use of cannulas or catheters to deliver IV therapies has origins in the 17th century, when a quill and pig's bladder were first used by Christopher Wren to instill a mixture of ale, opium, liver, and wine into a dog's vein. This method later was replaced by metal needles and plastic tubing, which were reused following cleaning and sterilization.
   B. Through extensive advances in technology, the plastic peripheral intravenous (PIV) catheter was introduced in 1950 by Dr. Davis Massa, an anesthesia resident who took a 16-gauge needle, shortened it, and inserted another steel needle within to act as an inner stylet. A polyvinyl chloride catheter was fitted over the top, and the tip of the catheter hardened, which then was shrunk to fit the needle. This "Rochester plastic needle" could be threaded directly into a blood vessel following venipuncture, revolutionizing IV therapy (Rivera, Strauss, van Zundert, & Mortier, 2005).
   C. Up to 70% of hospital inpatients require a PIV at some point during their admission (Bernatchez, 2014).
II. Device characteristics
   A. A PIV catheter is a small, hollow catheter inserted into a peripheral vein and used for the delivery of IV therapy (McCallum & Higgins, 2012).
   B. PIVs are used for short durations (Chopra et al., 2015; O'Grady et al., 2011). In children, PIVs can be inserted into the scalp (neonates) and foot (toddlers).
   C. Three main types of PIV administration exist: IV push, intermittent infusion, and continuous infusion.
III. Device features (Helm, Klausner, Klemperer, Flint, & Huang, 2015)
   A. Catheters are further defined by their gauge and length.
      1. Gauges range from 14–28 with single-lumen designs.
      2. Lengths range from ⅝–2 inches.
   B. Catheter material is made of polymers, including polyurethane and polyvinyl chloride. Latex-free catheters are available (see Appendix 3).
      1. Teflon® (DuPont): Stiff material that can damage the vein intima (inner lining) during insertion. It is associated with fewer infectious complications than catheters made of polyvinyl chloride (O'Grady et al., 2011).
      2. Polyurethane: Firm, not stiff, material that softens and becomes more pliable in the vein in response to the body's core temperature
         a) Provides exceptional tensile (physical) strength and flexible endurance, which permits the catheter to be constructed with a thinner wall and greater internal diameter for high flow rates
         b) Associated with less trauma for easier percutaneous insertion and decreased risk of phlebitis and other infectious complications
   C. Specific peripheral infusion devices
      1. Steel-tipped, winged infusion (butterfly) needles
      2. Over-the-needle: Catheter sheath externally located over the needle stylet
   D. Safety devices are available for PIVs to reduce the potential for needlesticks, exposure to bloodborne pathogens, and catheter-related complications, and also to comply with regulatory guidelines.
      1. Needle encapsulation/protection: Shielded butterfly needles, stylet protective devices, and needleless IV access systems
      2. Closed IV catheter systems: Integrate catheter, extension set, and securement device. The use of closed IV catheter systems has shown increased dwell times with lower

rates of phlebitis and infiltration (González-López et al., 2014).

    3. Passive safety catheters: A protective shield that automatically covers the needle point during its withdrawal from the catheter top without any physical intervention by the nurse. This design differs from active safety devices, which require pressing a button to trigger the withdrawal of the needle into a plastic sleeve using a spring. Use of passive safety catheters for PIV catheter insertion has been shown to reduce the number of needlestick injuries in the hospital setting (Hoffmann, Buchholz, & Schnitzler, 2013) (see Figure 2-1).

  E. Available in radiopaque design

IV. Device advantages and disadvantages (see Figure 2-2)

V. Patient selection criteria (Dychter et al., 2012; Polovich, Olsen, & LeFebvre, 2014)

  A. A patient's age, in general, does not restrict the use of PIVs.

  B. Indications for PIVs

    1. Short duration for nonirritating infusions and for fewer than seven days

    2. Best used for simple, onetime-use IV therapies such as IV push administration of a vesicant or nonvesicant chemotherapy. Sclerosing of veins can occur over time.

    3. Infusions such as antimicrobials, analgesics, blood components, fluid and electrolyte replacement, nonvesicant chemotherapy, and drugs that cannot be given orally because the molecules are too large to be absorbed or are destroyed by digestion

    4. Patients with a short life expectancy

  C. Contraindicated for continuous vesicant therapy or solutions with a pH less than 5 or greater than 9, glucose greater than 10%, protein greater

---

Figure 2-2. Advantages and Disadvantages of Peripheral Intravenous Catheters

Advantages	Disadvantages
• May be inserted by an RN	• Have a shorter life span than other types of venous access devices
• Can be easy to insert and maintain	• May involve discomfort with insertion
• Provide quick, simple access to vascular system	• Can be difficult to insert and maintain in young children, older adults, and those with fragile or sclerotic veins
• May be used in all patient care settings	• Can be cumbersome and restrictive, especially when inserted near a joint or in a dominant limb
• Involve minimal insertion costs compared to other venous access procedures	• Require daily care and maintenance
• Rarely associated with catheter-related bloodstream infections	• Can lead to peripheral vessels quickly becoming irritated from infusions of blood components, concentrated dextrose solutions, chemotherapy, and parenteral medications, including antimicrobial agents and electrolyte infusions
	• Less desirable access for infusions of vesicant agents (e.g., certain chemotherapy, calcium gluconate), electrolytes, and vasoconstrictors
	• Could be more costly if used long term and with repeated access, especially in the home environment
	• Can lead to exhaustion of all suitable peripheral veins because of frequent site changes

---

than 5%, or osmolarity greater than 900 mOsm/L (Boullata et al., 2014; Chopra et al., 2015; Cotogni & Pittiruti, 2014)

  D. No definitive recommendation can be made regarding blood specimen collection from PIVs. A meta-analysis demonstrated a significantly higher risk of hemolysis of blood samples drawn via PIVs (Danielis, 2014).

VI. Insertion techniques (Boyd, Aggarwal, Davey, Logan, & Nathwani, 2011; Helm et al., 2015; Infusion Nurses Society [INS], 2016; Institute for Healthcare Improvement, 2015; O'Grady et al., 2011; Polovich et al., 2014; Sabri, Szalas, Holmes, Labib, & Mussivand, 2013)

  A. Implement care bundles similar to those used with central venous access devices (VADs) to reduce risk of infection (see Appendices 3, 4, and 5).

  B. Perform patient assessment and preparation before insertion procedure.

Figure 2-1. Peripheral Needles With Passive Safety Catheter Features in Sizes 18g, 20g, and 22g

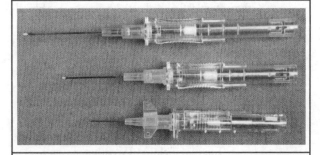

1. Consider any special needs regarding age, physical condition, or type of fluid being infused. Explain the insertion procedure to the patient, and answer any questions the patient and caregiver may have.
2. Older adult patients have fragile veins and less subcutaneous (SC) support tissue because of fragile skin.
3. Use minimal tourniquet pressure over clothing or no tourniquet with older adults; venous distention may take longer because of slower venous return.
4. Children's veins are smaller in diameter and may be covered by a layer of SC fat, which can make veins difficult to access.
5. Access sites for infants and toddlers include scalp and feet. Access in older children usually is achieved through hands or arms. Use of the antecubital fossa in the pediatric population is highly correlated with device failure (Malyon et al., 2014).
6. Studies have shown that it may be reasonable to use a lower extremity vein in older adults with poor venous access in the upper extremity. Incidence of phlebitis was 6% in the upper extremity compared to 9.4% in the lower extremity (Benaya, Schwartz, Kory, Yinnon, & Ben-Chetrit, 2015).

C. Implement interventions to reduce the pain of IV insertion, especially if interventions increase the chance of success (Burke, Vercler, Bye, Desmond, & Rees, 2011; Fink et al., 2009; Kiger et al., 2014) (see Appendices 6 and 7).

D. Vein selection (see Figures 2-3 and 2-4)
   1. Select vein based on type of fluid to be infused and the rate and duration of infusion. Ideally, it should not interfere with the patient's comfort or mobility.
   2. Preferred sites (Dychter et al., 2012; Helm et al., 2015; O'Grady et al., 2011)
      a) Upper extremity veins in adults include superficial dorsal and metacarpal veins on the dorsum of the hand and cephalic, basilic, and median veins on the upper arm.
      b) Upper or lower extremities in pediatric patients: The scalp can be used in neonates or young infants.
      c) Select the most distal site possible but proximal to previous venipuncture.
   3. Sites to avoid (Benaya et al., 2015; Helm et al., 2015; McCallum & Higgins, 2012; O'Grady et al., 2011)
      a) Avoid extremities or sites with impaired circulation or injury.

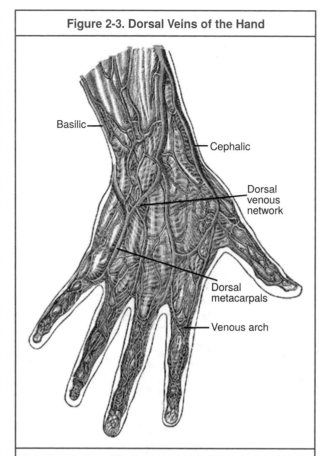

Figure 2-3. Dorsal Veins of the Hand

Basilic

Cephalic

Dorsal venous network

Dorsal metacarpals

Venous arch

Note. From *Anatomy of the Human Body* (plate 573), by H. Gray, 1918, Philadelphia, PA: Lea and Febiger. This file is licensed under the Creative Commons Attribution 2.5 Generic license (https://creativecommons .org/licenses/by/2.5/deed.en). Retrieved from https://commons.wikimedia .org/wiki/Gray%27s_Anatomy_plates.

         (1) Lymphedema or axillary lymph node dissection
         (2) Postoperative swelling
         (3) Recent trauma or hematoma
         (4) Local infection, phlebitis, or open wounds
         (5) Decreased sensation or paresthesia
      b) Avoid extremities where venipuncture has been performed within the past 24 hours, if possible.
      c) Prior to selecting a lower extremity vein, consult with the provider regarding VAD placement or other alternatives. Lower extremities are associated with a higher risk of thrombophlebitis. Obtain an order to use a lower extremity vein and replace as soon as possible.
      d) Avoid antecubital veins because of the difficulty in detecting infiltration and location in an area of flexion. In an

emergency situation, the use of these veins may be appropriate.

e) Avoid placing the cannula over a joint, such as the wrist or elbow, as joint

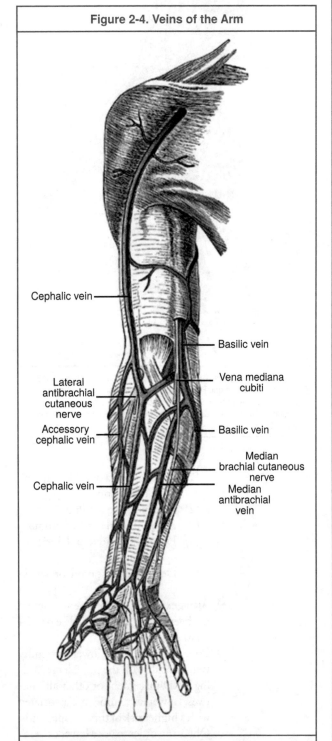

Figure 2-4. Veins of the Arm

Cephalic vein

Lateral antibrachial cutaneous nerve

Accessory cephalic vein

Cephalic vein

Basilic vein

Vena mediana cubiti

Basilic vein

Median brachial cutaneous nerve

Median antibrachial vein

Note. From *Anatomy of the Human Body* (plate 574), by H. Gray, 1918, Philadelphia, PA: Lea and Febiger. This file is licensed under the Creative Commons Attribution 2.5 Generic license (https://creativecommons .org/licenses/by/2.5/deed.en). Retrieved from https://commons.wikimedia .org/wiki/Gray%27s_Anatomy_plates.

movement may produce mechanical phlebitis and increase the risk of catheter kinking.

f) If possible, avoid venipuncture or IV insertion on the ipsilateral extremity of a mastectomy site (Fu, Deng, & Armer, 2014).

E. Device selection (Dychter et al., 2012; Hadaway, 2012; Helm et al., 2015; O'Grady et al., 2011)

1. Use the smallest gauge device and shortest length that will successfully deliver the prescribed therapy at the desired rate.

2. Select catheter based on intended purpose, expected length of therapy, viscosity of fluid, fluid components, presence of infection, condition of vein, and experience of the individual inserting the device.

3. Avoid the use of steel needles for administration of fluids and medications that may cause tissue necrosis if extravasation occurs; limit the use of steel needles to short-term or single-dose administration or onetime infusion and IV push.

4. A short length and small gauge is less traumatizing, reduces irritation, and permits better blood flow; 24 gauge can infuse up to 250 ml of fluid per hour. Considerations for gauge selection include

a) 16–18 gauge for major surgery

b) 18–20 gauge for rapid infusion of IV fluids, blood components, or viscous medications

c) 20 gauge for most IV applications and for blood products

d) 22–24 gauge with ¾-inch catheter for older adult and pediatric patients

5. Adequate gauge and length of needle decreases the risk of chemical phlebitis (irritation of the vein wall by medications) by providing good blood flow through the cannula, dispersing the medication into the bloodstream (Washington & Barrett, 2012).

6. Special consideration: Obese patients with deep veins in the SC tissue may need slightly longer PIV catheters; consider use of alternative VADs.

F. Procedure

1. Wash hands: Good hand hygiene and standard precautions are used for PIV insertion and maintenance; a new pair of disposable, nonsterile gloves is used in conjunction with an aseptic no-touch technique (ANTT) for PIV insertion.

a) ANTT: The planned insertion site is not palpated after skin cleansing unless sterile gloves were worn during cleansing. No definitive recommendations can be made regarding sterile versus nonsterile gloves (see Chapter 1).

b) ANTT is used to prevent microorganisms from hands, surfaces, and equipment from being introduced to the insertion site.

2. Organize equipment (see Appendix 6 for PIV clinical practicum).

a) Prepare IV fluid, attach administration set, and prime if PIV is to be connected to continuous fluids.

b) If administering medication for PIV push, prepare IV medication and connect short extension tubing, if needed.

c) If using PIV as a saline lock, prepare needleless connector and 0.9% normal saline (NS) flush.

3. Examine veins on both extremities by visual inspection and palpation, keeping in mind the purpose of IV therapy and any physical limitations of the patient (e.g., stroke limiting mobility on one side, axillary node dissection). Assess distal veins, and then move proximally.

a) Technology such as guidance with near-infrared light can assist in the location and insertion of PIVs and has been shown to facilitate first-attempt success rates with an associated decrease in patient perception of pain; however, this requires specialized training and equipment (Hadaway, 2012; Helm et al., 2015; Ismailoğlu, Zaybak, Akarca, & Kiyan, 2015; Maiocco & Coole, 2012; Sabri et al., 2013).

b) Feasibility testing of near-infrared spectroscopy using standard mobile device prototypes demonstrates superiority of vein visualization over simple visual inspection and palpation (Juric & Zalik, 2014).

c) Meta-analyses support use of ultrasound guidance for difficult peripheral access and in patients who have failed venous cannulation by standard methods; however, they do not strongly support use for routine PIV placement (Egan et al., 2013; Liu, Alsaawi, & Bjornsson, 2014).

4. Rewash hands and apply gloves.

5. Select appropriate IV needle or catheter. Administer local anesthetic, as needed (see Appendix 7).

6. Place tourniquet 5–6 inches above insertion site. Tourniquet should obstruct venous but not arterial flow. Check presence of distal pulse, and, if not felt, loosen tourniquet.

a) Select site: To assist in vein location, tap the vein, apply local warming, or have the patient place arm in dependent position (Helm et al., 2015; Kiger et al., 2014; Sabri et al., 2013; Washington & Barrett, 2012).

b) Remove tourniquet for the patient's comfort.

c) If a large amount of body hair is present at insertion site, clip the area. Avoid shaving, which can increase irritation and risk of infection.

7. Cleanse site and allow to air-dry before inserting catheter (see Appendix 2). Chlorhexidine gluconate is recommended for skin cleansing prior to insertion. If the patient has a known allergy to chlorhexidine, 70% alcohol or povidone-iodine can be used. Once skin is cleaned, do not palpate planned IV insertion site.

8. Reapply tourniquet.

9. Perform venipuncture: Insert needle at a 15°–30° angle with bevel up distal to actual site of venipuncture.

10. Observe blood return through tubing of butterfly needle or catheter, indicating successful venous access. A butterfly needle may be taped in place at this time or threaded into the vein. Thread the catheter in its entirety into the vein and simultaneously remove the stylet. Occlude tip of the catheter by pressing fingers of nondominant hand over vein to prevent retrograde bleeding.

11. Release tourniquet, then attach the catheter to the infusion set or syringe.

12. Flush the catheter with NS while holding the catheter or needle in place to remove retrograde blood. Watch the insertion site during initial flush to assess integrity of the

vein. Edema or pain and discomfort at site indicates an infiltration or ruptured vein. If this occurs, remove the device and restart in another location.

   a) If a second attempt is required, use the other extremity or select a site proximal to the previous venipuncture.

   b) When administering a vesicant chemotherapy agent, select a site proximal to the previous venipuncture or select a vein on the opposite extremity, if possible.

   c) To avoid unnecessary trauma to the patient, no more than two attempts at cannulation per nurse per patient should be performed. If unsuccessful after two nurses attempt, contact the provider to discuss alternative access device options.

13. Secure catheter or needle with a securement device, then apply occlusive dressing over insertion site. Do not put tape directly over insertion site.

   a) Catheter securement devices help to reduce dislodgment episodes and infection risk and increase dwell times of PIVs (Bausone-Gazda, Lafaiver, & Walters, 2010; Helm et al., 2015).

   b) For extremely short dwell times (e.g., less than 30 minutes, during a procedure), clean Micropore™ tape and gauze may be used; do not tape over the insertion site.

14. Discard used supplies; remove gloves.
15. Wash hands.
16. Label dressing with time, date of dressing change, and initials.
17. Document the number of attempts, location, type and gauge of catheter, dressing type, securement device, and the patient's response to the procedure.

VII. Unique maintenance and care: No definitive recommendations can be made regarding frequency of dressing changes or blood sampling techniques (Hadaway, 2012; Helm et al., 2015; INS, 2016; O'Grady et al., 2011; Stauss et al., 2012; Washington & Barrett, 2012) (see Appendices 2, 4, 5, 6, and 7).

A. Inspect catheter insertion site and palpate for tenderness daily through the intact dressing. Do not remove opaque (including gauze) dressings in the absence of clinical signs of infection. If signs of potential infection are present, remove opaque dressings and inspect site visually. Minimize manipulation of the catheter to prevent mechanical phlebitis.

B. When adherence to aseptic technique cannot be ensured, replace all PIVs inserted under emergency conditions as soon as possible.

C. Routine replacement of catheters (Abolfotouh, Salam, Bani-Mustafa, White, & Balkhy, 2014; Dychter et al., 2012; Ho & Cheung, 2012)

1. Studies from a variety of settings support the practice of changing PIVs only as clinically indicated. Studies show no difference in rates of phlebitis, occlusion, infiltration, infection, or mortality when PIVs are changed as clinically indicated versus every 72–96 hours (Helm et al., 2015; Pasalioglu & Kaya, 2014; Rickard et al., 2012; Webster, Osborne, Rickard, & New, 2015). This practice already is the standard of care in children (O'Grady et al., 2011).

2. Insert a new PIV when administering a vesicant, especially if more than 24 hours old (Polovich et al., 2014).

D. Dressing changes: Change dressing if wet, soiled, or nonocclusive. Dressing changes require ANTT.

E. Flushing: Use NS 1–3 ml every 8, 12, or 24 hours when the device is not in use to maintain patency in adults and in children aged one year or older (American Society of Health-System Pharmacists, 2012; Wang, Luo, He, Li, & Zhang, 2012).

F. Ensure all devices added onto catheter are Luer lock, including needleless connectors, stopcocks, short extensions, filters, and multisite connectors.

1. Needleless connectors allow for IV administration without use of a needle, thereby reducing the risk of needlestick. These devices also ensure that the IV system remains closed and can be left in place until the catheter is changed (if not contaminated or damaged).

2. Change administration sets when the PIV is replaced or when no longer intact.

3. Label all IVs and equipment with date, time, and initials.

G. Blood specimens: No definitive recommendation can be made regarding specific volume of blood discard or flush. Prior to policy development, the dead space volume of products used must be known (Danielis, 2014; Stauss et al., 2012).

1. In general, within certain limitations of infusates, PIVs flushed with NS are simple and safe for collecting blood samples for most laboratory tests (Baker et al., 2013; Ortells-Abuye, Busquets-Puigdevall, Díaz-Bergara, Paguina-Marcos, & Sánchez-Pérez, 2014).

2. Specimens collected from PIVs have an increased risk for hemolysis (Danielis, 2014; Lippi, Cervellin, & Mattiuzzi, 2013).
3. Discard 1 ml of waste to promote accurate laboratory testing results (Baker et al., 2013).
4. No definitive recommendation can be made on blood sampling from PIVs; more research is needed. Weighing the benefits and risks of safety, costs, and comfort may aid decision making (Danielis, 2014).

H. Administration types (Dychter et al., 2012)
1. IV push: Following flushing procedure, cleanse needleless connector, allow to air-dry, attach syringe containing medication, infuse over a short period of time (usually three to five minutes), and flush with 1–3 ml of NS following infusion.
2. Intermittent infusions: Used for drugs that require dilution or slow administration. Following flushing procedure, cleanse needleless connector, allow to air-dry, attach administration set of infusion to be administered, infuse over specified time, and flush with 1–3 ml of NS following completion of infusion.
3. Continuous infusion: Most common method of administering IV fluids and peripheral total parenteral nutrition. Follow flushing procedure, cleanse hub of catheter, allow to air-dry, attach administration set of infusion to be administered, and infuse at specified rate.

VIII. Removal technique (Hadaway, 2012; Helm et al., 2015; INS, 2016; O'Grady et al., 2011)
A. Indications: Remove catheter when signs and symptoms of infection, infiltration, or phlebitis are present, or when no longer required for therapy.
B. Procedure
1. Verify order and indication for removal.
2. Explain procedure to the patient.
3. Place the patient in chair or bed to stabilize extremity.
4. Inspect the general condition of the catheter pathway.
5. Discontinue all infusions into the device.
6. Apply gloves; remove dressing and observe site for edema, erythema, or discharge.
7. Change gloves; grasp device by the hub and, while stabilizing the skin and vein with sterile gauze in the nondominant hand, slowly and steadily pull out at the same angle of insertion.
8. If removal is due to infection, send catheter tip for culture, if ordered.
9. Apply constant, firm pressure to exit site until bleeding stops (longer in patients with coagulopathies, thrombocytopenia, or on anticoagulants).
10. Apply dressing or adhesive bandage; monitor as necessary.
11. Instruct the patient or caregiver to report any discomfort or signs of bleeding, bruising, redness, swelling, or drainage.
12. Inspect the device for defects: Report any defects to the manufacturer and regulatory agencies. Examine distal tip for signs of jagged, uneven edges suggestive of breakage.
13. Document observations and actions.

IX. Complications (Abolfotouh et al., 2014; Dychter et al., 2012; Hadaway, 2012; O'Grady et al., 2011; Polovich et al., 2014; Sabri et al., 2013; Vallecoccia et al., 2015; Washington & Barrett, 2012)
A. Insertion complications include bleeding, vein injury, nerve injury, infiltration, phlebitis, and thrombosis.
B. Vein injury from catheters can result in pain, tenderness, edema, erythema (vasodilation), thrombosis, sclerosis, and infiltration.
C. Phlebitis: most common complication, resulting in inflammation of the vein
1. Etiology: Insufficient vessel size to accommodate the catheter to allow hemodilution, traumatic insertion, or mechanical or chemical irritation
2. Risk factors
   a) Prolonged dwell time
   b) Mechanical irritation: Movement of the catheter, multiple IV attempts, catheter too large for vein, location of the catheter (hand, antecubital fossa, and wrist areas), or catheter material
   c) Chemical irritation: Tonicity of infusate, number and dosage of medications, pH of medication, or skin not allowed to fully dry after cleansing prior to insertion (Cotogni & Pittiruti, 2014)
   d) Increases with age of device or advanced age of the patient
3. Prevention: Use strict aseptic technique and careful placement for insertion and maintenance care. Regularly assess for signs of phlebitis.
4. Signs and symptoms: Pain, erythema, streak formation, palpable cord, and edema
   a) Older adult patients may not experience pain from phlebitis or infiltration because of a decrease in sensory perception; monitoring for complications through observation is important.

_____
_____
_____
_____
_____
_____
_____
_____

    b) Children, older adults, or those with communication limitations may not be able to voice pain.
  5. Diagnostic tests: Not indicated
  6. Management: Remove device, apply heat, and give analgesic, as needed.
D. Infiltration: Second most common complication (Dychter et al., 2012; Helm et al., 2015; Sabri et al., 2013)
  1. Etiology: Mechanical (e.g., injury during insertion, catheter malposition following insertion) or physiologic (e.g., preexisting or developing vein problems such as sclerosis). Because of penetration of the catheter into or through the venous wall, infiltration leads to infusion of fluids or medications into the surrounding soft tissue.
  2. Risk factors: Placement in joint regions (e.g., wrist, antecubital fossa), inadequate catheter securement, traumatic injury to vessel wall on insertion, older or younger age, dehydration, and obesity
  3. Prevention: Assess for infiltration. Occlude the vessel at the tip of the catheter with digital pressure. If the infusion continues, the fluid is probably infiltrating.
    a) Use of appropriately sized syringes to prevent vein rupture
    b) The larger the syringe, the less pressure is generated when force is applied and the more force is required to create a vacuum. Less force is generated in either infusion or aspiration with larger syringes, thereby reducing or preventing complications.
    c) Do not use a 1 ml syringe with PIVs. Use at least a 3 ml syringe or larger for all flushing and administration of medications.
  4. Signs and symptoms: Leaking fluid around insertion site; cool, pale skin; possible decreased infusion rate; edema at inser-

tion site; tenderness; and skin tightness or discomfort
  5. Diagnostic tests: Not indicated
  6. Management: Remove device, apply heat or cold (depending on the agent infiltrated), elevate extremity, and give analgesic, as needed.
E. Infection
  1. Etiology: Microorganisms enter through a PIV by the external catheter upon insertion, the interior of the catheter, the contamination of connectors, the repalpation of a proposed puncture site prior to insertion, excessive catheter manipulation, or by contaminated infusion.
    a) PIVs historically have been rarely associated with bloodstream infections. The reported rate of colonized peripheral catheters at the time of removal is 5%–25% (Abolfotouh et al., 2014; Dychter et al., 2012; Hadaway, 2012; Helm et al., 2015).
    b) Emerging data suggest that the rate of catheter-related bloodstream infections from peripheral catheters may be higher than once thought (Trinh et al., 2011); more research is needed to fully evaluate.
    c) The most common organism is *Staphylococcus aureus.*
  2. Risk factors: Inadequate cleansing technique, poor skills of the nurse, an immunocompromised patient, older or younger age, comorbidities (e.g., diabetes, cancer, heart disease), or a malnourished patient
  3. Prevention: Use strict aseptic technique for insertion and maintenance care.
  4. Signs and symptoms: Depend on type of infection
    a) Local: Erythema, purulent drainage, warmth, induration, or palpable cord
    b) Phlebitis: Pain, erythema, streak formation, palpable cord, or edema
    c) Bloodstream: Pain, erythema, streak formation, palpable cord, edema, or fever
  5. Diagnostic tests: Wound and blood cultures, as ordered
  6. Management: Remove device, apply heat, and administer antibiotics systemically per culture result.
F. Extravasation: The leaking or escape of infusate from the vessel into the surrounding tissue (Coyle, Griffie, & Czaplewski, 2014; Dychter

et al., 2012; Le & Patel, 2014; Molas-Ferrer et al., 2015; Polovich et al., 2014)

1. Etiology: Peripheral vein wall puncture, administration of a vesicant in a vein below a recent venipuncture, or an inadequately secured IV catheter causes leaking of vesicant agent into the surrounding tissue. Damage is dependent on specific factors:
    a) Mechanism of action and properties of drug
    b) Amount of drug extravasated
2. Risk factors: Inadequate IV insertion technique, small fragile veins, history of multiple venipunctures, limited extremity vein selection, decreased sensation or circulatory impairments, patient with altered mental status
3. Prevention
    a) Use aseptic technique when accessing peripheral vein.
    b) Avoid multiple attempts in establishing access.
    c) Avoid areas of impairment, previous IV sites, and inserting above previous venipuncture sites.
    d) Use transparent dressing over IV to visualize the site throughout vesicant administration.
    e) Verify blood return prior to, during, and after administration. Do not give vesicant through PIV without a blood return.
    f) Instruct the patient to promptly report symptoms of extravasation.
4. Signs and symptoms: Burning/stinging at site; pain; erythema; difficulty infusing solution; leaking around the insertion site; absence of blood return during or following infusion, followed by blistering, tissue necrosis, and ulceration; decreased IV flow
5. Diagnostic tests: Not indicated
6. Management
    a) Stop infusion and aspirate residual drug from the catheter using a 3 ml syringe.
    b) Assess the site and estimate amount of vesicant extravasated.
    c) Administer antidote through IV catheter, as indicated; remove peripheral catheter.
    d) Apply cold or heat, as indicated.
    e) Determine the cause of extravasation, notify the provider, measure and photograph the site, document actions, and provide patient education and follow-up.

X. Practicum on PIV insertion and care (see Appendix 6)
XI. Education and documentation (see Chapter 17)
XII. Vascular teams (see Figure 2-5)

Figure 2-5. Vascular Teams

Function
- Specially trained RNs or advanced practice nurses that insert or maintain peripheral intravenous (PIV), midline, non-tunneled catheters, or peripherally inserted central catheters (PICCs)
- Research demonstrates that insertion and/or care of catheters by vascular teams reduces the incidence of bloodstream infections and other complications associated with PIVs, midline catheters, and PICCs.
- Many institutions have disbanded or downsized teams to perform only PICC insertion or PIV insertions in the pediatric population.
- Limited studies exist to guide the implementation of infusion teams.

Models
- RN: assumes full responsibility of all insertions and care
- Insertion teams: insert PICCs; may insert nontunneled catheters with specialized training
- Infusion teams/IV therapy teams: insertion and care of PIVs, midline catheters, and PICCs

Roles of Dedicated Teams
PIVs, midline catheters, and PICCs:
- Insertion and removal
- Daily management
- Infection surveillance
- Evaluation for necessity
- Education of nurses on new technology and evidence-based research
- Development of policies and procedures
- Data collection and analysis for quality improvement

Note. Based on information from Hadaway et al., 2013; Harpel, 2013; O'Grady et al., 2011; Sabri et al., 2013.

References

Abolfotouh, M.A., Salam, M., Bani-Mustafa, A., White, D., & Balkhy, H.H. (2014). Prospective study of incidence and predictors of peripheral intravenous catheter-induced complications. *Therapeutics and Clinical Risk Management, 10,* 993–1001. doi:10.2147/TCRM.S74685

American Society of Health-System Pharmacists. (2012). ASHP therapeutic position statement on the institutional use of 0.9% sodium chloride injection to maintain patency of peripheral indwelling intermittent infusion devices. *American Journal of Health-System Pharmacy, 69,* 1252–1254. doi:10.2146/ajhp120076

Baker, R.B., Summer, S.S., Lawrence, M., Shova, A., McGraw, C., & Khoury, J. (2013). Determining optimal waste volume from an intravenous catheter. *Journal of Infusion Nursing, 36,* 92–96. doi:10.1097/NAN.0b013e318282a4c2

Bausone-Gazda, D., Lafaiver, C.A., & Walters, S.-A. (2010). A randomized controlled trial to compare the complications of 2 peripheral intravenous catheter-stabilization systems. *Journal of Infusion Nursing, 33,* 371–384. doi:10.1097/NAN.0b013e3181f85be2

Benaya, A., Schwartz, Y., Kory, R., Yinnon, A.M., & Ben-Chetrit, E. (2015). Relative incidence of phlebitis associated with peripheral intravenous catheters in the lower versus upper extremities. *European Journal of Clinical Microbiology and Infectious Diseases, 34*, 913–916. doi:10.1007/s10096-014-2304-7

Bernatchez, S.F. (2014). Care of peripheral venous catheter sites: Advantages of transparent film dressings over tape and gauze. *Journal of the Association of Vascular Access, 19*, 256–261. doi:10.1016/j.java.2014.09.001

Boullata, J.I., Gilbert, K., Sacks, G., Labossiere, R.J., Crill, C., Goday, P., ... American Society for Parenteral and Enteral Nutrition. (2014). A.S.P.E.N. clinical guidelines: Parenteral nutrition ordering, order review, compounding, labeling, and dispensing. *Journal of Parenteral and Enteral Nutrition, 38*, 334–377. doi:10.1177/0148607114521833

Boyd, S., Aggarwal, I., Davey, P., Logan, M., & Nathwani, D. (2011). Peripheral intravenous catheters: The road to quality improvement and safer patient care. *Journal of Hospital Infection, 77*, 37–41. doi:10.1016/j.jhin.2010.09.011

Burke, S.D., Vercler, S.J., Bye, R.O., Desmond, P.C., & Rees, Y.W. (2011). Local anesthesia before IV catheterization. *American Journal of Nursing, 111*(2), 40–45. Retrieved from http://www.nursingcenter.com/cearticle?an=00000446-201102000-00027&Journal_ID=54030&Issue_ID=1177299#P19 P28 P29 P47

Chopra, V., Flanders, S.A., Saint, S., Woller, S.C., O'Grady, N.P., Safdar, N., ... Bernstein, S.J. (2015). The Michigan Appropriateness Guide for Intravenous Catheters (MAGIC): Results from a multispecialty panel using the RAND/UCLA Appropriateness Method. *Annals of Internal Medicine, 163*(Suppl. 6), S1–S40. doi:10.7326/M15-0744

Cotogni, P., & Pittiruti, M. (2014). Focus on peripherally inserted central catheters in critically ill patients. *World Journal of Critical Care Medicine, 3*, 80–94. doi:10.5492/wjccm.v3.i4.80

Coyle, C.E., Griffie, J., & Czaplewski, L.M. (2014). Eliminating extravasation events: A multidisciplinary approach. *Journal of Infusion Nursing, 37*, 157–164. doi:10.1097/NAN.0000000000000034

Danielis, M. (2014). Risk of hemolysis in blood sampling from peripheral intravenous catheter: A literature review. *Professioni Infermieristiche, 67*, 166–172.

Dychter, S.S., Gold, D.A., Carson, D., & Haller, M. (2012). Intravenous therapy: A review of complications and economic considerations of peripheral access. *Journal of Infusion Nursing, 35*, 84–91. doi:10.1097/NAN.0b013e31824237ce

Egan, G., Healy, D., O'Neill, H., Clarke-Moloney, M., Grace, P.A., & Walsh, S.R. (2013). Ultrasound guidance for difficult peripheral venous access: Systematic review and meta-analysis. *Emergency Medicine Journal, 30*, 521–526. doi:10.1136/emermed-2012-201652

Fink, R.M., Hjort, E., Wenger, B., Cook, P.F., Cunningham, M., Orf, A., ... Zwink, J. (2009). The impact of dry versus moist heat on peripheral IV catheter insertion in a hematology-oncology outpatient population [Online exclusive]. *Oncology Nursing Forum, 36*, E198–E204. doi:10.1188/09.ONF.E198-E204

Fu, M.R., Deng, J., & Armer, J.M. (2014). Putting evidence into practice: Cancer-related lymphedema: Evolving evidence for treatment and management from 2009–2014. *Clinical Journal of Oncology Nursing, 18*(Suppl. 6), 68–79. doi:10.1188/14.CJON.S3.68-79

González-López, J.L., Vilela, A.A., del Palacio, E.F., Corral, J.O., Martí, C.B., & Portal, P.H. (2014). Indwell times, complications and costs of open vs closed safety peripheral intravenous catheters: A randomized study. *Journal of Hospital Infection, 86*, 117–126. doi:10.1016/j.jhin.2013.10.008

Hadaway, L. (2012). Short peripheral intravenous catheters and infections. *Journal of Infusion Nursing, 35*, 230–240. doi:10.1097/NAN.0b013e31825af099

Hadaway, L., Dalton, L., & Mercanti-Erieg, L. (2013). Infusion teams in acute care hospitals: Call for a business approach: An Infusion Nurses Society white paper. *Journal of Infusion Nursing, 36*, 356–360. doi:10.1097/NAN.0b013e3182a123a9

Harpel, J. (2013). Best practices for vascular resource teams. *Journal of Infusion Nursing, 36*, 46–50. doi:10.1097/NAN.0b013e3182798862

Helm, R.E., Klausner, J.D., Klemperer, J.D., Flint, L.M., & Huang, E. (2015). Accepted but unacceptable: Peripheral IV catheter failure. *Journal of Infusion Nursing, 38*, 189–203. doi:10.1097/NAN.0000000000000100

Ho, K.H.M., & Cheung, D.S.K. (2012). Guidelines on timing in replacing peripheral intravenous catheters. *Journal of Clinical Nursing, 21*, 1499–1506. doi:10.1111/j.1365-2702.2011.03974.x

Hoffmann, C., Buchholz, L., & Schnitzler, P. (2013). Reduction of needlestick injuries in healthcare personnel at a university hospital using safety devices. *Journal of Occupational Medicine and Toxicology, 8*, 20. doi:10.1186/1745-6673-8-20

Infusion Nurses Society. (2016). *Infusion therapy standards of practice.* Norwood, MA: Author.

Institute for Healthcare Improvement. (2015). Evidence-based care bundles. Retrieved from http://www.ihi.org/Topics/Bundles/Pages/default.aspx

Ismailoğlu, E.G., Zaybak, A., Akarca, F.K., & Kiyan, S. (2015). The effect of the use of ultrasound in the success of peripheral venous catheterisation. *International Emergency Nursing, 23*, 89–93. doi:10.1016/j.ienj.2014.07.010

Juric, S., & Zalik, B. (2014). An innovative approach to near-infrared spectroscopy using a standard mobile device and its clinical application in the real-time visualization of peripheral veins. *BMC Medical Informatics and Decision Making, 14*, 100. doi:10.1186/s12911-014-0100-z

Kiger, T., Knudsen, E.A., Curran, W., Hunter, J., Schaub, A., Williams, M.J., ... Kwekkeboom, K. (2014). Survey of heat use during peripheral IV insertion by health care workers. *Journal of Infusion Nursing, 37*, 433–440. doi:10.1097/NAN.0000000000000074

Le, A., & Patel, S. (2014). Extravasation of noncytotoxic drugs: A review of the literature. *Annals of Pharmacotherapy, 48*, 870–886. doi:10.1177/1060028014527820

Lippi, G., Cervellin, G., & Mattiuzzi, C. (2013). Critical review and meta-analysis of spurious hemolysis in blood samples collected from intravenous catheters. *Biochemia Medica, 23*, 193–200. doi:10.11613/BM.2013.022

Liu, Y.T., Alsaawi, A., & Bjornsson, H.M. (2014). Ultrasound-guided peripheral venous access: A systematic review of randomized-controlled trials. *European Journal of Emergency Medicine, 21*, 18–23.

Maiocco, G., & Coole, C. (2012). Use of ultrasound guidance for peripheral intravenous placement in difficult-to-access patients: Advancing practice with evidence. *Journal of Nursing Care Quality, 27*(1), 51–55. doi:10.1097/NCQ.0b013e31822b4537

Malyon, L., Ullman, A.J., Phillips, N., Young, J., Kleidon, T., Murfield, J., & Rickard, C.M. (2014). Peripheral intravenous catheter duration and failure in paediatric acute care: A prospective cohort study. *Emergency Medicine Australasia, 26*, 602–608. doi:10.1111/1742-6723.12305

McCallum, L., & Higgins, D. (2012). Care of peripheral venous cannula sites. *Nursing Times, 10*, 12–15.

Molas-Ferrer, G., Farré-Ayuso, E., doPazo-Oubiña, F., deAndrés-Lázaro, A., Guell-Picazo, J., Borrás-Maixenchs, N., ... Creus-Baró, N. (2015). Level of adherence to an extravasation protocol over 10 years in a tertiary care hospital [Online exclusive]. *Clinical Journal of Oncology Nursing, 19*, E25–E30. doi:10.1188/15.cjon.e25-e30

O'Grady, N.P., Alexander, M., Burns, L.A., Dellinger, E.P., Garland, J., Heard, S.O., ... Healthcare Infection Control Practices Advisory Committee. (2011). Guidelines for the prevention of intravascular catheter-related infections. *Clinical Infectious Diseases, 52*, E162–E193. doi:10.1093/cid/cir257

Ortells-Abuye, N., Busquets-Puigdevall, T., Díaz-Bergara, M., Paguina-Marcos, M., & Sánchez-Pérez, I. (2014). A cross-sectional study to compare two blood collection methods: Direct venous puncture and peripheral venous catheter. *BMJ Open, 4,* e004250. doi:10.1136/bmjopen-2013-004250

Pasalioglu, K.B., & Kaya, H. (2014). Catheter indwell time and phlebitis development during peripheral intravenous catheter administration. *Pakistan Journal of Medical Sciences, 30,* 725–730. doi:10.12669/pjms.304.5067

Polovich, M., Olsen, M., & LeFebvre, K.B. (Eds.). (2014). *Chemotherapy and biotherapy guidelines and recommendations for practice* (4th ed.). Pittsburgh, PA: Oncology Nursing Society.

Rickard, C.M., Webster, J., Wallis, M.C., Marsh, N., McGrail, M.R., French, V., ... Whitby, M. (2012). Routine versus clinically indicated replacement of peripheral intravenous catheters: A randomised controlled equivalence trial. *Lancet, 380,* 1066–1074. doi:10.1016/S0140-6736(12)61082-4

Rivera, A.M., Strauss, K.W., van Zundert, A., & Mortier, E. (2005). The history of peripheral intravenous catheters: How little plastic tubes revolutionized medicine. *Acta Anaesthesiologica Belgica, 56,* 271–282.

Sabri, A., Szalas, J., Holmes, K.S., Labib, L., & Mussivand, T. (2013). Failed attempts and improvement strategies in peripheral intravenous catheterization. *Bio-Medical Materials and Engineering, 23,* 93–108. doi:10.3233/BME-120735

Stauss, M., Sherman, B., Pugh, L., Parone, D., Looby-Rodriguez, K., Bell, A., & Reed, C.R. (2012). Hemolysis of coagulation specimens: A comparative study of intravenous draw methods. *Journal of Emergency Nursing, 38,* 15–21. doi:10.1016/j.jen.2010.08.011

Trinh, T.T., Chan, P.A., Edwards, O., Hollenbeck, B., Huang, B., Burdick, N., ... Mermel, L.A. (2011). Peripheral venous catheter-related *Staphylococcus aureus* bacteremia. *Infection Control and Hospital Epidemiology, 32,* 579–583. doi:10.1086/660099

Vallecoccia, M.S., De Pascale, G., Taraschi, C., De Angelis Durante, R., Dolcetti, L., Pittiruti, M., & Scoppettuolo, G. (2015). Closed vs. open systems: When should short peripheral intravenous catheters be the first choice? *Journal of Hospital Infection, 89,* 72–73. doi:10.1016/j.jhin.2014.09.010

Wang, R., Luo, O., He, L., Li, J.-X., & Zhang, M.-G. (2012). Preservative-free 0.9% sodium chloride for flushing and locking peripheral intravenous access device: A prospective controlled trial. *Journal of Evidence-Based Medicine, 5,* 205–208. doi:10.1111/jebm.12004

Washington, G.T., & Barrett, R. (2012). Peripheral phlebitis. *Journal of Infusion Nursing, 35,* 252–258. doi:10.1097/NAN.0b013e31825af30d

Webster, J., Osborne, S., Rickard, C.M., & New, K. (2015). Clinically-indicated replacement versus routine replacement of peripheral venous catheters. *Cochrane Database of Systematic Reviews, 2015*(8). doi:10.1002/14651858.cd007798.pub4

Chapter 3

Midline Catheters

Diane G. Cope, PhD, ARNP-BC, AOCNP®

I. History (Dawson & Moureau, 2013)
   A. Midline catheters were first introduced in the 1950s for surgical patients and intended for subclavian access. In the 1980s, the split-away plastic introducer was developed to facilitate midline catheter placement.
   B. Extensive use of midline catheters has been controversial, with little evidence-based research supporting risks and benefits.
   C. Limited prospective research has recently supported midline catheters as a safe alternative to central devices, with complication rates comparable to those of other short- and long-term devices (Dumont, Getz, & Miller, 2014).
II. Device characteristics (Cotogni & Pittiruti, 2014; Dawson & Moureau, 2013; Giuliani et al., 2013) (see Figure 3-1)
   A. Short-term peripheral device: Research suggests replacing short-term central catheters, when feasible, with midline catheters to reduce the incidence of central line–associated bloodstream infections.
   B. A prospective randomized trial comparing short-term low pH vancomycin infusions through a novel midline device versus peripherally inserted central catheters (PICCs) demonstrated no significant difference in complications or safety; midline insertions proved more cost-effective compared to PICCs (Caparas & Hu, 2014).
   C. Considered a peripheral line because the tip is not located in the central circulation. The midline catheter tip terminates in the axillary vein in the upper arm (Bortolussi et al., 2015; Infusion Nurses Society [INS], 2013).
III. Device features (Cotogni & Pittiruti, 2014; Deutsch, Sathyanarayana, Singh, & Nicastro, 2014; Pathak et al., 2015; Scoppettuolo et al., 2016)
   A. Catheter material: Silicone, polyurethane, and available with latex-free design
   B. Available as radiopaque
   C. Available in single and double lumens with open- or closed-valve tip
   D. Range from 2 Fr (23 gauge) to 6 Fr (18 gauge)

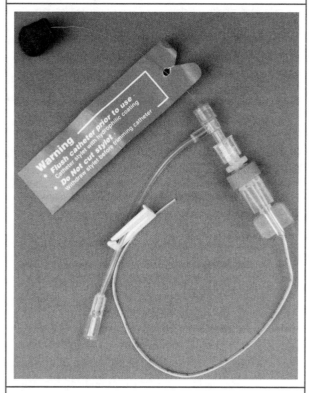

Figure 3-1. Midline Venous Catheter With Guidewire

   E. Range from 8–25 cm in length
   F. Prime volume of 0.5–1.5 ml
   G. Available in power-injectable design
IV. Device advantages and disadvantages (see Figure 3-2)
V. Patient selection criteria (Chopra et al., 2015; Cotogni & Pittiruti, 2014)
   A. Patients with limited peripheral veins for venous access
   B. Patients with need for venous access for a limited length of time (at least six weeks and potentially for months) (Scoppettuolo et al., 2016)
   C. Patients or caregivers who are willing and able to follow instructions to properly care for a midline device in the home setting

---

Figure 3-2. Advantages and Disadvantages of Midline Catheters

Advantages	Disadvantages
• Considered peripheral lines; chest x-ray not required for tip placement verification • Can be placed at the bedside by a specially trained nurse • Dwell time of 1–8 weeks • Ideal for those with limited peripheral access but who require prolonged IV therapy • Available in single and double lumens, radiopaque, and power-injectable versions • Can be used for most IV solutions • Possible reduction in central line–associated bloodstream infections when used to replace central catheters when feasible • Do not require routine replacement (only replaced as is indicated) • Associated with lower rates of phlebitis than peripheral IVs and lower rates of infection than central venous access devices • Can be removed at the bedside • Relatively economical compared to more permanent lines	• Cannot be used for continuous infusion of vesicants • May limit a patient's overall mobility or comfort if necessary to insert into contralateral limb due to compromised alternate limb (e.g., lymphedema, axillary dissection) • May decrease ability to draw blood because of size and flexible nature • Contraindicated for continuous infusions of vesicants, infusates with pH < 5 or > 9, parenteral nutrition, infusates with glucose concentrations > 10%, solutions with protein concentrations > 5%, or hyperosmolar solutions > 900 mOsm/L • Require a patient to have adequate peripheral veins • Require adequate patient support to maintain catheter in homecare setting • Not available as a triple lumen

---

D. Patients receiving IV therapy that is appropriate for a midline catheter. Contraindications include the following (Boullata et al., 2014; Chopra et al., 2015; Cotogni & Pittiruti, 2014; INS, 2016):
   1. Continuous infusion of vesicants
   2. Infusates with pH less than 5 or greater than 9
   3. Parenteral nutrition
   4. Solutions with glucose concentration greater than 10%
   5. Solutions with protein concentration greater than 5%
   6. Solutions with osmolarity greater than 900 mOsm/L
E. Patient preference for this type of device over more permanent devices
F. Patients with limited life expectancy
G. For patients scheduled to receive IV therapy for more than a week, a plan should be followed to maximize comfort and preserve the integrity of the veins.
H. Contraindicated in an extremity affected by a mastectomy, lymph node dissection, or lymphedema. Contraindicated in patients with severe renal dysfunction who may require an arteriovenous fistula formation. Avoid use in patients with a history of thrombosis or hypercoagulability.

VI. Insertion techniques (Bortolussi et al., 2015; Scoppettuolo et al., 2016)
A. Implement care bundles to reduce the chance of infection. Care bundles are a group of evidence-based interventions aimed at improving the processes of care and patient outcomes (Institute for Healthcare Improvement, n.d.) (see Appendices 3 and 4).
B. Before the insertion procedure, verify scope of practice with the individual state board of nursing and institutional guidelines.
C. Perform a patient assessment and preparation before the procedure.
   1. Consider any special needs regarding age, physical condition, or type of fluid being infused. Explain the insertion procedure to the patient, and answer any questions the patient and significant others may have.
   2. Older adult patients have fragile veins and less subcutaneous (SC) support tissue because of thinning of the skin.
   3. Use minimal tourniquet pressure over clothing or no tourniquet with older adults. Venous distention may take longer because of slower venous return.
   4. Children's veins are smaller in diameter and may be covered by a layer of SC fat, which can make veins difficult to access.
D. Implement interventions to reduce the pain of IV insertion, especially if they increase the chance of success (see Appendix 7).
E. Vein selection: Insert in an antecubital vein, terminating in the upper arm or axilla (see Figure 2-4 in Chapter 2). Appropriate veins include
   1. Basilic
   2. Cephalic
   3. Median cubital
F. Insertion procedure
   1. Organize equipment and wash hands.
   2. Examine veins on both extremities, taking into account the purpose of the IV therapy, the most comfortable exit site for the patient, and any physical issues the patient may have that may limit the use of one arm (INS, 2016).

3. Use local anesthetic, as ordered. Be aware that anesthetic may obscure the vein secondary to vasoconstriction and vasospasm or may prevent the patient from sensing infiltration (see Appendix 7).

4. Place the midline catheter per the manufacturer's guidelines; the nurse inserting should be skilled regarding the specifics of the individual product.

5. Can use ultrasound guidance at the bedside to facilitate effective placement (Bortolussi et al., 2015; Deutsch et al., 2014).

6. Anticipate the insertion site to be 1–1.5 inches above or below antecubital fossa. Extend the patient's arm, and abduct the arm at a 45° angle.

7. Place a tourniquet 5–6 inches above the insertion site at the mid-upper arm area. The tourniquet should obstruct venous but not arterial flow. Check for the presence of a distal pulse. Remove the tourniquet for the patient's comfort.

8. Clip the area if a large amount of body hair is present at insertion site. Avoid shaving, which can cause increased irritation and risk of infection.

9. Cleanse the site, and allow to air-dry without fanning (see Appendix 2). Reapply tourniquet. Apply sterile gloves. Drape the arm with sterile drapes for sterile field. Flush the catheter with 0.9% normal saline (NS) solution.

10. Stabilize the vein below the access site with nondominant hand. Perform venipuncture by inserting the needle at a 15°–30° angle with bevel up distal to actual venipuncture site.

11. Observe blood return through tubing of the catheter, indicating the needle has entered the vein. Advance to the length of the needle, and remove the tourniquet.

12. Once venipuncture is complete, retract the needle into the needle safety tube on the external end of the catheter. The tip of the catheter is advanced slowly for several inches to the desired initial length through the introducer. Remove the guidewire slowly while stabilizing the midline catheter at the insertion site. Remove the introducer, and break away or peel away from the catheter by pulling apart at the wings. Flush with NS to verify patency.

13. Secure catheter with securement device, and apply dressing over insertion site. X-ray verification of tip placement is not indicated.

14. Document insertion, including type of line used, length of catheter, and patient tolerance.

15. Change the dressing 24 hours after insertion to assess for complications and then per protocol for transparent film or gauze dressing (see Appendices 2, 4, and 5).

VII. Unique maintenance and care (Boullata et al., 2014; Chopra et al., 2015; Cotogni & Pittiruti, 2014; O'Grady et al., 2011) (see Appendices 2, 4, 5, and 6): No definitive recommendations can be made regarding flushing solution, volume, and frequency; frequency of dressing and needleless connector changes; or blood sampling technique.

A. Inspect the catheter insertion site and palpate for tenderness daily through the intact dressing. If signs of potential infection are present, remove dressing and inspect the site visually. Minimize manipulation of the catheter to prevent mechanical phlebitis.

B. Replace midline catheters only when there is a specific indication (Abolfotouh, Salam, Bani-Mustafa, White, & Balkhy, 2014; Dychter, Gold, Carson, & Haller, 2012; Ho & Cheung, 2012). Midline catheters are associated with lower rates of phlebitis than peripheral IVs and lower rates of infection than central venous catheters (O'Grady et al., 2011).

C. Dressing changes: Change dressing if it becomes wet, soiled, or nonocclusive.
   1. Dressing changes require an aseptic no-touch technique.
   2. Remove existing dressing and securement device while stabilizing midline catheter with nondominant hand.

D. Flushing: Flush catheter prior to use with 3 ml NS. Use NS 1–3 ml every 8, 12, or 24 hours when device is not in use to maintain patency in adults and children aged one year or older (American Society of Health-System Pharmacists, 2012; Wang, Luo, He, Li, & Zhang, 2012).

E. Blood specimens: No definitive recommendation can be made regarding specific volume of blood discard or flush. Prior to policy development, the dead space volume of the products used must be known. Using midline catheters for blood specimens continues to be debated (Scoppettuolo et al., 2016; Stauss et al., 2012).

　　1. In general, within certain limitations of infusate, midlines flushed with NS are simple and safe for collecting blood samples for most laboratory tests (Baker et al., 2013; Ortells-Abuye et al., 2014).

　　2. Discard 1–3 ml or more of waste to promote accurate laboratory testing results (Baker et al., 2013).

F. Administration practices (Dychter et al., 2012)

　　1. IV push: Following the flushing procedure, cleanse the needleless connector, allow the solution to dry, attach the syringe containing the medication, infuse over a short period of time, and flush with 1–3 ml NS following completion of infusion.

　　2. Intermittent infusions: Used for drugs that require dilution or slow administration. Following the flushing procedure, cleanse needleless connector, allow solution to dry, attach administration set of infusion to be administered, infuse over specified time, and flush with 1–3 ml NS following completion of infusion.

　　3. Continuous infusions: Most common method of administering IV fluids, drugs, and peripheral nutrition. Following the flushing procedure, cleanse needleless connector or hub, allow solution to dry, attach administration set of infusion to be administered, and infuse at specified rate.

　　4. If used for intermittent vesicant administration, exercise caution and carefully monitor, as a risk of extravasation exists, which may go undetected because the line may be misidentified as a central line. The midline catheter is a peripheral venous device.

VIII. Removal technique (Hadaway, Dalton, & Mercanti-Erieg, 2013; Helm, Klausner, Klemperer, Flint, & Huang, 2015; INS, 2016; O'Grady et al., 2011; Scoppettuolo et al., 2016)

A. Prior to removal, verify scope of practice with the individual state board of nursing and institutional guidelines. Credentialing and ongoing competency validation are required.

B. Indications: Remove the catheter when signs and symptoms of infection, infiltration, or phlebitis exist, or when no longer required for therapy.

C. Procedure

　　1. Verify order and indication for removal when IV therapy is discontinued.

　　2. Explain procedure to the patient.

　　3. Place the patient in a chair or bed to stabilize the extremity.

　　4. Inspect the general condition of the catheter pathway.

　　5. Discontinue all infusions into the device.

　　6. Put on gloves; remove dressing; remove securement device; and observe site for any pain, edema, redness, or discharge.

　　7. Change gloves; grasp device by the hub; and while stabilizing the skin and vein with sterile gauze in the nondominant hand, slowly and steadily pull until device is completely removed.

　　8. If removal of the catheter is indicated for infection, send the catheter tip for culture, if ordered.

　　9. Apply constant, firm pressure to the exit site until bleeding stops (longer in patients with coagulopathies or thrombocytopenia and those on anticoagulants). Apply dressing or adhesive bandage; monitor as necessary.

　　10. Instruct the patient or caregiver to report any discomfort or signs of bleeding, bruising, redness, swelling, or drainage.

　　11. Measure the catheter for appropriate length and catheter integrity. Inspect the device for defects, and report any to the manufacturer and regulatory agencies. Examine distal tip for signs of jagged, uneven edges suggestive of breakage.

　　12. Document observations and actions.

IX. Complications (Coyle, Griffie, & Czaplewski, 2014; O'Grady et al., 2011; Polovich, Olsen, & LeFebvre, 2014; Sabri, Szalas, Holmes, Labib, & Mussivand, 2013; Scoppettuolo et al., 2016)

A. Insertion complications: Bleeding, vein injury, nerve injury, infiltration, phlebitis, or thrombosis

B. Vein injury: Pain, tenderness, edema, redness (vasodilation), thrombosis, sclerosis, or infiltration

C. Phlebitis: Most common complication, resulting in inflammation of the vein

　　1. Etiology: Insufficient vessel size to accommodate the catheter and allow hemodilution, traumatic insertion, or mechanical or chemical irritation

　　2. Risk factors

　　　　a) Prolonged dwell time

　　　　b) Mechanical irritation: Movement of the catheter, multiple cannulation attempts, catheter too large for vein, location of the catheter, or catheter material

c) Chemical irritation: Tonicity of fluid, number and dosage of medications, pH of the medications, or skin not allowed to dry after cleaning and prior to insertion

d) Increases with age of device or advanced age of the patient

3. Signs and symptoms: Pain, erythema, streak formation, or palpable cord edema

   a) Older adult patients may not experience pain from phlebitis or infiltration because of a decrease in sensory perception; monitoring for complications through observation is important.

   b) Children, older adults, or those with communication limitations may not be able to verbalize pain.

4. Diagnostic tests: Not indicated

5. Management: Remove device, apply heat, and give analgesic, as needed.

D. Infiltration: Second most common complication

1. Etiology: Mechanical (e.g., injury during insertion, catheter malposition following insertion) or physiologic (e.g., preexisting or developing vein problems such as sclerosis). From the penetration of the catheter into or through the venous wall, infiltration leads to infusion of fluids or medications into the surrounding soft tissue.

2. Risk factors: Insertion into antecubital fossa, inadequate catheter securement, traumatic injury to vessel wall on insertion, older or younger age, dehydration, and obesity

3. Prevention: Assess for infiltration by occluding the vessel at the tip of the catheter with digital pressure. If infusion continues, the fluid is likely infiltrating.

   a) Use of appropriately sized syringes will prevent vein rupture or infiltration with IV push administration or a vacuum on blood aspiration.

   b) The larger the syringe, the less pressure is generated when force is applied and the more force is required to create a vacuum. Less force is generated in either infusion or aspiration with larger syringes, thereby reducing or preventing complications.

   c) Do not use a 1 ml syringe with midline catheters. Use a syringe 3 ml or greater for all flushing and administration of medications.

4. Signs and symptoms: Leaking fluid around insertion site, cool and pale skin, possibly decreased infusion rate, edema at insertion site, tenderness, or skin tightness or discomfort

5. Diagnostic tests: Not indicated

6. Management: Remove device, apply heat, and give analgesic, as needed.

E. Infection

1. Etiology: Microorganisms enter by migration at insertion site, the interior of the catheter, contamination of connectors, excessive catheter manipulation, repalpation of a proposed puncture site prior to insertion, or by contaminated infusion. The most common organism is *Staphylococcus aureus*.

2. Risk factors: Inadequate cleansing technique, contamination of insertion site or supplies, immunocompromised patient, older or younger age, comorbidities (e.g., diabetes, cancer, heart disease), or malnourishment

3. Prevention: Use strict aseptic technique for insertion and maintenance care.

4. Signs and symptoms: Depend on type of infection

   a) Local: Erythema, purulent drainage, warmth, induration, or palpable cord

   b) Phlebitis: Pain, erythema, streak formation, palpable cord, or edema

   c) Bloodstream: Pain, erythema, streak formation, palpable cord, edema, fever, or chills

5. Diagnostic tests: Wound and blood cultures, as ordered

6. Management: Remove device, apply heat or cold (depending on agent infiltrated), and administer antibiotics systemically, per culture result.

F. Extravasation: The leaking or escape of infusate from the vessel into the surrounding tissue (Coyle et al., 2014; Le & Patel, 2014; Molas-Ferrer et al., 2015; Polovich et al., 2014)

1. Etiology: Peripheral vein wall puncture; administration of a vesicant in a vein below a recent venipuncture; or inadequately secured IV catheter, which results in leaking of vesicant agent into surrounding tissue. Damage is dependent on specific factors.

   a) Mechanism of action or properties of drug

   b) Amount of drug extravasated

2. Risk factors: Inadequate insertion technique, small fragile veins, history of multiple venipunctures, limited extremity vein selection, decreased sensation or circulatory impairments, and patient with altered mental status

3. Prevention
   a) Use clean technique in accessing peripheral vein, and avoid multiple attempts in establishing access.
   b) Avoid areas of impairment, previous IV sites, and insertion above previous venipuncture sites.
   c) Use transparent dressing over IV to visualize the site throughout vesicant administration.
   d) Verify blood return prior to, during, and after administration. Do not give vesicant through midline without a blood return.
   e) Instruct the patient to promptly report symptoms of extravasation.
4. Signs and symptoms: Burning or stinging at site; pain; erythema; difficulty infusing solution; leaking around the insertion site; absence of blood return during or following infusion, followed by blistering, tissue necrosis, and ulceration; decreased IV flow
5. Diagnostic tests: Not indicated
6. Management
   a) Stop infusion and aspirate residual drug from the catheter using a 3 ml syringe.
   b) Remove midline catheter, unless antidote is given through existing midline; in that case, remove after administration of antidote.
   c) Assess site and estimate amount of vesicant extravasated.
   d) Administer antidote or extravasation treatment, as indicated.
   e) Apply cold or heat, as indicated.
   f) Determine the cause of extravasation, notify the physician, measure and photograph the site, document patient assessment and nursing care, and provide patient education and follow-up.
X. Practicum on midline insertion and care (see Appendix 6)

XI. Education and documentation (See Appendix 6 and Chapter 17 for competency.)
XII. Special considerations for pediatrics and older adults
   A. Pediatrics: Available in 24- and 22-gauge sizes in 6–8 cm in length
   B. Pediatric insertion sites: Basilic and cephalic vein in the upper extremity
   C. Older adults: Avoid tourniquet use in older adults with fragile veins and thin skin. Excessive antiseptic can dry already compromised skin (INS, 2013).
XIII. Infusion teams (Hadaway et al., 2013; Harpel, 2013; O'Grady et al., 2011, Sabri et al., 2013) (see Figure 2-5 in Chapter 2)

References

Abolfotouh, M.A., Salam, M., Bani-Mustafa, A., White, D., & Balkhy, H.H. (2014). Prospective study of incidence and predictors of peripheral intravenous catheter-induced complications. *Therapeutics and Clinical Risk Management, 10,* 993–1001. doi:10.2147/TCRM.S74685

American Society of Health-System Pharmacists. (2012). ASHP therapeutic position statement on the institutional use of 0.9% sodium chloride injection to maintain patency of peripheral indwelling intermittent infusion devices. *American Journal of Health-System Pharmacy, 69,* 1252–1254. doi:10.2146/ajhp120076

Baker, R.B., Summer, S.S., Lawrence, M., Shova, A., McGraw, C.A., & Khoury, J. (2013). Determining optimal waste volume from an intravenous catheter. *Journal of Infusion Nursing, 36,* 92–96. doi:10.1097/NAN.0b013e318282a4c2

Bortolussi, R., Zotti, P., Conte, M., Marson, R., Polesel, J., Colussi, A., … Spazzapan, S. (2015). Quality of life, pain perception, and distress correlated to ultrasound-guided peripherally inserted central venous catheters in palliative care patients in a home or hospice setting. *Journal of Pain and Symptom Management, 50,* 118–123. doi:10.1016/j.jpainsymman.2015.02.027

Boullata, J.I., Gilbert, K., Sacks, G., Labossiere, R.J., Crill, C., Goday, P., … American Society for Parenteral and Enteral Nutrition. (2014). A.S.P.E.N. clinical guidelines: Parenteral nutrition ordering, order review, compounding, labeling, and dispensing. *Journal of Parenteral and Enteral Nutrition, 38,* 334–377. doi:10.1177/0148607114521833

Caparas, J.V., & Hu, J.P. (2014). Safe administration of vancomycin through a novel midline catheter: A randomized, prospective clinical trial. *Journal of Vascular Access, 15,* 251–256. doi:10.5301/jva.5000220

Chopra, V., Flanders, S.A., Saint, S., Woller, S.C., O'Grady, N.P., Safdar, N., … Bernstein, S.J. (2015). The Michigan Appropriateness Guide for Intravenous Catheters (MAGIC): Results from a multispecialty panel using the RAND/UCLA Appropriateness Method. *Annals of Internal Medicine, 163*(Suppl. 6), S1–S40. doi:10.7326/M15-0744

Cotogni, P., & Pittiruti, M. (2014). Focus on peripherally inserted central catheters in critically ill patients. *World Journal of Critical Care Medicine, 3,* 80–94.

Coyle, C., Griffie, J., & Czaplewski, L.M. (2014). Eliminating extravasation events: A multidisciplinary approach. *Journal of Infusion Nursing, 37,* 157–164. doi:10.1097/NAN.0000000000000034

Dawson, R.B., & Moureau, N.L. (2013). Midline catheters: An essential tool in CLABSI reduction. Retrieved from http://www.infectioncontroltoday.com/articles/2013/03/midline-catheters-an-essential-tool-in-clabsi-reduction.aspx

Deutsch, G.B., Sathyanarayana, S.A., Singh, N., & Nicastro, J. (2014). Ultrasound-guided placement of midline catheters in the surgical intensive care unit: A cost-effective proposal for timely central line removal. *Journal of Surgical Research, 191,* 1–5. doi:10.1016/j.jss.2013.03.047

Dumont, C., Getz, O., & Miller, S. (2014). Evaluation of midline vascular access: A descriptive study. *Nursing, 44*(10), 60–66. doi:10.1097/01.NURSE.0000453713.81317.52

Dychter, S.S., Gold, D.A., Carson, D., & Haller, M. (2012). Intravenous therapy: A review of complications and economic considerations of peripheral access. *Journal of Infusion Nursing, 35,* 84–91. doi:10.1097/NAN.0b013e31824237ce

Giuliani, J., Andreetta, L., Mattioli, M., Melotto, A., Zuliani, S., Zanardi, O., & Borese, B. (2013). Intravenous midline catheter usage: Which clinical impact in homecare patients? *Journal of Palliative Medicine, 16,* 598. doi:10.1089/jpm.2012.0615

Hadaway, L., Dalton, L., & Mercanti-Erieg, L. (2013). Infusion teams in acute care hospitals: A call for a business approach: An Infusion Nurses Society white paper. *Journal of Infusion Nursing, 36,* 356–360. doi:10.1097/NAN.0b013e3182a123a9Harpel, J. (2013). Best practices for vascular resource teams. *Journal of Infusion Nursing, 36,* 46–50. doi:10.1097/NAN.0b013e3182798862

Helm, R.E., Klausner, J.D., Klemperer, J.D., Flint, L.M., & Huang, E. (2015). Accepted but unacceptable: Peripheral IV catheter failure. *Journal of Infusion Nursing, 38,* 189–203. doi:10.1097/NAN.0000000000000100

Ho, K.H.M., & Cheung, D.S.K. (2012). Guidelines on timing in replacing peripheral intravenous catheters. *Journal of Clinical Nursing, 21,* 1499–1506. doi:10.1111/j.1365-2702.2011.03974.x

Infusion Nurses Society. (2013). *Policies and procedures for infusion nursing of the older adult.* Norwood, MA: Author.

Infusion Nurses Society. (2016). *Infusion therapy standards of practice.* Norwood, MA: Author.

Institute for Healthcare Improvement. (n.d.). Evidence-based care bundles. Retrieved from http://www.ihi.org/Topics/Bundles/Pages/default.aspx

Le, A., & Patel, S. (2014). Extravasation of noncytotoxic drugs. A review of the literature. *Annals of Pharmacotherapy, 48,* 870–886. doi:10.1177/1060028014527820

Molas-Ferrer, G., Farré-Ayuso, E., doPazo-Oubiña, F., deAndrés-Lázaro, A., Guell-Picazo, J., Borrás-Maixenchs, N., … Creus-Baró, N. (2015). Level of adherence to an extravasation protocol over 10 years in a tertiary care hospital [Online exclusive]. *Clinical Journal of Oncology Nursing, 19,* E25–E30. doi:10.1188/15.cjon.e25-e30

O'Grady, N.P., Alexander, M., Burns, L.A., Dellinger, E.P., Garland, J., Heard, S.O., … Healthcare Infection Control Practices Advisory Committee. (2011). Guidelines for the prevention of intravascular catheter-related infections. *Clinical Infectious Diseases, 52,* E162–E193. doi:10.1093/cid/cir257

Ortells-Abuye, N., Busquets-Puigdevall, T., Díaz-Bergara, M., Paguina-Marcos, M., & Sánchez-Pérez, I. (2014). A cross-sectional study to compare two blood collection methods: Direct venous puncture and peripheral venous catheter. *BMJ Open, 4,* e004250. doi:10.1136/bmjopen-2013-004250

Pathak, R., Patel, A., Enuh, H., Adekunle, O., Shrisgantharajah, V., & Diaz, K. (2015). The incidence of central line–associated bacteremia after the introduction of midline catheters in a ventilator unit population. *Infectious Diseases in Clinical Practice, 23,* 131–134. doi:10.1097/IPC.0000000000000237

Polovich, M., Olsen, M., & LeFebvre, K.B. (Eds.). (2014). *Chemotherapy and biotherapy guidelines and recommendations for practice* (4th ed.). Pittsburgh, PA: Oncology Nursing Society.

Sabri, A., Szalas, J., Holmes, K.S., Labib, L., & Mussivand, T. (2013). Failed attempts and improvement strategies in peripheral intravenous catheterization. *Bio-Medical Materials and Engineering, 23,* 93–108. doi:10.3233/BME-120735

Scoppettuolo, G., Pittiruti, M., Pitoni, S., Dolcetti, L., Emoli, A., Mitidieri, A., … Annetta, M.G. (2016). Ultrasound-guided "short" midline catheters for difficult venous access in the emergency department: A retrospective analysis. *International Journal of Emergency Medicine, 9,* 3. doi:10.1186/s12245-016-0100-0

Stauss, M., Sherman, B., Pugh, L., Parone, D., Looby-Rodriguez, K., Bell, A., & Reed, C.R. (2012). Hemolysis of coagulation specimens: A comparative study of intravenous draw methods. *Journal of Emergency Nursing, 38,* 15–21. doi:10.1016/.j.jen.2010.08.011

Wang, R., Luo, O., He, L., Li, J.X., & Zhang, M.G. (2012). Preservative-free 0.9% sodium chloride for flushing and locking peripheral intravenous access device: A prospective controlled trial. *Journal of Evidence-Based Medicine, 5,* 205–208. doi:10.1111/jebm.12004

Chapter 4

Nontunneled Central Venous Lines

Dawn Camp-Sorrell, RN, MSN, FNP, AOCN®, and Laurl Matey, MSN, RN, CHPN

I. History (Aubaniac, 1990; Cheung, Baerlocher, Asch, & Myers, 2009; Gallieni, Pittiruti, & Biffi, 2008)
   A. Nontunneled catheters have continued to evolve since 1945, when polyurethane material was beginning to be used in catheter development.
   B. By 1949, access was mainly accomplished through the femoral and external jugular veins.
   C. In 1952, the subclavian vein was used for central line access to allow for rapid resuscitation for injured war victims.
   D. Total parenteral nutrition (TPN) was being administered successfully with available central line access in dogs in 1966, proving this method safe and effective.
   E. Newer polyurethane and power-injectable models were introduced in the mid-2000s.
II. Device characteristics (see Figures 4-1 and 4-2)
   A. Short-term catheter
   B. Can be used for immediate access for all types of therapy, including emergencies
   C. Often used for rapid resuscitation or pressure monitoring
III. Device features (Gentile et al., 2013)
   A. Size: Ranges from 14–24 gauge, 4–8.5 Fr, and 10–30 cm length in single-lumen and multilumen designs. Four- and five-lumen catheter designs recently have become available.
   B. Catheter material: Polyurethane and silicone with available options, including latex free, radiopaque, chlorhexidine-sulfadiazine impregnated, and heparin coated
   C. Distal tip opening design
   D. Distal tip openings on multilumen catheters may be side by side or staggered.
   E. Power-injectable design
   F. Clamps attached per lumen
IV. Device advantages and disadvantages (see Figure 4-3)
V. Patient selection criteria (Alexandrou et al., 2014; Chung & Beheshti, 2011; Dassinger et al., 2015; Gibson & Bodenham, 2013; Villalta-García et al., 2015)
   A. Use a catheter with the smallest gauge necessary for indicated therapy to decrease the incidence of venous thrombosis.
   B. Patients receiving short-term treatment with no need for extended therapy
   C. Patients with poor peripheral venous access
   D. Patients who require treatment with fluids that are hyperosmolar, alkaline, or acidic
   E. Patients who require frequent venous access for infusion or blood specimens
   F. Patients who are poor surgical candidates for long-term catheter placement
   G. Critically ill patients requiring multilumen access or central venous pressure monitoring
   H. Patients needing emergent central access
   I. Absolute contraindication is a combative patient.
VI. Insertion techniques (Brass, Hellmich, Kolodziej, Schick, & Smith, 2015; Chung & Beheshti, 2011; Dassinger et al., 2015; Gibson & Bodenham, 2013; Kim et al., 2012; Lennon, Zaw, Pöpping, & Wenk, 2012; Perbet et al., 2014; Youn et al., 2015)
   A. Only healthcare professionals who have successfully completed a specialized training course should insert nontunneled central venous access devices (CVADs) (Alexandrou et al., 2014). In the United States, state boards of nursing govern who may insert and remove nontunneled CVADs; laws governing this practice vary widely from state to state.

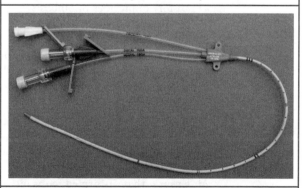

Figure 4-1. Triple-Lumen, Nontunneled Catheter With Open Distal Tip

Figure 4-2. Triple-Lumen, Nontunneled Catheter

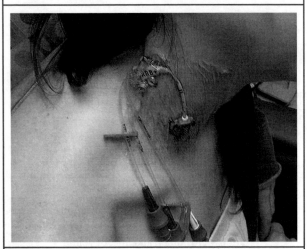

Note. Public domain image by Jsonp. Retrieved from https://commons.wikimedia.org/wiki/File:Triple-Lumen.jpg.

B. Prior to placement, ensure that contraindications do not exist, informed consent is obtained, preplacement assessment is completed, laboratory studies are verified, and the medication/chemotherapy order is reviewed (see Appendix 4).

C. Vein selection
   1. Use the right internal jugular vein because it follows a fairly straight course to the subclavian.
   2. The left subclavian vein is an acceptable choice, as it has a smooth curve to the superior vena cava without an acute turn.
   3. If the right internal jugular is not available, the left internal jugular, the external jugular, or the right subclavian vein may be used. The following conditions may require femoral placement:
      a) Enlarged axillary or subclavian nodes
      b) Tumor mass of neck or chest region
      c) Previous surgery or radiation therapy to the axillary or subclavian area
      d) History of previous thrombosis
      e) Presence of cardiac pacemaker
      f) Superior vena cava syndrome
   4. Femoral insertion with the tip in the inferior vena cava is possible but has an increased risk of infection and thrombotic complications.

D. Insertion procedure (Tang et al., 2014)
   1. Prepreparation
      a) Explain the insertion procedure to the patient and answer any questions the patient or caregiver may have.
      b) Ensure that informed consent is obtained.

   c) Determine if the patient has allergies to cleansing agents or tape products, and inform the practitioner placing the line.
   d) Evaluate prior to placement for obesity, coagulation disorders, short neck stature (limited space to access vein in the neck region), acute respiratory failure, thrombocytopenia, and history of central venous catheter insertions.
   2. Position the patient.
      a) Unless contraindicated, place the patient in the Trendelenburg position, which distends the vein selected for cannulation and decreases the risk of air embolism.
      b) Position the patient's neck and shoulders to increase venous distention (e.g., placing a rolled towel beneath the area).
   3. Use maximum sterile barrier precautions, including mask, cap, sterile gown, and sterile gloves, for all practitioners involved with the insertion procedure, and cover the patient with a sterile drape to reduce infection risk.

Figure 4-3. Advantages and Disadvantages of Nontunneled Central Venous Lines

Advantages	Disadvantages
• May be used to infuse all IV therapies and draw blood • May be inserted at the bedside or in ambulatory surgery using sterile technique • May be inserted without general anesthesia or procedural sedation • May be used to monitor central venous pressure • May be placed in an emergency situation and used immediately • Does not require needle access for use after insertion • Designed for short-term use • Available in a variety of gauges, in single, double, triple, quad, and five lumens, and as power-injectable versions • Can be used for multiple, incompatible solutions concurrently (multilumen) • Available antimicrobial-impregnated catheters may decrease risk of infection. • Available heparin-coated catheters may decrease risk of venous thrombosis.	• May be associated with discomfort at insertion • More prone to infection because of a lack of tunnel/cuff, the external portion, and insertion at bedside • Require diligent aseptic care to prevent infection and maintain line function • May require checking of placement with x-ray prior to use • Not used for long-term venous access

4. Cleanse the insertion site (see Appendix 2). If necessary, clip (do not shave) long hair to decrease contamination.
5. Use local anesthetic to decrease insertion discomfort (see Appendix 7).
6. Percutaneous placement
   a) Ultrasound guidance: Decreases the risk of arterial puncture and hematoma formation
   b) Landmark approach: Uses anatomic areas to locate and access the central vein without imaging studies. A triangle of landmarks (clavicle and the two heads of the sternocleidomastoid muscle) identifies the insertion site.
   c) Electrocardiogram and fluoroscopy guidance techniques have been used with success in nontunneled placement (Rossetti et al., 2015; Wang et al., 2015).
7. Insert the needle percutaneously into the vein with a stylet and guidewire, using the clavicle as a guide, according to the Seldinger technique.
   a) When a flashback is observed, remove the syringe and advance the guidewire into the vein. To minimize complications, the guidewire is not advanced further than 18 cm.
   b) Advance the catheter over the guidewire into the subclavian vein until it reaches the superior vena cava.
   c) Remove the guidewire and flush each lumen with saline.
8. Avoid suturing; secure catheter with a securement device. Apply an occlusive dressing over the exit site (O'Grady et al., 2011).
9. Confirm correct placement prior to use to determine proper location of tip and to detect pneumothorax. When ultrasound guidance is used for placement, a chest x-ray is not necessary. Proper catheter tip location is just above or in the lower third of the superior vena cava at the cavoatrial junction or in inferior vena cava, if placed femorally.
10. Document the length of the catheter, the presence of blood return, and the patient's condition.
11. To minimize infection, replace catheters inserted during an emergency or in the femoral vein as soon as possible.

VII. Unique maintenance and care: No definitive recommendations can be made for flushing solution, volume, and frequency; frequency of dressing and needleless connector changes; or blood sampling technique (see Appendices 2, 3, 4, 5, and 8).

A. Dressing: Change 24 hours after insertion.
B. Flushing: Use heparin 10–100 IU/ml, 2–3 ml/day per lumen; heparin lock after use for intermittent infusions after flushing with 0.9% normal saline (NS). When flushed every eight hours, 10 ml NS has been effective in maintaining lumen patency (Gorji, Rezaei, Jafari, & Cherati, 2015). Clamps are used when accessing or deaccessing nontunneled VADs.
C. Needleless connector: Change connector after each use, if damaged, or if contaminated with blood.
D. Blood sampling: Discard 3–5 ml of blood, obtain specimen, and flush with 10–20 ml NS.
   1. A recent study revealed accurate complete blood count, chemistry panel, and coagulation tests compared to peripheral samples when a 2 ml discard volume was used from the proximal lumen.
   2. Researchers proposed to use middle and distal lumens for drugs and TPN and proximal lumens for fluid therapy, electrolyte replacement, and blood sampling (Villalta-García et al., 2015).

VIII. Removal technique
A. Remove nontunneled lines when therapy is completed, when the line is no longer functional because of thrombus or mechanical failure, or when the line is infected.
B. Do not routinely replace (O'Grady et al., 2011).
C. Verify order for removal and indication. Prior to removal, verify scope of practice with the individual state board of nursing and institutional guidelines.
D. Explain the procedure to the patient.
E. Place the patient in a reclining position.
F. Inspect the general condition of the catheter.
G. Discontinue all infusions into the device.
H. Put on gloves, remove the dressing, remove the securement device, and inspect the exit site for redness, pain, swelling, exudate, or other problems.
I. Change gloves and remove sutures, if present.
J. Have the patient perform the Valsalva maneuver. Performing the Valsalva maneuver decreases the risk of an air embolism during catheter removal.
   1. Instruct the patient to take a deep breath and hold it.
   2. Instruct the patient to "bear down" for 10 seconds.
K. Grasp the hub of the catheter, and gently and steadily retract catheter until it is completely removed.
L. Apply constant, firm pressure to the exit site until bleeding stops (longer in patients with coagulopathies or decreased platelet count). Apply sterile,

occlusive dressing; monitor the patient for discomfort, bleeding, bruising, redness, swelling, or drainage; and advise the patient and caregiver to report these symptoms if they occur.

M. Visually inspect the CVAD for appropriate length and defects, such as holes, tears, or jagged edges suggesting breakage. If the length is shorter than expected or the edges appear broken, notify the provider.

N. Document observations, actions, and patient teaching.

IX. Complications (Alexandrou et al., 2014; Gentile et al., 2013; Gibson & Bodenham, 2013; Lennon et al., 2012) (see Chapter 9)

A. Insertion complications: Pneumothorax, migration, malposition, and bleeding

B. Removal complications: Venous air embolism, dyspnea, pain, bleeding from the insertion site, and arrhythmias

X. Education and documentation (see Chapter 17)

XI. Practicum on short-term, nontunneled venous catheter care (see Appendix 8)

The authors would like to acknowledge Susan A. Ezzone, MS, RN, CNP, AOCNP®, and Misty Lamprecht, MS, RN, CNS, AOCN®, for their contribution to this chapter that remains unchanged from the previous edition of this book.

References

Alexandrou, E., Spencer, T.R., Frost, S.A., Mifflin, N., Davidson, P.M., & Hillman, K.M. (2014). Central venous catheter placement by advanced practice nurses demonstrates low procedural complication and infection rates: A report from 13 years of service. *Critical Care Medicine, 42,* 536–543. doi:10.1097/CCM.0b013e3182a667f0

Aubaniac, R. (1990). The subclavian vein puncture—Advantages and technique. 1952. *Nutrition, 6,* 139–140.

Brass, P., Hellmich, M., Kolodziej, L., Schick, G., & Smith, A.F. (2015). Ultrasound guidance versus anatomical landmarks for subclavian or femoral vein catheterization. *Cochrane Database of Systematic Reviews, 2015*(1). doi:10.1002/14651858.CD011447

Cheung, E., Baerlocher, M.O., Asch, M., & Myers, A. (2009). Venous access: A practical review for 2009. *Canadian Family Physician, 55,* 494–496.

Chung, H.-Y., & Beheshti, M.V. (2011). Principles of non-tunneled central venous access. *Techniques in Vascular and Interventional Radiology, 14,* 186–191. doi:10.1053/j.tvir.2011.05.005

Dassinger, M.S., Renaud, E.J., Goldin, A., Huang, E.Y., Russell, R.T., Streck, C.J., ... Blakely, M.L. (2015). Use of real-time ultrasound during central venous catheter placement: Results of an APSA survey. *Journal of Pediatric Surgery, 50,* 1162–1167. doi:10.1016/j.pedsurg.2015.03.003

Gallieni, M., Pittiruti, M., & Biffi, R. (2008). Vascular access in oncology patients. *CA: A Cancer Journal for Clinicians, 58,* 323–346. doi:10.3322/ca.2008.0015

Gentile, A., Petit, L., Masson, F., Cottenceau, V., Bertrand-Barat, J., Freyburger, G., ... Sztark, F. (2013). Subclavian central venous catheter-related thrombosis in trauma patients: Incidence, risk factors and influence of polyurethane type. *Critical Care, 17,* R103. doi:10.1186/cc12748

Gibson, F., & Bodenham, A. (2013). Misplaced central venous catheters: Applied anatomy and practical management. *British Journal of Anaesthesia, 110,* 333–346. doi:10.1093/bja/aes497

Gorji, M.A.H., Rezaei, F., Jafari, H., & Cherati, J.Y. (2015). Comparison of the effects of heparin and 0.9% sodium chloride solutions in maintenance of patency of central venous catheters. *Anesthesiology and Pain Medicine, 5,* e22595. Retrieved from http://www.ncbi.nlm.nih.gov/pmc/articles/PMC4389103

Kim, W.Y., Lee, C.W., Sohn, C.H., Seo, D.W., Yoon, J.C., Koh, J.W., ... Koh, Y. (2012). Optimal insertion depth of central venous catheters: Is a formula required? A prospective cohort study. *Injury, 43,* 38–41. doi:10.1016/j.injury.2011.02.007

Lennon, M., Zaw, N.N., Pöpping, D.M., & Wenk, M. (2012). Procedural complications of central venous catheter insertion. *Minerva Anestesiologica, 1234*–1240.

O'Grady, N.P., Alexander, M., Burns, L.A., Dellinger, E.P., Garland, J., Heard, S.O., ... Healthcare Infection Control Practices Advisory Committee. (2011). Guidelines for the prevention of intravascular catheter-related infections. *Clinical Infectious Diseases, 52,* E162–E193. doi:10.1093/cid/cir257

Perbet, S., Pereira, B., Grimaldi, F., Dualé, C., Bazin, J.-E., & Constantin, J.-M. (2014). Guidance and examination by ultrasound versus landmark and radiographic method for placement of subclavian central venous catheters: Study protocol for a randomized controlled trial. *Revista Latino-Americana de Enfermagem, 15,* 175. doi:10.1186/1745-6215-15-175

Rossetti, F., Pittiruti, M., Lamperti, M., Graziano, U., Celentano, D., & Capozzoli, G. (2015). The intracavitary ECG method for positioning the tip of central venous access devices in pediatric patients: Results of an Italian multicenter study. *Journal of Vascular Access, 16,* 137–143. doi:10.5301/jva.5000281

Tang, H.-J., Lin, H.-L., Lin, Y.-H., Leung, P.-O., Chuang, Y.-C., & Lai, C.-C. (2014). The impact of central line insertion bundle on central line-associated blood stream infection. *BMC Infectious Diseases, 14,* 356. doi:10.1186/1471-2334-14-356

Villalta-García, P., López-Herránz, M., Mazo-Pascual, S., Honrubia-Fernández, T., Jañez-Escalada, L., & Fernández-Pérez, C. (2015). Reliability of blood test results in samples obtained using a 2-mL discard volume from the proximal lumen of a triple-lumen central venous catheter in the critically ill patient. *Nursing in Critical Care.* Advance online publication. doi:10.1111/nicc.12220

Wang, G., Guo, L., Jiang, B., Huang, M., Zhang, J., & Qin, Y. (2015). Factors influencing intracavitary electrocardiographic P-wave changes during central venous catheter placement. *PLOS ONE, 10,* e0124846. doi:10.1371/journal.pone.0124846

Youn, S.H., Lee, J.C.J., Kim, Y., Moon, J., Choi, Y., & Jung, K. (2015). Central venous catheter-related infection in severe trauma patients. *World Journal of Surgery, 39,* 2400–2406. doi:10.1007/s00268-015-3137-y

Chapter 5

Peripherally Inserted Central Catheters

Diane G. Cope, PhD, ARNP-BC, AOCNP®

I. History
  A. First introduced in the 1980s and primarily used for venous access in homecare patients (Bowe-Geddes & Nichols, 2005; Cotogni & Pittiruti, 2014)
  B. Designed for long-term central venous access (six months or greater)
  C. Increased popularity in part due to lower insertion costs, lower risks of insertion complications, and the fact it is within the scope of nursing practice to have RNs trained to perform insertion procedure
II. Device characteristics (Chopra et al., 2015; Hagle & Cook, 2014; Park & Kim, 2015; Sekold, Walker, & Dwyer, 2015)
  A. Commonly used in intensive care units with the advent of power-injectable peripherally inserted central catheters (PICCs)
  B. Introduced percutaneously into a palpable peripheral vein above and below the antecubital fossa and terminated in the central venous system
III. Device features (Baskin et al., 2014; Park & Kim, 2015)
  A. Catheter material: Silicone, polyurethane, or elastomeric hydrogel; radiopaque
  B. Range from 3–6 Fr in single-, double-, and triple-lumen designs; pediatric sizes from 1.9–2.6 Fr in single-, double-, and triple-lumen designs
  C. Lengths range from 50–60 cm.
  D. Prime volume of 0.5–1.5 ml
  E. Valved or open-ended distal tips are available.
  F. Power-injectable PICCs (valved and nonvalved) are available for the delivery of power injection flow rates required for contrast-enhanced injections. A randomized study failed to demonstrate a significant functional, maintenance, or complication rate advantage with use of the more expensive valved PICC versus the nonvalved PICC (Pittiruti et al., 2014).
  G. Available with pressure-activated safety valves designed to prevent blood backflow
  H. Available with polymer infused into the catheter shaft material that remains present throughout the life of the catheter, providing long-term durability and decreased accumulation of catheter-related thrombosis
  I. Approved for use up to 12 months; however, evidence supports a longer duration if the device is functioning without complications (O'Grady et al., 2011).
IV. Device advantages and disadvantages (Johansson, Hammaskjöld, Lundberg, & Arnlind, 2013) (see Figure 5-1)
V. Patient selection criteria (Bourgeois, Lamagna, & Chiang, 2011; Chopra et al., 2015; Cotogni & Pittiruti, 2014; Gabriel, 2013; Green et al., 2015; Hagle & Cook, 2014; Wojnar & Beaman, 2013)
  A. Patients with poor, fragile, or small peripheral veins for administration of therapy with long-term duration
  B. Patients receiving administration of solutions that are irritants or vesicants or solutions with a pH less than 5 or greater than 9, glucose greater than 10%, protein greater than 5%, or osmolarity greater than 900 mOsm/L (Boullata et al., 2014; Chopra et al., 2015; Cotogni & Pittiruti, 2014)
  C. Patients who prefer this type of device over other venous access devices (VADs)
  D. In the home setting, patients who have a caregiver who can properly care for the device
  E. Patients with anatomic abnormality or tumor burden in the chest, chest wall, or neck that would contraindicate placement of an implantable port or tunneled catheter
  F. Contraindicated in patients with severe renal dysfunction who may require an arteriovenous fistula formation
VI. Insertion techniques (Chopra et al., 2015; Cotogni & Pittiruti, 2014; Johansson et al., 2013; Moureau et al., 2013; Park & Kim, 2015; Steele & Norris, 2014; Wang et al., 2015) (see Figure 5-2)
  A. Only healthcare professionals who have successfully completed a specialized training course should insert PICCs.
    1. In the United States, state boards of nursing govern who may insert, access, man-

---

Figure 5-1. Advantages and Disadvantages of Peripherally Inserted Central Catheters (PICCs)

Advantages
- May be used immediately after confirmed placement
- May be inserted by an RN with specialized training who has demonstrated clinical competence in insertion technique
- Insertion at the bedside or in an outpatient setting
- Provide a safe, economical means of vascular access for therapies
- Pose no risk of insertion-related pneumothorax or great vessel perforation
- If inserted properly and maintained, demonstrate a lower complication rate than other types of venous access devices
- Available in single-, double-, and triple-lumen; radiopaque; power-injectable; and valved and nonvalved designs
- Can be used for up to 12 months or longer with proper maintenance
- Ideal for those with poor, fragile, or small peripheral veins; those requiring vesicant or irritant medication infusions; or those requiring hyperosmolar solution infusions
- Can be used for blood sampling with proper technique
- Legitimate first choice for venous access in patients who are acutely or critically ill and who need intensive IV therapy and assurance of continuous venous access
- Ideal for patients with chest or neck tumor burden that would interfere with implantable port, tunneled, or nontunneled catheter placement
- Decrease stress exerted on the patient by reducing the number of venipunctures required to administer therapy
- Ideal in homecare settings if family member or caregiver is available to properly care for device
- Less expensive than nontunneled short-term catheters, long-term catheters, or implanted ports
- Repair kits available

Disadvantages
- Specialized educational preparation and confirmation of clinical competence required for RNs
- Laws governing RN practice vary widely from state to state in the United States.
- RNs must maintain a level of skill and competence.
- Limit arm movement
- May limit the patient's overall mobility if it is necessary to insert the catheter into contralateral limb because of compromised alternate limb (e.g., lymphedema, axillary dissection)
- May not be able to draw blood with small gauge PICCs
- Smaller French sizes not suitable for red blood cell transfusion
- More expensive than peripheral IVs
- Require adequate patient support and a caregiver to maintain catheter in homecare setting

---

age, and remove PICCs; laws governing this practice vary widely from state to state.

2. Research supports high insertion success rates and low malposition rates of bedside insertions performed by trained RNs, requiring minimal support from interventional radiology and substantially reducing insertion costs (Sainathan, Hempstead, & Andaz, 2014).

B. Pediatric considerations: Conscious or general sedation typically is used for insertion to ensure that the patient remains still for the procedure (Braswell, 2011; Cotogni & Pittiruti, 2014; Westergaard, Classen, & Walther-Larsen, 2013).

C. Insertion may be performed by skilled practitioners using ultrasound guidance or anatomic landmarks.

   1. Use of ultrasound versus anatomic landmarks reduces incidence of insertion failure, decreases the costs of multiple cannulations, and can confirm correct tip position. Research demonstrates that avoiding injury of the vein wall during placement via ultrasound guidance correlates positively with reduced rates of catheter-related thrombosis (Bowen, Mone, Nelson, & Scaife, 2014; Katheria, Fleming, & Kim, 2013; Lamperti et al., 2012; O'Grady et al., 2011; Teichgräber, Kausche, Nagel, & Gebauer, 2011).

   2. Studies demonstrate high technical success, low patient distress, and low early complication rates when ultrasound guidance is used (Bortolussi et al., 2015; Katheria et al., 2013).

   3. Electrocardiogram guidance techniques have been used with success for tip placement verification (Rossetti et al., 2015; Wang et al., 2015).

D. Prior to placement, ensure that contraindications do not exist, informed consent is obtained, the preplacement assessment is completed, laboratory studies have been verified, and the medication or chemotherapy order has been reviewed (see Appendix 4).

E. Insertion methods (Cotogni & Pittiruti, 2014)

   1. Peel-away sheath technique: Puncture vein with a needle/sheath device. Remove stylet and thread into the vein. Peel the sheath/

cannula down to the hub of the catheter, break away, and then remove from the catheter.

   a) Advantages: Risk of catheter damage is low, a variety of gauge sizes are available, and this technique can be performed virtually without blood spills.

   b) Disadvantages: A larger introducer unit is required. This technique has a higher incidence of thrombophlebitis than the modified Seldinger method and may cause more bleeding around the exit site during the first few hours after insertion.

2. Over-wire Seldinger method: Puncture vein with a smaller gauge steel needle. Observe for blood in the attached syringe. Remove syringe and thread guidewire through the needle into the vein. Remove needle and cannula. Thread peel-away sheath down to the skin over the guidewire introducer. Remove guidewire and advance the catheter to correct position and stabilize.

   a) Advantages: This method requires a smaller venipuncture, a variety of gauge sizes are available, and the risk of catheter damage is eliminated.

   b) Disadvantages: This method is more complex and may require a minor surgical incision, which increases cost.

F. Catheter tip is just above or in the lower third of the superior vena cava at the cavoatrial junction. European guidelines recommend tip location in the right atria. Most literature cites termination at the cavoatrial junction as optimal placement (Association for Vascular Access, 1998; Johnston, Bishop, Martin, See, & Streater, 2013; Moureau et al., 2013; Oliver & Jones, 2014; Perin & Scarpa, 2015; Pittiruti, Hamilton, Biffi, MacFie, & Pertkiewicz, 2009).

Figure 5-2. Venous Anatomy

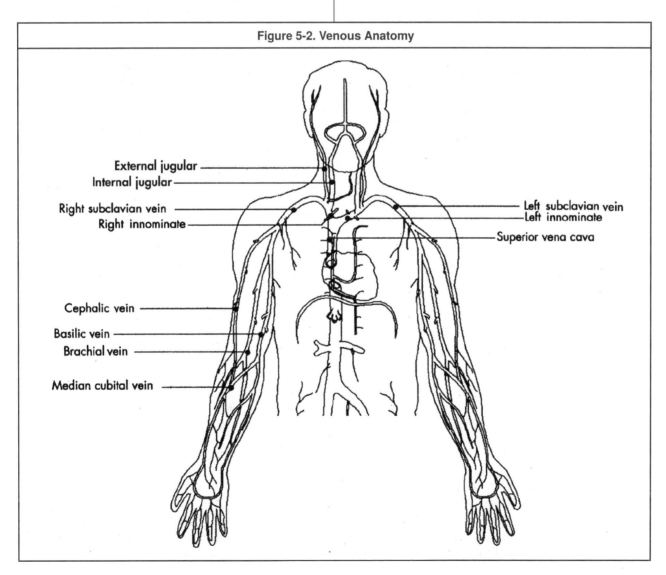

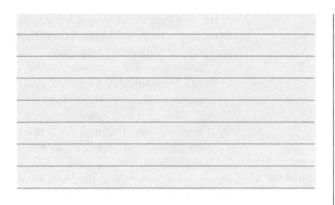

G. Guidance systems are available to identify the placement of PICCs.
   1. A Doppler method is used with internal physiologic parameters to accurately guide PICCs into the superior vena cava.
   2. Some PICCs have guidance systems that detect slight magnetic fields generated by the preloaded stylet to guide the catheter into position. Audible or visual signals indicate the location of tip position.
H. Insertion procedure (Baskin et al., 2014; Hagle & Cook, 2014; Infusion Nurses Society, 2013, 2016)
   1. Choose appropriate PICC size (diameter) and number of lumens, as indicated.
   2. Explain the insertion procedure to the patient and answer any questions the patient or significant others may have. Ensure that informed consent is obtained.
   3. Gather all necessary supplies, including any IV administration sets and medications or IV fluids to be used.
   4. Wash hands.
   5. Examine the patient's arms and select the best vein for cannulation.
      a) Avoid veins that are sclerotic on inspection and palpation.
      b) Select the patient's nondominant arm, if possible. If the patient has undergone axillary dissection, use the contralateral arm.
      c) Avoid extremities that may have compromised circulation, such as those with the presence of lymphedema or venous congestion secondary to superior vena cava syndrome.
      d) The basilic vein is the best choice, as it is the straightest and has the most direct route to the central venous system (Bourgeois et al., 2011; Hagle & Cook, 2014).
      e) The cephalic vein is the secondary choice because its abrupt angle that

joins to the axillary vein makes advancement of the line more difficult.
      f) Adult considerations: The preferred vein choices include cephalic, accessory cephalic, basilic, and median cubital.
      g) Geriatric considerations: Consider that fragile skin and veins can tear easily; use tourniquet with caution.
      h) Pediatric considerations
         (1) Three months of age: Superficial temporal, posterior auricular, saphenous, or median cubital veins are preferred.
         (2) Four months of age until ambulatory: Saphenous, cephalic, basilic, or median cubital veins are preferred.
         (3) Ambulatory child: Basilic, cephalic, brachial, or median cubital veins are preferred.
   6. Use local anesthetic with order (Bourgeois et al., 2011) (see Appendix 7).
   7. Use a measuring tape to determine appropriate catheter length.
      a) Measure from the point of venipuncture, over the course of the selected venous pathway, across the shoulder to the right side of the sternal notch, and down to the third intercostal space.
      b) The tip of the catheter should rest in the cavoatrial junction (see Figure 5-3).
      c) Add 2.5 cm (1 inch) onto this measurement to account for the length of the catheter outside of the insertion site (Sharp et al., 2013).
   8. Use maximum sterile barrier precautions, including mask, sterile gown, gloves, and drapes. Open the PICC tray and add additional supplies. The general insertion procedure may vary according to the type of PICC being used and institutional policy. Ensure familiarity and skill with the product selected and follow the manufacturer's directions (Bourgeois et al., 2011; O'Grady et al., 2011).
   9. Position the patient's arm at a 45°–90° angle from the body, below heart level, to aid in vein engorgement.
   10. Place a sterile drape under the patient's arm.
   11. Cleanse the area and allow to air-dry before initiating cannulation. Do not fan the area to facilitate drying (see Appendix 2).
   12. Fill two syringes with 0.9% normal saline (NS). Use one syringe to prime extension tubing, which may be needed during the procedure.

Figure 5-3. Peripherally Inserted Central Catheter Placement

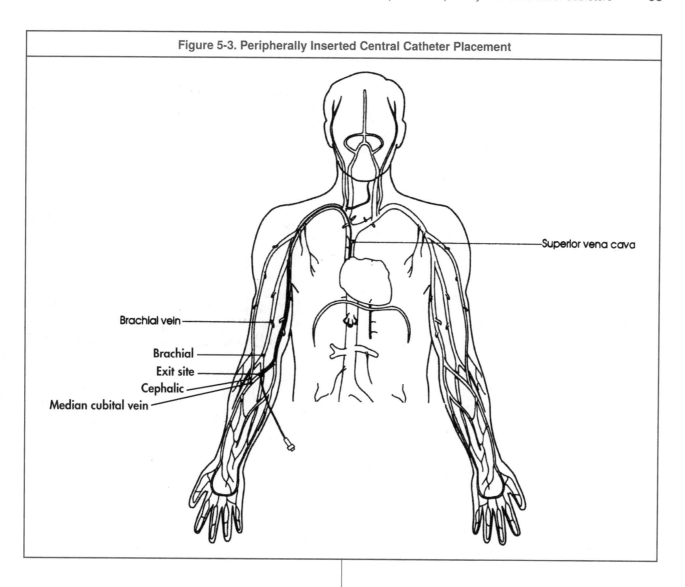

13. Place fenestrated (opened-center) sterile drape over the arm, leaving the insertion site exposed.
14. Prepare the catheter.
    a) Using sterile measuring tape, measure the length of catheter needed based on previous assessment.
    b) Pull the guidewire back half an inch from this distance.
    c) No definitive recommendation can be made regarding the catheter trim procedure. Trim the catheter with sterile scissors according to the manufacturer's recommendation.
       (1) Some PICC manufacturers do not recommend trimming the catheter. Others recommend trimming at a 45° or 90° angle.
       (2) Valved PICCs are trimmed proximally and not at the distal tip.

(3) Altering the PICC by cutting or trimming the tip prior to insertion may increase the occurrence of deep vein thrombosis (Steele & Norris, 2014).
(4) Apply a tourniquet approximately four inches above selected site. Check distal pulse to ensure that arterial circulation has not been compromised. Change sterile gloves.
(5) While stabilizing the vein, perform venipuncture and observe blood return.
(6) Release the tourniquet and continue to advance the catheter.
(7) Attach prefilled syringe, and flush with NS. Ensure adequate blood return. Primed exten-

sion tubing may be attached at this time.

(8) After securing the catheter hub with a securement device, flush with heparin solution.

(9) Place an occlusive dressing over the insertion site and external part of the catheter up to the hub. Change the dressing 24 hours after initial insertion to a transparent occlusive dressing (see Appendix 5).

(10) Check catheter placement.

(a) If catheter is placed under ultrasound guidance, placement has been confirmed after insertion. A follow-up chest x-ray is not necessary.

(b) Tip placement must be confirmed prior to use. Some institutions may require that the guidewire be left in place to aid in PICC line verification during radiographic study because the small size of PICCs makes radiographic visualization challenging; this can be facilitated with the guidewire in place. Extreme caution should be used during the radiographic study to prevent catheter puncture. Guidewires should not be left in place for long periods of time.

(11) Document the number of attempts, location, type and gauge of catheter, dressing type, securement method, and the patient's response.

VII. Insertion complications (see Table 9-1 in Chapter 9)

VIII. Unique maintenance and care (see Appendices 2, 4, 5, and 9): No definitive recommendations can be made for flushing solution, volume, and frequency; frequency of dressing and needleless connector changes; or blood sampling technique (see Figure 5-4).

A. Dressing changes

1. Change initial dressing 24 hours after insertion.

2. Remove the dressing over exit site toward the upper extremity to prevent catheter dislodgment.

3. Change securement devices at the time of dressing changes.

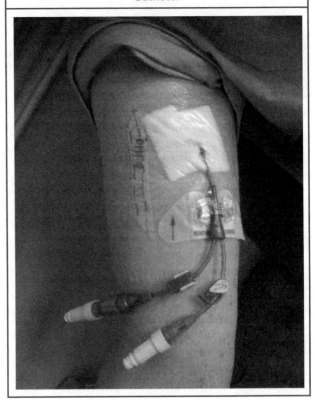

Figure 5-4. Peripherally Inserted Central Venous Catheter

B. Change needleless connectors with each use, if damaged, or if contaminated with blood.

C. Flushing: Flush with NS 5–10 ml after each use. Use 3 ml of 10–100 IU/ml heparin daily, every other day, or three times weekly, per lumen. Use 5–10 ml NS flush with valved PICCs daily, every other day, or three times weekly, per lumen.

D. Blood sampling: Smaller gauge PICCs may not yield blood return. A recent study revealed that vancomycin and tobramycin antibiotic levels can be drawn from PICCs in children with accurate results compared with peripheral catheters. A 3–5 ml discard was used, the blood sample was obtained, and the catheter was flushed with NS then flushed with heparin (Green et al., 2015).

IX. Removal technique (Costa, Dorea, Kimura, Yamamoto, & Damiani, 2014; Hagle & Cook, 2014; Park & Kim, 2015; Wojnar & Beaman, 2013)

A. Indications (Chopra et al., 2015)

1. Completion of therapy

2. Infection not responsive to treatment

3. Radiologically confirmed thrombosis not responsive to fibrinolytic therapy

4. Catheter fracture

5. Phlebitis not responsive to treatment

B. Prior to removal, verify scope of practice with the individual state board of nursing and institutional guidelines.

1. Verify order for removal of catheter.
2. Gather materials needed, including measuring tape, gauze, and occlusive dressing.
3. Wash hands and put on gloves.
4. Remove existing dressing. Remove contaminated gloves and put on a new pair.
5. Grasp PICC at the insertion site and slowly pull outward about one inch, pulling parallel to the skin.
6. Release it and grasp again at insertion site, continuing to pull the PICC out in short increments.
7. When the PICC is completely removed, place gauze over the site and apply light pressure until bleeding stops, then apply occlusive dressing. Remove the dressing in 24 hours and observe site. Apply new dressing, if needed.
8. Observe catheter tip for integrity, and measure length and compare it to the length documented at insertion. If the catheter is not intact, notify the provider. If the PICC is removed for infection, send the tip for culture, if ordered.
9. Removal complications
   a) Venospasm
      (1) Stop the procedure if resistance is felt. Reposition the patient's arm and attempt again.
      (2) If resistance continues, apply warm compress to the upper arm for 15–20 minutes and reattempt gentle removal.
      (3) If resistance persists and the catheter has been removed far enough to do so, apply a tourniquet above the proximal end of the catheter and reattempt removal. This causes internal pressure that may release the venospasm and allow the catheter to be removed.
      (4) If resistance persists, apply a gauze and tape dressing to the insertion site for 12–24 hours, then reattempt removal.
   b) Thrombosis
      (1) Thrombosis in the lumen can cause the catheter to adhere to the vessel wall during removal.
      (2) If the catheter is difficult to remove, stop the procedure.
      (3) Use interventions recommended for venospasm.
      (4) If these attempts fail, notify the provider for possible radiologic studies to rule out thrombosis.
   c) Catheter fracture
      (1) Damage can occur prior to removal or if excessive force is applied during the removal process.
      (2) If fracture occurs during removal but sufficient catheter length distal to insertion site exists, clamp the catheter and continue removal.
      (3) If fracture occurs at the insertion site, clamp the catheter and apply a tourniquet around the upper arm to prevent migration of the fragment. The tourniquet should not impede the arterial flow; check radial pulse.
      (4) Notify the provider immediately.
      (5) If complete fracture occurs within the vein proximal to the insertion site, immediately apply the tourniquet at the highest point possible on the arm; risk of fragment embolus is present.
      (6) Place the patient in the Trendelenburg position; contact the provider immediately. Closely monitor the patient for shortness of breath, tachycardia, confusion, pallor, or hypotension. Prepare the patient for removal by an interventional radiologist, thoracic surgeon, or vascular surgeon.

X. Complications (see Chapter 9)
XI. Practicum on long-term VAD insertion and care (see Appendix 9)
XII. Education and documentation

    A. Patient education unique to PICCs (Park & Kim, 2015)
        1. Inform the patient that a central VAD has been inserted and describe any features (e.g., power-injectable PICC, valved).
        2. Instruct the patient on the use of an ice pack for comfort if the PICC insertion site is tender.
        3. Instruct the patient to carry a PICC identification card.
        4. Instruct the patient to avoid allowing peripheral blood sampling or blood pressure monitoring in the arm where the PICC is placed.
    B. Documentation (see Chapter 17)
XIII. Infusion teams (see Figure 2-5 in Chapter 2)

References

Association for Vascular Access. (1998). NAVAN position statement on terminal tip placement. *Journal of Vascular Access Devices, 3,* 8–10.

Baskin, K.M., Hunnicutt, C., Beck, M.E., Cohen, E.D., Crowley, J.J., & Fitz, C.R. (2014). Long-term central venous access in pediatric patients at high risk: Conventional versus antibiotic-impregnated catheters. *Journal of Vascular and Interventional Radiology, 25,* 411–418. doi:10.1016/j.jvir.2013.11.024

Bortolussi, R., Zotti, P., Conte, M., Marson, R., Polesel, J., Colussi, A., … Spazzapan, S. (2015). Quality of life, pain perception, and distress correlated to ultrasound-guided peripherally inserted central venous catheters in palliative care patients in a home or hospice setting. *Journal of Pain and Symptom Management, 50,* 118–123. doi:10.1016/j.jpainsymman.2015.02.027

Boullata, J.I., Gilbert, K., Sacks, G., Labossiere, R.J., Crill, C., Goday, P., … American Society for Parenteral and Enteral Nutrition. (2014). A.S.P.E.N. clinical guidelines: Parenteral nutrition ordering, order review, compounding, labeling, and dispensing. *Journal of Parenteral and Enteral Nutrition, 38,* 334–377. doi:10.1177/0148607114521833

Bourgeois, F.C., Lamagna, P., & Chiang, V.W. (2011). Peripherally inserted central catheters. *Pediatric Emergency Care, 27,* 556–561. doi:10.1097/PEC.0b013e31821dc9b6

Bowe-Geddes, L.A., & Nichols, H.A. (2005). An overview of peripherally inserted central catheters. *Topics in Advanced Practice Nursing eJournal, 5*(3). Retrieved from http://www.medscape.com/viewarticle/508939

Bowen, M.E., Mone, M.C., Nelson, E.W., & Scaife, C.L. (2014). Image-guided placement of long-term central venous catheters reduces complications and cost. *American Journal of Surgery, 208,* 937–941. doi:10.1016/j.amjsurg.2014.08.005

Braswell, L.E. (2011). Peripherally inserted central catheter placement in infants and children. *Techniques in Vascular and Interventional Radiology, 14,* 204–211. doi:10.1053/j.tvir.2011.05.004

Chopra, V., Flanders, S.A., Saint, S., Woller, S.C., O'Grady, N.P., Safdar, N., … Bernstein, S.J. (2015). The Michigan Appropriateness Guide for Intravenous Catheters (MAGIC): Results from a multispecialty panel using the RAND/UCLA Appropriateness Method. *Annals of Internal Medicine, 163*(Suppl. 6), S1–S40. doi:10.7326/M15-0744

Costa, P., Dorea, E.P., Kimura, A.F., Yamamoto, L.Y., & Damiani, L.P. (2014). Incidence of nonelective removal of single-lumen silicone and dual-lumen polyurethane percutaneously inserted central catheters in neonates. *Journal of the Association for Vascular Access, 19,* 35–41. doi:10.1016/j.java.2013.11.001

Cotogni, P., & Pittiruti, M. (2014). Focus on peripherally inserted central catheters in critically ill patients. *World Journal of Critical Care Medicine, 3,* 80–94. doi:10.5492/wjccm.v3.i4.80

Gabriel, J. (2013). Long-term central venous access device selection. *Nursing Times, 109*(39), 12–15.

Green, M.E., Sullivan, K.J., Wells, S., Board, R., Feldman, H.A., & McCabe, M. (2015). A comparison of antibiotic serum concentrations drawn simultaneously from peripherally inserted central catheters and peripheral veins in children with respiratory infection. *Journal of Pediatric Nursing, 30,* 868–876. doi:10.1016/j.pedn.2015.07.011

Hagle, M.E., & Cook, A.M. (2014). Central venous access. In S.M. Weinstein & M.E. Hagle (Eds.), *Plumer's principles and practice of infusion therapy* (9th ed., pp. 335–390). Philadelphia, PA: Wolters Kluwer Health/Lippincott Williams & Wilkins.

Infusion Nurses Society. (2013). *Policies and procedures for infusion nursing of the older adult.* Norwood, MA: Author.

Infusion Nurses Society. (2016). *Infusion therapy standards of practice.* Norwood, MA: Author.

Johansson, E., Hammarskjöld, F., Lundberg, D., & Arnlind, M.H. (2013). Advantages and disadvantages of peripherally inserted central venous catheters (PICC) compared to other central venous lines: A systematic review of the literature. *Acta Oncologica, 52,* 886–892. doi:10.3109/0284186X.2013.773072

Johnston, A.J., Bishop, S.M., Martin, L., See, T.C., & Streater, C.T. (2013). Defining peripherally inserted central catheter tip position and an evaluation of insertions in one unit. *Anaesthesia, 68,* 484–491. doi:10.1111/anae.12188

Katheria, A.C., Fleming, S.E., & Kim, J.H. (2013). A randomized controlled trial of ultrasound-guided peripherally inserted central catheters compared with standard radiograph in neonates. *Journal of Perinatology, 33,* 791–794.

Lamperti, M., Bodenham, A.R., Pittiruti, M., Blaivas, M., Augoustides, J.G., Elbarbary, M., … Verghese, S.T. (2012). International evidence-based recommendations on ultrasound-guided vascular access. *Intensive Care Medicine, 38,* 1105–1117. doi:10.1007/s00134-012-2597-x

Moureau, N., Lamperti, M., Kelly, L.J., Dawson, R., Elbarbary, M., van Baxtel, A.J., & Pittiruti, M. (2013). Evidence-based consensus on the insertion of central venous access devices: Definition of minimal requirements for training. *British Journal of Anaesthesia, 110,* 347–356. doi:10.1093/bja/aes499

O'Grady, N.P., Alexander, M., Burns, L.A., Dellinger, E.P., Garland, J., Heard, S.O., … Healthcare Infection Control Practices Advisory Committee. (2011). Guidelines for the prevention of intravascular catheter-related infections. *Clinical Infectious Diseases, 52,* E162–E193. doi:10.1093/cid/cir257

Oliver, G., & Jones, M. (2014). ECG or x-ray as the "gold standard" for establishing PICC-tip location? *British Journal of Nursing, 23*(Suppl. 19), S10–S16. doi:10.12968/bjon.2014.23(Suppl. 19).S10

Park, J.Y., & Kim, H.L. (2015). A comprehensive review of clinical nurse specialist-led peripherally inserted central catheter placement in Korea: 4,101 cases in a tertiary hospital. *Journal of Infusion Nursing, 38,* 122–128. doi:10.1097/NAN.0000000000000093

Perin, G., & Scarpa, M.-G. (2015). Defining central venous line position in children: Tips for the tip. *Journal of Vascular Access, 16,* 77–86. doi:10.5301/jva.5000285

Pittiruti, M., Emoli, A., Porta, P., Marche, B., DeAngelis, R., & Scoppettuolo, G. (2014). A prospective, randomized comparison of three different types of valved and non-valved peripherally inserted central catheters. *Journal of Vascular Access, 15,* 519–523. doi:10.5301/jva.5000280

Pittiruti, M., Hamilton, H., Biffi, R., MacFie, J., & Pertkiewicz, M. (2009). ESPEN Guidelines on parenteral nutrition: Central venous catheters (access, care, diagnosis and therapy of complications). *Clinical Nutrition, 28,* 365–377. doi:10.1016/j.clnu.2009.03.015

Rossetti, F., Pittiruti, M., Lamperti, M., Graziano, U., Celentano, D., & Capozzoli, G. (2015). The intracavitary ECG method for positioning the tip of central venous access devices in pediatric patients: Results of an Italian multicenter study. *Journal of Vascular Access, 16,* 137–143. doi:10.5301/jva.5000281

Sainathan, S., Hempstead, M., & Andaz, S. (2014). A single institution experience of seven hundred consecutively placed peripherally inserted central venous catheters. *Journal of Vascular Access, 15,* 498–502. doi:10.5301/jva.5000248

Sekold, T.L., Walker, S., & Dwyer, T. (2015). A comparison of silicone and polyurethane PICC lines and postinsertion complication rates: A systematic review. *Journal of Vascular Access, 16,* 167–177. doi:10.5301/jva.5000330

Sharp, R., Gordon, A., Mikocka-Walus, A., Childs, J., Grech, C., Cummings, M., & Esterman, A. (2013). Vein measurement by peripherally inserted central catheter nurses using ultrasound: A reliability study. *Journal of the Association for Vascular Access, 18,* 234–238. doi:10.1016/j.java.2013.08.001

Steele, D., & Norris, C.M. (2014). Cutting peripherally inserted central catheters may lead to increased rates of catheter-related deep vein thrombosis. *Journal of Infusion Nursing, 37,* 466–472. doi:10.1097/NAN.0000000000000073

Teichgräber, U.K.M., Kausche, S., Nagel, S.N., & Gebauer, B. (2011). Outcome analysis in 3,160 implantations of radiologically guided placements of totally implantable central venous port systems. *European Radiology, 21,* 1224–1232. doi:10.1007/s00330-010-2045-7

Wang, G., Guo, L., Jiang, B., Huang, M., Zhang, J., & Qin, Y. (2015). Factors influencing intracavitary electrocardiographic P-wave changes during central venous catheter placement. *PLOS ONE, 10,* e0124846. doi:10.1371/journal.pone.0124846

Westergaard, B., Classen, V., & Walther-Larsen, S. (2013). Peripherally inserted central catheters in infants and children: Indications, techniques, complications and clinical recommendations. *Acta Anaesthesiologica Scandinavica, 57,* 278–287. doi:10.1111/aas.12024

Wojnar, D.G., & Beaman, M.L. (2013). Peripherally inserted central catheter: Compliance with evidence-based indications for insertion in an inpatient setting. *Journal of Infusion Nursing, 36,* 291–296. doi:10.1097/NAN.0b013e318297c1a8

Chapter 6

Tunneled Central Venous Catheters

Heather Thompson Mackey, RN, MSN, ANP-BC, AOCN®

I. History (Heberlein, 2011; Weinstein, 2014)
  A. The first tunneled venous access device (VAD), the Broviac® catheter, was introduced in 1973 for administration of long-term hyperalimentation in children. It was inserted into the subclavian vein and tunneled under the subcutaneous (SC) tissue to increase the longevity of the catheter and to decrease infection.
  B. A larger bore catheter, the Hickman® catheter, was introduced in 1976 to expand the applications and patient populations for tunneled catheters.
II. Device characteristics (Hagle & Cook, 2014; Heberlein, 2011; O'Grady et al., 2011)
  A. Flexible catheter inserted into central vein with the tip lying in the superior vena cava. External portion pulled (or tunneled) through the SC skin to exit distally from the insertion site.
  B. Used for longer-term therapy (typically greater than six months)
  C. Typically has lower rates of infection when compared to nontunneled VADs
III. Device features (Hagle & Cook, 2014; Infusion Nurses Society [INS], 2016; O'Grady et al., 2011; Schiffer et al., 2013) (see Figures 6-1 and 6-2)
  A. Lengths range from 47–97 cm.
  B. Sizes range from 2.7–12.5 Fr.
  C. Internal diameters range from 0.5–1.6 mm.
  D. Available in single-, double-, and triple-lumen designs
  E. Prime volume of 0.6–1.8 ml, allowing variable flow rates, including high flow (in excess of 300 ml/min) for hemodialysis
  F. Designed with polyurethane, silicone, or a combination of the two materials
  G. Power-injectable design available
  H. Designed with cuffs to aid in securing the device and reducing risk of infection
    1. Positioned in the SC tunnel 1–2 inches from the exit site. Cuff becomes enmeshed with fibrous SC tissue within several weeks after insertion; SC tissue aids in securing the catheter. Cuff can minimize but cannot guarantee that dislodgment is avoided.
    2. The cuff potentially minimizes the risk of ascending infection from the exit site into the tunnel.
    3. An antimicrobial cuff design is available, which releases an antimicrobial agent for approximately four to six weeks or until the catheter is embedded into tissue.
  I. Heparin coating available
    1. Promotes biocompatibility within the vein, thereby reducing fibrin formation
    2. Heparin is intended to decrease fibrin buildup and decrease occurrence of organisms adhering to fibrin, resulting in an infection.
    3. May cause heparin-induced thrombocytopenia, increased risk of bleeding, or allergic reactions
    4. Although more research on heparin coating is needed, limited studies show that heparinization reduces the frequency of catheter-related bloodstream infections at a relatively low cost over a short time period (Abdelkefi et al., 2007; Shah & Shah, 2014).

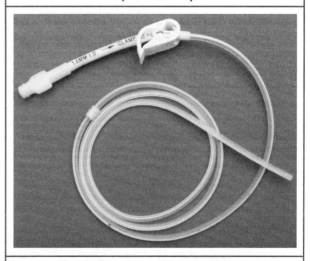

Figure 6-1. Single-Lumen Tunneled Catheter With Open Distal Tip

Note. Copyright 2015 by Oncology Nursing Society. All rights reserved.

Figure 6-2. Triple-Lumen Tunneled Catheter With Closed Distal Tip

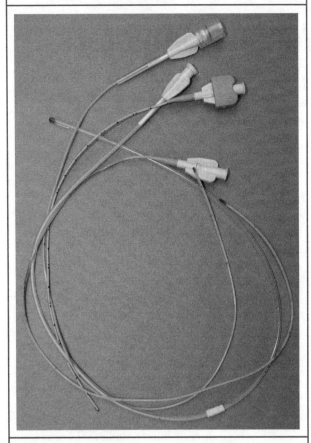

J. Distinguished by type of distal tips
1. Open-ended distal tip catheters: Most common
   a) Catheters require clamping when not in use with release of clamp ("unclamping") prior to infusion and aspiration.
   b) Catheters may have clamps located directly on fortified areas.
2. Closed-ended distal tip catheters
   a) Rounded, closed-tip catheters with an internal three-way, pressure-sensitive valve that opens inwardly with aspiration and outwardly with flushing or infusion. The valve remains closed when not in use.
   b) Does not require clamping or unclamping
3. Available with three-way, pressure-activated safety valves (PASVs) located in the catheter hub
   a) Designed to permit fluid infusion and reduce the risk of blood backflow into the catheter lumen during increases in

central venous pressure that can occur with exercise or involuntary responses, such as coughing
   b) The three-way safety valve resists fluid or blood backflow, reducing need for clamps and potentially reducing the risk of occlusion and infection.
   c) Pressure activated and direction specific, generally eliminating the need for heparin flush. It opens with minimal positive pressure during infusion and requires up to four times as much negative pressure for aspiration.
   K. Radiopaque markings along the catheter for identification during radiographic imaging
IV. Device advantages and disadvantages (see Figure 6-3)
V. Patient selection criteria (Albuquerque, 2015; Keeler, 2014; Lopez et al., 2014; Newman et al., 2012; O'Grady et al., 2011; Schiffer et al., 2013)
   A. Patient's age, in general, does not restrict use of tunneled central VAD.
   B. Indications for tunneled VAD include the following:

Figure 6-3. Advantages and Disadvantages of Tunneled Central Venous Access Devices

Advantages	Disadvantages
• Can be used immediately after placement once radiographic confirmation is made • Preserve peripheral veins • Provide a means for rapid hemodilution of infused solutions • Provide a reliable source of IV access • Designed for long-term IV therapy for frequent venous access and are functional for years • Available in single-, double-, and triple-lumen designs • Provide preattached clamps, except for valved catheters • Decrease risk of microorganisms entering the venous system through tunneling because of anatomic distance between insertion and exit sites • Repair kits for external segments available for tunneled catheters • Come in a variety of sizes to accommodate pediatric and adult patients • Available in power-injectable design	• Require routine exit-site care • Require routine flushing of catheter lumens • Pose risk of complications, such as catheter-related infection and thrombosis • Cost of maintenance supplies • Body image changes • Surgical procedure (insertion)

1. Any patient population that requires long-term IV access, such as hematopoietic stem cell transplant recipients, those with hematologic disease, or those with malignant diseases requiring IV chemotherapy that will result in a prolonged nadir of blood counts
2. Drugs that cannot be given orally because the molecules are too large to be absorbed, or because they are destroyed by digestion
3. Administration of solutions that are irritants, vesicants, solutions with a pH less than 5 or greater than 9, glucose greater than 10%, protein greater than 5%, or osmolarity greater than 900 mOsm/L (Boullata et al., 2014; Chopra et al., 2015; Cotogni & Pittiruti, 2014)

C. Contraindications (Heberlein, 2011; Kugler et al., 2015)
1. Systemic infection or sepsis
2. Infection overlying the insertion site; presence of coagulopathies and platelet defects. Coagulopathies and thrombocytopenia should be corrected, when possible, prior to catheter insertion.

VI. Insertion techniques (Albuquerque, 2015; Bowen, Mone, Nelson, & Scaife, 2014; Dierickx & Macken, 2015; Hagle & Cook, 2014; Heberlein, 2011; Institute for Healthcare Improvement, n.d.; Lewis, Crapo, & Williams, 2013; Newman et al., 2012; O'Grady et al., 2011)
A. Inserted by surgeon or interventional radiologist using ultrasound or fluoroscopy
B. Prior to placement, ensure that contraindications do not exist, informed consent is obtained, pre-placement assessment has been completed, laboratory studies are verified, and a medication/chemotherapy order is reviewed (see Appendix 4).
C. Vein selection
1. Selected according to patient's anatomic structure, type and purpose of catheter, and vessel used
2. No definitive recommendation can be made regarding a preferred vein (except femoral vein) for insertion of tunneled VADs to minimize infection risk (O'Grady et al., 2011).
3. Most common veins used for insertion (see Figure 6-4)
   a) Internal jugular vein: The right internal jugular is preferred due to ease of insertion into the junction of the superior vena cava and right atrium.
   b) Subclavian vein
   c) Femoral vein: Avoid in adult patients (O'Grady et al., 2011) and in patients with cancer (Schiffer et al., 2013).
D. Procedure description

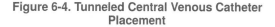

Figure 6-4. Tunneled Central Venous Catheter Placement

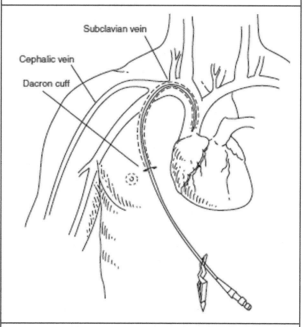

Note. From "Chemotherapy: Principles of Administration" (p. 450), by G.M. Wilkes in C.H. Yarbro, D. Wujcik, and B.H. Gobel (Eds.), *Cancer Nursing: Principles and Practice* (8th ed.), 2018, Burlington, MA: Jones & Bartlett Learning. Copyright 2018 by Jones & Bartlett Learning. Reprinted with permission.

1. Depending on the type of catheter and indication for placement, the insertion site will vary.
   a) Most commonly inserted via the percutaneous insertion technique using the internal jugular or subclavian vein
      (1) Once vein is cannulated, the guidewire is advanced into the vein.
      (2) A pull-apart sheath introducer is threaded over the guidewire and the guidewire is removed. The catheter is advanced through the introducer into the vein.
      (3) The catheter is tunneled through the SC tissue, with the tunnel created from the vein entry site to the exit site.
      (4) The catheter is pulled from the exit site through the tunnel to the vein entry site and trimmed via an anterograde technique. For a valved or closed distal tip catheter, the retrograde technique is used, where the catheter is pulled from the vein entry site to the exit site and trimmed.

(5) The exit site depends on male or female anatomy; however, usually it is above the nipple line midway between the sternum and clavicle.
  b) Catheters also can be inserted using the cut-down insertion method.
    (1) Greatly reduces risk of hemothorax or pneumothorax
    (2) Is more time consuming and difficult to perform than other methods
    (3) Requires more manipulation of skin and SC tissue, thereby increasing infection rate
    (4) Veins used: Axillary, external jugular, internal jugular, cephalic, and subclavian
  2. Catheter tip must be confirmed prior to use. The catheter tip is just above or in the lower third of the superior vena cava at the cavoatrial junction. A retrospective analysis concluded that tunneled catheters placed with ultrasound or fluoroscopy do not require postoperative chest x-ray to confirm placement (Bowen et al., 2014).
  3. Secure catheter with sutures.
    a) Exit-site sutures remain in place until healing occurs, which can range from 10 days to 6 weeks (or longer if immunosuppression is present).
    b) Sutures are removed after healing in order to prevent irritation and infection at the exit site.
E. Postprocedure care
  1. Label dressing with time, date of dressing placement, and initials.
  2. Monitor the patient's vital signs every 15 minutes for the first hour and then PRN based on organizational policy and procedure. Monitor for bleeding at insertion and exit site.
  3. Document the catheter type and size, date, time, provider name, and the patient's response in the medical record.
F. Insertion complications: Pneumothorax, arterial injury, catheter malposition, bleeding, arrhythmia, and air embolism (Bowen et al., 2014) (see Chapter 9)
VII. Unique maintenance and care: No definitive recommendations can be made for flushing solution, volume, and frequency; frequency of dressing and needleless connector changes; or blood sampling technique (Hagle & Cook, 2014; INS, 2016; Keeler, 2014; O'Grady et al., 2011; Schiffer et al., 2013) (see Appendices 4 and 5 and Figure 6-5).

A. General care
  1. Clamps are used when accessing or deaccessing open-ended distal tip tunneled VADs to prevent air embolism or blood backflow.
    a) Never use a hemostat or sharp-edged clamp that could damage or cut the catheter. Keep toothless plastic clamps available for emergency use. Do not use scissors near the catheters.
    b) If clamping is not possible, have the patient perform the Valsalva maneuver (forcefully exhale and hold breath) whenever the catheter is open to air.
  2. Valved, closed-ended distal tip catheters or catheters with PASV do not require clamping if the valve is functioning properly. Clamping will damage the catheter.
  3. Catheter material weakens if exposed to alcohol and iodine-containing products with long-term use.
  4. Instruct the patient to completely cover the exit site and external catheter with a waterproof covering while swimming or showering. Some providers prefer that patients

Figure 6-5. Tunneled Central Venous Catheter

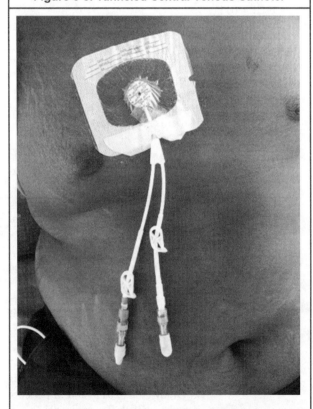

Note. Image courtesy of Dawn Camp-Sorrell. Used with permission.

with external catheters refrain from swimming entirely. Little evidence is available regarding the increased risk of infection when swimming (Miller et al., 2014).

B. Dressing changes
  1. Change dressing 24 hours after insertion. Change dressing if wet, soiled, contaminated, or nonocclusive.
  2. Use an aseptic no-touch technique.
  3. No definitive recommendation can be made regarding the need for a dressing over well-healed exit sites of long-term, tunneled VADs (O'Grady et al., 2011).

C. Flushing
  1. Solution
    a) Open-ended distal tip catheters: Use heparin 10–100 IU/ml; 3 ml/day or every other day; or 5 ml three times a week or 5 ml weekly, per lumen.
    b) Closed-ended distal tip tunneled VAD: Use 5–10 ml 0.9% normal saline after each use; 5 ml daily, every other day, or three times weekly.
  2. Technique
    a) Flush vigorously using a pulsatile (push-pause motion) technique, maintaining pressure at the end of the flush to prevent backflow.
    b) Maintain a positive pressure technique while flushing a tunneled central VAD by clamping the extension tubing while still flushing the line. This will help prevent the development of fibrin sheath, leading to withdrawal or infusion occlusions and contributing to the development of venous thrombosis.
    c) Flush tunneled central VADs that do not have a clamp with positive pressure by disconnecting the syringe from the needleless connector while continuing to push fluid.

D. Blood sampling
  1. Stop the infusion and clamp all lumens not being used for blood withdrawal on open-ended distal tip tunneled central VADs.
  2. Discard 3–5 ml of blood, obtain specimen, and flush vigorously using pulsating (push-pause motion) technique with 10–20 ml of normal saline after blood withdrawal.
  3. If using a vacutainer with a closed-ended distal tip or PASV catheter, the procedure may not yield a blood sample because the pressure may collapse the catheter.

E. Needleless connector: Change with each use, every week if not in use, or if damaged or contaminated with residual blood.

VIII. Removal technique (Boddi et al., 2015; INS, 2016; Keeler, 2014; O'Grady et al., 2011; Schiffer et al., 2013)
  A. Prior to removal, verify scope of practice with the individual state board of nursing and institutional guidelines.
  B. Indications
    1. Remove when no longer required for therapy.
    2. Remove if systemic infection does not respond to antibiotics, if tunnel becomes infected, or if thrombosis is occluding or is a source of infection.
  C. Procedure
    1. Verify order for removal and indication.
    2. Note length of catheter on insertion.
    3. Gather required equipment.
    4. Explain procedure to the patient.
    5. Wash hands.
    6. Place the patient in a reclining position.
    7. Inspect the general condition of the catheter and tunneled pathway.
    8. Discontinue all infusions into the device.
    9. Put on gloves, remove dressing, and observe site for edema, erythema, or other problems.
    10. Change gloves and remove sutures as needed.
    11. Have the patient perform the Valsalva maneuver.
    12. Grasp the hub of device and gently and steadily retract the catheter until completely removed.
    13. Send the catheter tip for culture with provider order if infection is suspected.
    14. Apply constant, firm pressure to exit site until bleeding stops (longer in patients with coagulopathies, thrombocytopenia, or those on anticoagulant therapy). Apply occlusive dressing. Change dressing after 24 hours and assess site.
    15. Instruct the patient or caregiver to report any discomfort or signs of bleeding, bruising, erythema, edema, and drainage.
    16. Inspect the device for defects. Report any defects to the manufacturer and regulatory agencies. Examine the distal tip for signs of jagged, uneven edges suggestive of breakage.
    17. Discard used supplies and remove gloves.
    18. Wash hands.
    19. Document observations and actions in the patient's medical record.
    20. Contact the provider immediately if difficulty occurs in retrieving the cuff or removing the catheter.

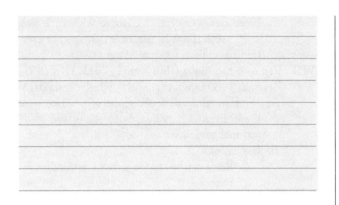

21. If tunnel infection is suspected, a cut-down procedure may be performed to remove the cuff, based on provider preference.

22. If questions exist concerning incomplete device removal, call the provider immediately. A chest x-ray or cathetergram is recommended.

IX. Complications (Albuquerque, 2015; Boddi et al., 2015; Heberlein, 2011; Lipitz-Snyderman et al., 2014; Newman et al., 2012) (see Chapter 9)

X. Education and documentation (Heberlein, 2011) (see Chapter 17)

XI. Competency documentation for tunneled VAD care (see Appendix 9)

The author would like to acknowledge Susan A. Ezzone, MS, RN, CNP, AOCNP®, and Misty Lamprecht, MS, RN, CNS, AOCN®, for their contribution to this chapter that remains unchanged from the previous edition of this book.

References

Abdelkefi, A., Achour, W., Ben Othman, T., Ladeb, S., Torjman, L., Lakhal, A., ... Ben Abdeladhim, A. (2007). Use of heparin-coated central venous lines to prevent catheter-related bloodstream infection. *Journal of Supportive Oncology, 5,* 273–278.

Albuquerque, M.P. (2015). The surgery of the long-term central venous accesses in oncology. *Surgical Oncology, 24,* 153–161. doi:10.1016/j.suronc.2015.06.015

Boddi, M., Villa, G., Chiostri, M., De Antoniis, F., DeFanti, I., Spinelli, A., ... Pelagatti, C. (2015). Incidence of ultrasound-detected asymptomatic long-term central vein catheter-related thrombosis and fibrin sheath in cancer patients. *European Journal of Haematology, 95,* 472–479. doi:10.1111/ejh.12519

Boullata, J.I., Gilbert, K., Sacks, G., Labossiere, R.J., Crill, C., Goday, P., ... American Society for Parenteral and Enteral Nutrition. (2014). A.S.P.E.N. clinical guidelines: Parenteral nutrition ordering, order review, compounding, labeling, and dispensing. *Journal of Parenteral and Enteral Nutrition, 38,* 334–377. doi:10.1177/0148607114521833

Bowen, M.E., Mone, M.C., Nelson, E.W., & Scaife, C.L. (2014). Image-guided placement of long-term central venous catheters reduces complications and cost. *American Journal of Surgery, 208,* 937–941. doi:10.1016/j.amjsurg.2014.08.005

Chopra, V., Flanders, S.A., Saint, S., Woller, S.C., O'Grady, N.P., Safdar, N., ... Bernstein, S.J. (2015). The Michigan Appropriateness Guide for Intravenous Catheters (MAGIC): Results from a multispecialty panel using the RAND/UCLA Appropriateness Method. *Annals of Internal Medicine, 163*(Suppl. 6), S1–S40. doi:10.7326/M15-0744

Cotogni, P., & Pittiruti, M. (2014). Focus on peripherally inserted central catheters in critically ill patients. *World Journal of Critical Care Medicine, 3,* 80–94. doi:10.5492/wjccm.v3.i4.80

Dierickx, D., & Macken, E. (2015). The ABC of apheresis. *Acta Clinica Belgica, 70,* 95–99. doi:10.1179/2295333714Y.0000000096

Hagle, M.E., & Cook, A.M. (2014). Central venous access. In S.M. Weinstein & M.E. Hagle (Eds.), *Plumer's principles and practice of infusion therapy* (9th ed., pp. 335–390). Philadelphia, PA: Wolters Kluwer Health/Lippincott Williams & Wilkins.

Heberlein, W. (2011). Principles of tunneled cuffed catheter placement. *Techniques in Vascular and Interventional Radiology, 14,* 192–197. doi:10.1053/j.tvir.2011.05.008

Infusion Nurses Society. (2016). *Infusion therapy standards of practice.* Norwood, MA: Author.

Institute for Healthcare Improvement. (n.d.). Evidence-based care bundles. Retrieved from http://www.ihi.org/Topics/Bundles/Pages/default.aspx

Keeler, M. (2014). Central line practice in Canadian blood and marrow transplant. *Canadian Oncology Nursing Journal, 24,* 67–71. doi:10.5737/1181912x2426771

Kugler, E., Levi, A., Goldberg, E., Zaig, E., Raanani, P., & Paul, M. (2015). The association of central venous catheter placement timing with infection rates in patients with acute leukemia. *Leukemia Research, 39,* 311–313. doi:10.1016/j.leukres.2014.12.017

Lewis, G.C., Crapo, S.A., & Williams, J.G. (2013). Critical skills and procedures in emergency medicine: Vascular access skills and procedures. *Emergency Medicine Clinics of North America, 31,* 59–86. doi:10.1016/j.emc.2012.09.006

Lipitz-Snyderman, A., Sepkowitz, K.A., Elkin, E.B., Pinheiro, L.C., Sima, C.S., Son, C.H., ... Bach, P.B. (2014). Long-term central venous catheter use and risk of infection in older adults with cancer. *Journal of Clinical Oncology, 32,* 2351–2356. doi:10.1200/JCO.2013.53.3018

Lopez, P.-J., Troncoso, B., Grandy, J., Reed, F., Ovalle, A., Celis, S., ... Zubieta, R. (2014). Outcome of tunnelled central venous catheters used for haemodialysis in children weighing less than 15 kg. *Journal of Pediatric Surgery, 49,* 1300–1303. doi:10.1016/j.jpedsurg.2014.02.043

Miller, J., Dalton, M.K., Duggan, C., Lam, S., Iglesias, J., Jaksic, T., & Gura, K.M. (2014). Going with the flow or swimming against the tide: Should children with central venous catheters swim? *Nutrition in Clinical Practice, 29,* 97–109. doi:10.1177/0884533613515931

Newman, N., Issa, A., Greenberg, D., Kapelushnik, J., Cohen, Z., & Leibovitz, E. (2012). Central venous catheter-associated bloodstream infections. *Pediatric Blood and Cancer, 59,* 410–414. doi:10.1002/pbc.24135

O'Grady, N.P., Alexander, M., Burns, L.A., Dellinger, E.P., Garland, J., Heard, S.O., ... Healthcare Infection Control Practices Advisory Committee. (2011). Guidelines for the prevention of intravascular catheter-related infections. *Clinical Infectious Diseases, 52,* E162–E193. doi:10.1093/cid/cir257

Schiffer, C.A., Mangu, P.B., Wade, J.C., Camp-Sorrell, D., Cope, D.G., El-Rayes, B.F., ... Levine, M. (2013). Central venous catheter care for the patient with cancer: American Society of Clinical Oncology clinical practice guideline. *Journal of Clinical Oncology, 31,* 1357–1370. doi:10.1200/JCO.2012.45.5733

Shah, P.S., & Shah, N. (2014). Heparin-bonded catheters for prolonging the patency of central venous catheters in children. *Cochrane Database of Systematic Reviews, 2014*(2). doi:10.1002/14651858.CD005983.pub3

Weinstein, S. (2014). History of infusion therapy. In S.M. Weinstein & M.E. Hagle (Eds.), *Plumer's principles and practice of infusion therapy* (9th ed., pp. 3–12). Philadelphia, PA: Wolters Kluwer Health/Lippincott Williams & Wilkins.

Chapter 7

Implanted Venous Ports

Lisa Schulmeister, RN, MN, ACNS-BC, FAAN

I. History
    A. First introduced in 1982 (Gyves et al., 1982)
    B. Totally implanted venous access device
    C. Intended to reduce the risk of infection, improve quality of life, reduce maintenance care, and provide an alternative to external catheters
    D. Designed for long-term use
II. Device characteristics (Biffi, Toro, Pozzi, & Di Carlo, 2014; Bonciarelli et al., 2011) (see Figures 7-1 and 7-2)
    A. Completely implanted device
    B. Placement locations (O'Grady et al., 2011; Schiffer et al., 2013)
        1. Usually placed in anterior chest wall or peripheral ports placed in upper arm

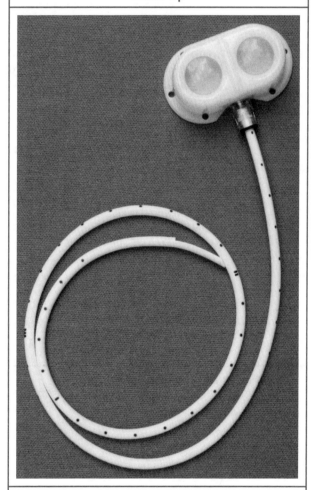

Figure 7-2. Double-Lumen Venous Port With Open Distal Tip

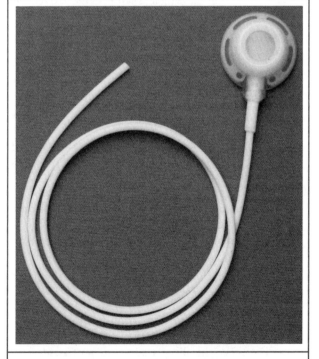

Figure 7-1. Single-Lumen Venous Port With Open Distal Tip

        2. Less commonly placed in abdomen in patients with central vein occlusions, with catheter tip in the inferior vena cava at the level of the diaphragm (Goltz, Janssen, Petritsch, & Kickuth, 2014)
    C. Has evolved over the past three decades (Biffi, Toro, et al., 2014; Zaghal et al., 2012)

1. Smaller and lighter, with additional features
2. Available as valved and open-ended catheters
3. Plastic polymer and titanium designs permit magnetic resonance imaging.
4. Power-injectable ports (also called CT-injectable or power ports) allow injection of contrast media at high infusion pressures (Goltz et al., 2012).

III. Device features (Indrajit et al., 2015; Walser, 2012) (see Figure 7-3)
  A. Portal body
    1. Consists of septum and reservoir within the portal body
    2. Made of plastic polymers, stainless steel, titanium, or a combination of materials
    3. Has several suture holes to secure portal body in the port pocket
    4. Available in full size, intermediate, and low profiles in single or dual chambers to accommodate patient's size
    5. Reservoir volume varies with size of reservoir and usually is 0.4–1.5 ml. (Consult the manufacturer's website for reservoir volumes for specific brands and types of implanted ports.)
    6. Power-injectable portal bodies have different configurations (e.g., palpation bumps, triangular or angled shapes) than round or rectangular nonpower-injectable venous ports to facilitate proper identification. These portal bodies are imprinted or engraved with manufacturer identifiers (Goltz et al., 2012).
    7. A peripheral port also is available for placement distal or proximal to antecubital fossa in single-port designs. The portal body is approximately half the size of a standard port. The peripheral port features a longer catheter (open ended, valve ended, or pressure-activated safety valve [PASV]).
  B. Septum of portal body
    1. Comprised of self-sealing silicone
    2. Must only be accessed using a noncoring needle. Hollow-bore needles will "core" or damage the silicone, resulting in leakage.
    3. Able to withstand hundreds of noncoring needle punctures. Consult the manufacturer's website for data for specific brands and types of implanted portal septum.
    4. PASV design available; the valve is located in the portal body and designed to open for infusion and close after blood sampling or infusion.
  C. Catheter attached to portal body
    1. Available as a preattached catheter or attached during implantation using a locking mechanism (sleeve or collar)
    2. Made of radiopaque silicone or polyurethane to ensure tip placement confirmation with imaging studies
    3. Range in length from 50–90 cm (preinsertion) and in circumference (size) from 4–12 Fr
    4. Typically trimmed upon insertion; priming volume dependent on length
    5. Available in polymer design infused throughout the catheter shaft material and remains present throughout the life of the catheter, providing long-term durability and decreased accumulation of catheter-related thrombus

IV. Device advantages and disadvantages (see Figure 7-4)
V. Patient selection criteria
  A. Any patient population that requires long-term IV access, such as hematopoietic stem cell transplant recipients, those with hematologic disease, or those with malignant diseases requiring IV chemotherapy that will result in a prolonged nadir of blood counts
  B. Drugs that cannot be given orally because the molecules are too large to be absorbed or because they are destroyed by digestion
  C. Administration of solutions that are irritants, vesicants, solutions with a pH less than 5 or greater than 9, glucose greater than 10%, protein greater than 5%, or osmolarity greater than 900 mOsm/L (Boullata et al., 2014; Chopra et al., 2015; Cotogni & Pittiruti, 2014)
  D. Poor peripheral veins
  E. A peripherally placed (arm) port is ideal for patients who are not candidates for chest wall

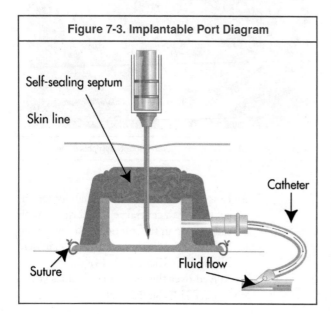

Figure 7-3. Implantable Port Diagram

Figure 7-4. Advantages and Disadvantages of Implanted Venous Ports

Advantages	Disadvantages
• Long-term device • Ideal for intermittent access or continuous IV therapies, including vesicants • Less potential for infection than external catheters • No dressing required when not accessed; ideal for patients with tape sensitivities and active lifestyles and occupations • Require infrequent maintenance when not in use • Can be used to draw blood • Have less effect on body image than external catheters; newer models are lower profile. • The power-injectable model allows the injection of contrast media at high infusion pressures.	• Insertion and removal are performed by a surgeon or interventional radiologist. • Most expensive venous access devices to insert • Must be accessed with a specialized noncoring needle • Catheter can disconnect from port and migrate, causing extravasation. • May interfere with sleep • Over time, "sludge" (e.g., clotted blood, drug precipitates) may collect in port reservoir and decrease flow efficiency. • Require a skilled nurse to access and deaccess • Not available in triple lumen • If infection cannot be successfully treated, surgical removal is required. • Peripheral port use limits access for blood sampling, IVs, and blood pressure monitoring to the contralateral limb.

placement, such as those who have one or more of the following:

1. An open chest wound
2. Impaired skin integrity
3. Tumor involvement of the chest wall
4. Excessive adipose tissue that obviates the ability to suture the port to the muscle or locate septum

F. Special population considerations
   1. Pediatric patients must have sufficient chest wall muscle to support an implanted port (i.e., older than 6 months to 1 year of age).
   2. Metallic ports in radiation fields (e.g., chest wall) have resulted in dose perturbation (alteration and deflection or increased absorption) due to electrons emerging from the metallic portion of the port. Plastic ports or peripherally placed ports should be considered (Chatzigiannis et al., 2011; Gossman et al., 2009).

VI. Insertion techniques (Biffi, Pozzi, et al., 2014; Granziera et al., 2014; Iorio & Cavallaro, 2015; Teichgräber, Kausche, Nagel, & Gebauer, 2011; Walser, 2012) (see Figure 7-5)

A. Prior to placement, ensure that contraindications do not exist, informed consent is obtained, preplacement assessment is completed, laboratory studies are verified, and medication/chemotherapy order is reviewed (see Appendix 4).

B. Location of portal body placement is ideally determined prior to insertion procedure in a consultation with the patient and nurse.
   1. The portal body should be located over a rib for stability and placed in a nonobstructed area (e.g., away from bra straps and/or pacemaker).
   2. Sternal placement in obese patients may facilitate access.
   3. Deeply placed portal bodies and portal bodies in the axilla, breast tissue, or soft tissue of the abdomen may be difficult to access and should be avoided.
   4. Femoral placement for central vein occlusion (Goltz et al., 2014)

C. An implanted port placement is inserted by a surgeon or interventional radiologist under conscious or general anesthesia.

D. Ultrasound-guided insertion by skilled practitioners should be used to decrease number of cannulation attempts, reduce complications, and guide correct catheter tip placement by those trained and skilled in this technique (Bowen, Mone, Nelson, & Scaife, 2014; Brass, Hellmich, Kolodziej,

Figure 7-5. Radiographic Placement Confirmation of Implanted Port

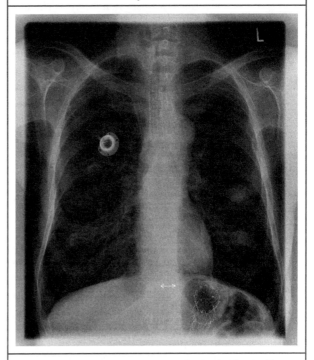

Schick, & Smith, 2015; Lamperti et al., 2012; O'Grady et al., 2011; Sofue et al., 2015; Teichgräber et al., 2011; Thomopoulos et al., 2014). Electrocardiogram and fluoroscopy guidance techniques have been used with success (Rossetti et al., 2015; Wang et al., 2015).

1. Subclavian approach: An incision is made under the clavicle, and a subcutaneous (SC) pocket is created. The SC vein is percutaneously entered and a guidewire is passed into the superior vena cava (SVC). A dilator and peel-away sheath are passed over the guidewire, and the guidewire and dilator are removed. The catheter is threaded into place, and the peel-away sheath is removed.

2. Internal jugular (IJ) approach: The IJ vein is identified using ultrasound. A small incision is made in the patient's neck, and a guidewire is passed into the SVC via the IJ. A tunnel is created in the SC tissue between the neck incision and the port pocket incision. A dilator and peel-away sheath are passed over the guidewire, the guidewire and dilator are removed, the catheter is threaded into place, and the peel-away sheath is removed.

3. Cut-down approach: The skin overlying the deltopectoral groove is cut to visualize the cephalic vein, the cephalic vein is cannulated, and a guidewire is placed in the vein. A dilator and peel-away sheath are passed over the guidewire, the guidewire and dilator are removed, the catheter is threaded into place, and the peel-away sheath is removed; alternately, a cut-down approach to the external jugular vein may be used (Iorio & Cavallaro, 2015).

4. Peripheral implantation: A port pocket site in upper arm is identified; the cephalic, basilic, or median cubital basilic vein is accessed using an introducer needle attached to a syringe; a blood return is confirmed and the syringe is removed; the tapered end of a J-wire is inserted into the needle; the guidewire is advanced to the SVC; the needle is withdrawn; the dilator and peel-away sheath are advanced over the guidewire; the dilator and guidewire are removed; the catheter is inserted into the sheath and advanced to the cavoatrial junction; and the peel-away sheath is removed (Wildgruber et al., 2015).

5. For all insertion approaches, a nonattached catheter is trimmed to the appropriate length and attached to the portal body. The appropriate length of an attached catheter is estimated prior to insertion and trimmed to desired length.

6. The length of a catheter is based on the distance from the planned catheter tip position to the planned location of the portal body.

7. Mathematical formulas assist in determining appropriate catheter lengths in children and adults (Shin et al., 2015; Stroud et al., 2014).

8. Venous access ports with catheter tips that are too high (above the cavoatrial junction) are at higher risk for further malposition and thrombosis; tips that are too low (in the right atrium) increase the risk of arrhythmia (Linnemann, 2014; Moureau et al., 2013).

9. For all insertion approaches, the portal body is sutured into the fascia and the exit site is sutured closed.

10. A noncoring needle is inserted into the portal body, blood is aspirated, and the device is flushed.

11. Implanted ports with confirmed placement and patency can be used immediately and the noncoring needle is left intact. The catheter tip is just above or in the lower third of the SVC at the cavoatrial junction; consensus guidelines support these preferred tip locations (Ahn & Chung, 2015; Gonda & Li, 2011; Moureau et al., 2013).

12. A retrospective analysis of 1,378 patient electronic medical records concluded no significant increase in infection rates when used on the same day as insertion for outpatient therapy (Young, Young, Vogel, Sutkowski, & Venkaterupumal, 2016).

13. A retrospective analysis concluded that if a port is placed with ultrasound or fluoroscopy, a postoperative chest x-ray is not needed to confirm placement (Bowen et al., 2014).

14. Multicenter research revealed that intracavitary electrocardiography is a safe and accurate alternative method of positioning the catheter tip in the pediatric popu-

lation (Rossetti et al., 2015); similar findings have been noted in adult patient populations (Wang et al., 2015).
  E. Insertion complications (see Chapter 9, Table 9-1)
VII. Unique maintenance and care (see Appendices 2, 4, 5, 7, and 10). No definitive recommendations can be made for flushing solution, volume, and frequency; frequency of dressing and needleless connector changes; or blood sampling technique (see Figure 7-6).
  A. Peripheral ports
    1. Do not obtain blood pressure measurements from the arm with the peripheral port.
    2. Do not attempt to draw blood or insert a peripheral IV catheter above the peripheral portal body.
  B. Accessing and deaccessing implanted ports (see Appendix 10)
    1. Patient assessment (Bustos, Aguinaga, Carmona-Torre, & Del Pozo, 2014)
      a) Wash hands.
      b) Examine the skin integrity overlying the portal body for redness, edema, or bruising.
      c) Palpate the area around the portal body for warmth and tenderness, and ask the patient about a fever or other signs of infection.
      d) Assess for potential or actual portal body erosion through the skin (Burris & Weis, 2014). Risk is higher in patients with portal bodies implanted close to the skin surface and in patients with significant weight loss.
      e) Inspect the anterior chest wall for collateral veins (dilated superficial veins), which may be a sign of catheter occlusion.
      f) Observe the face and neck for edema, which may be a sign of catheter-related thrombosis or SVC syndrome.
    2. Use only noncoring needles.
      a) A specially designed needle tip separates the silicone septum and prevents "coring," which could lead to debris in the reservoir and leakage.
      b) An offset bevel allows the tip of the needle to be flush with the bottom of the portal body without impeding the flow of solution.
      c) Needle lengths range from 0.5–2 inches.
      d) The most commonly used gauges range from 19–22.

      e) Configuration is straight for flushing and immediate deaccess or bent at a 90° angle for intermittent or continuous infusions.
      f) Available with short pieces of extension tubing, with and without clamps (Extension tubing also may have a Y-site.)
      g) Most include needlestick prevention features.
      h) Power needles are available in 19, 20, and 22 gauge with 0.75–1.5 inch lengths used with power-injectable design ports (e.g., contrast media) (Goltz et al., 2012; Indrajit et al., 2015).
    3. Accessing procedure (O'Grady et al., 2011; Schiffer et al., 2013)
      a) Assess need for a topical anesthetic (see Appendix 7).
      b) Determine appropriate noncoring needle size and length based on the patient's prior use, type and duration of therapy, and patient assessment findings. Ideally, the 90° turn of the noncoring needle should rest as close to the skin as possible; a gap greater than quarter of an inch indicates that a shorter needle should be used.
      c) Palpate the outline of the port body.
      d) Wash hands.
      e) Apply gloves and cleanse the implanted port site (see Appendix 2). Current

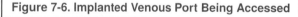
Figure 7-6. Implanted Venous Port Being Accessed

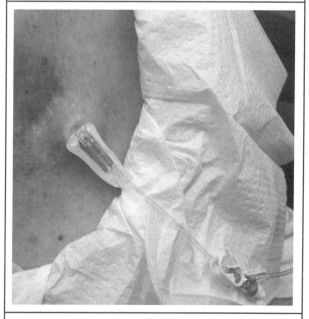

Note. Image courtesy of Diane G. Cope. Used with permission.

research is insufficient to support routine use of sterile gloves during accessing and deaccessing procedures (see Chapter 1 for controversial issues).

f) Remove the cap on the distal end of the noncoring needle connection tubing and prime the tubing with saline.

g) Stabilize the portal body with one hand and insert the noncoring needle into the center of the portal body until the bottom of the portal body is felt. For obese patients and those with deeply implanted ports, a second person may be helpful in locating and stabilizing the port and a longer needle may be needed (see Figures 7-6 and 7-7).

h) In vitro research has suggested that orienting the noncoring needle bevel opening toward the bottom of the port increases flushing efficiency (Guiffant, Durussel, Flaud, Vigier, & Merckx, 2012).

i) Aspirate to confirm a blood return and flush with 5 to 10 ml of 0.9% normal saline (NS).

j) Secure the noncoring needle using a transparent dressing or a securement device. For short-term use, gauze and tape may be used if properly secured (Webster, Gillies, O'Riordan, Sherriff, & Rickard, 2016) (see Appendix 5).

k) Instruct the patient to report tugging or pulling on the infusion tubing and any activity that may cause the noncoring needle to dislodge. Use a tension loop to prevent needle dislodgment. Consider use of a secondary securement device, if needed, to ensure that the needle is secured.

4. Deaccessing procedure

a) Wash hands and apply gloves.

b) Flush the noncoring needle with NS and follow with a heparin flush solution for open-ended catheters. Valved catheters may be flushed with NS only.

c) Remove the dressing.

d) Use nondominant hand to stabilize portal body.

e) Use dominant hand to gently remove noncoring needle and engage the safety mechanism that encloses the needle point, if present.

f) Discard the noncoring needle in a sharps container.

g) Apply adhesive bandage, as needed.

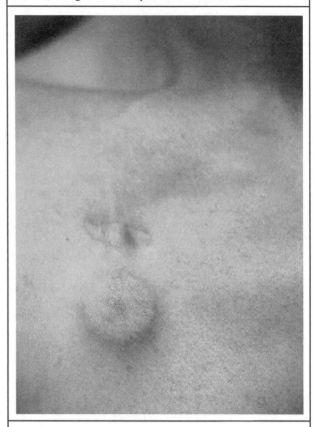

Figure 7-7. Implanted Venous Port

Note. Image courtesy of Diane G. Cope. Used with permission.

C. Flushing (Dal Molin et al., 2014; Kefeli et al., 2009; Odabas et al., 2014; Schiffer et al., 2013) (see Appendix 5)

1. No definitive recommendation can be made for flushing volume, solution, or frequency.

2. Research has suggested that the use of NS for intermittent locking of ports may be as effective as using heparinized solution (Bertoglio et al., 2012; Dal Molin et al., 2014; Goossens et al., 2013; Gorji, Rezaei, Jafari, & Cherati, 2015; López-Briz et al., 2014).

3. Heparin flush: Use 10–100 IU/ml, 5 ml after each use, per lumen; every 4–8 weeks if not in use.

4. For valved ports not in use, flush with 5 ml saline every 4–8 weeks to maintain patency.

5. Evidence has suggested that flushing intervals can approach up to three months without severe complications when flushing with 10 ml NS and 3 ml (100 IU/ml) heparinized saline (Odabas et al., 2014).

6. Due to the potential for an increased risk of microbial antibiotic resistance, no definitive recommendation can be made regard-

ing the routine use of antibiotic lock techniques for the prevention of catheter-associated infection (van de Wetering, van Woensel, & Lawrie, 2013).

   7. Consider the use of antibiotic lock therapy once a port-related infection is diagnosed, or if the patient is at high risk of infection; however, the frequency, length of dwell time, and whether or not to discard or flush antibiotic dwell have not been determined. Sensitivities of the organism dictate antibiotic use (Chesshyre, Goff, Bowen, & Carapetis, 2015; Fernández-Hidalgo & Almirante, 2014; Justo & Bookstaver, 2014; Raad & Chaftari, 2014; van de Wetering et al., 2013; Zhang, Gowardman, Morrison, Runnegar, & Rickard, 2016).

   D. Blood sampling: Discard 3–5 ml and flush with 10–20 ml NS (Conway, McCollom, & Bannon, 2014; Dailey, Berger, & Dabu, 2014; Rosenbluth et al., 2014) (see Appendix 5).

   E. Dressing changes: Remove dressing 24 hours after insertion. No dressing is needed unless being used for therapy; following chlorhexidine (CHG) skin preparation, use a CHG-impregnated sponge dressing for any long-term infusion exceeding 4–6 hours or if the port remains accessed for intermittent infusion for greater than 4–6 hours (O'Grady et al., 2011; Schiffer et al., 2013) (see Appendix 5).

VIII. Removal technique
   A. Indications (Granziera et al., 2014; Kim, Oh, Chang, & Jeong, 2012)
      1. Completion of therapy
      2. Infection (port pocket or catheter-related sepsis) not responsive to treatment
      3. Radiologically confirmed thrombosis not responsive to fibrinolytic therapy
      4. Dehiscence of port pocket incision
      5. Portal body erosion through the skin
      6. Catheter fracture or malposition
      7. Port body separation from catheter
   B. Removed by surgeon or interventional radiologist
IX. Complications (Ignatov et al., 2009; Klösges et al., 2015) (see Chapter 9)
X. Education and documentation (see Chapter 17)
XI. Unique patient education
   A. Inform the patient that a venous access port has been implanted, and describe any features (e.g., power port, dual lumen, open ended, valved).
   B. Instruct the patient to use an ice pack for comfort if the port is used prior to the resolution of postoperative edema and tenderness.
   C. Instruct the patient to carry a port identification card.

   D. If the patient has a metal port, inform the patient to alert radiology staff if an MRI is scheduled.
   E. Remind the patient to avoid manipulating the portal body; twiddler's syndrome occurs when a portal body is rotated by the patient and may result in malposition of the portal body or a catheter fracture near the catheter or portal body connection area (Busch et al., 2012).
   F. Instruct the patient to not allow peripheral blood sampling or blood pressure monitoring in the arm where the peripheral port is placed.
XII. Competency documentation for implanted port care (see Appendix 10)

The author would like to acknowledge Debra J. McCorkindale, RN, BSN, for her contribution to this chapter that remains unchanged from the previous edition of this book.

References

Ahn, S., & Chung, J.H. (2015). Proper tip position of central venous catheter in pediatric patients. *Journal of Vascular Access, 16*, 399–402. doi:10.5301/jva.5000393

Bertoglio, S., Solari, N., Meszaros, P., Vassalio, F., Bonvento, M., Pastorino, S., & Bruzzi, P. (2012). Efficacy of normal saline versus heparinized saline solution for locking catheters of totally implantable long-term ventral vascular access devices in adult cancer patients. *Cancer Nursing, 35*, E35–E42. doi:10.1097/NCC.0b013e31823312b1

Biffi, R., Pozzi, S., Bonomo, G., Della Vigna, P., Monfardini, L., Radice, D., … Orsi, F. (2014). Cost effectiveness of different central venous approaches for port placement and use in adult oncology patients: Evidence from a randomized three-arm trial. *Annals of Surgical Oncology, 21*, 3725–3731. doi:10.1245/s10434-014-3784-5

Biffi, R., Toro, A., Pozzi, S., & Di Carlo, I. (2014). Totally implantable vascular access devices 30 years after the first procedure. What has changed and what is still unsolved? *Supportive Care in Cancer, 22*, 1705–1714. doi:10.1007/s00520-014-2208-1

Bonciarelli, G., Batacchi, S., Biffi, R., Buononato, M., Damascelli, B., Ghibaudo, F., … Gruppo Aperto di Studio Accessi Venosi Centrali a Lungo Termine. (2011). GAVeCeLT consensus statement on the correct use of totally implantable venous access devices for diagnostic radiology procedures. *Journal of Vascular Access, 12*, 292–305. doi:10.5301/JVA.2011.7736

Boullata, J.I., Gilbert, K., Sacks, G., Labossiere, R.J., Crill, C., Goday, P., … American Society for Parenteral and Enteral Nutrition. (2014). A.S.P.E.N. clinical guidelines: Parenteral nutrition ordering, order review, compounding, labeling, and dispensing. *Journal of Parenteral and Enteral Nutrition, 38*, 334–377. doi:10.1177/0148607114521833

Bowen, M.E., Mone, M.C., Nelson, E.W., & Scaife, C.L. (2014). Image-guided placement of long-term central venous catheters reduces complications and cost. *American Journal of Surgery, 208*, 937–941. doi:10.1016/j.amjsurg.2014.08.005

Brass, P., Hellmich, M., Kolodziej, L., Schick, G., & Smith, A.F. (2015). Ultrasound guidance versus anatomical landmarks for internal jugular vein catheterization. *Cochrane Database of Systematic Reviews, 2015*(1). doi:10.1002/14651858.cd006962.pub2

Burris, J., & Weis, M.P. (2014). Reduction of erosion risk in adult patients with implanted venous access ports. *Clinical Journal of Oncology Nursing, 18*, 403–405. doi:10.1188/14.CJON.403-405

Busch, J.D., Herrmann, J., Heller, F., Derlin, T., Koops, A., Adam, G., & Habermann, C.R. (2012). Follow-up of radiologically totally implanted central venous access ports of the upper arm: Long-term complications in 127,750 catheter-days. *American Journal of Roentgenology, 199,* 447–452. doi:10.2214/AJR.11.7970

Bustos, C., Aguinaga, A., Carmona-Torre, F., & Del Pozo, J.L. (2014). Long-term catheterization: Current approaches in the diagnosis and treatment of port-related infections. *Infection and Drug Resistance, 7,* 25–35. doi:10.2147/IDR.S37773

Chatzigiannis, C., Lymperopoulou, G., Sandilos, P., Dardoufas, C., Yakoumakis, E., Georgiou, E., & Karaiskos, P. (2011). Dose perturbation in the radiotherapy of breast cancer patients implanted with the Magna-Site: A Monte Carlo study. *Journal of Applied Clinical Medical Physics, 12,* 3295.

Chesshyre, E., Goff, Z., Bowen, A., & Carapetis, J. (2015). The prevention, diagnosis and management of central venous line infections in children. *Journal of Infection, 71*(Suppl. 1), S59–S75. doi:10.1016/j.jinf.2015.04.029

Chopra, V., Flanders, S.A., Saint, S., Woller, S.C., O'Grady, N.P., Safdar, N., ... Bernstein, S.J. (2015). The Michigan Appropriateness Guide for Intravenous Catheters (MAGIC): Results from a multispecialty panel using the RAND/UCLA Appropriateness Method. *Annals of Internal Medicine, 163*(Suppl. 6), S1–S40. doi:10.7326/M15-0744

Conway, M.A., McCollom, C., & Bannon, C. (2014). Central venous catheter flushing recommendations: A systematic evidence-based practice review. *Journal of Pediatric Oncology Nursing, 31,* 185–190. doi:10.1177/1043454214532028

Cotogni, P., & Pittiruti, M. (2014). Focus on peripherally inserted central catheters in critically ill patients. *World Journal of Critical Care Medicine, 3,* 80–94. doi:10.5492/wjccm.v3.i4.80

Dailey, M.S., Berger, B., & Dabu, F. (2014). Activated partial thromboplastin times from venipuncture versus central venous catheter specimens in adults receiving continuous heparin infusions. *Critical Care Nurse, 34*(5), 27–41. doi:10.4037/ccn2014933

Dal Molin, A., Allara, E., Montani, D., Milani, S., Frassati, C., Cossu, S., ... Rasero, L. (2014). Flushing the central venous catheter: Is heparin necessary? *Journal of Vascular Access, 15,* 241–248. doi:10.5301/jva.5000225

Fernández-Hidalgo, N., & Almirante, B. (2014). Antibiotic-lock therapy: A clinical viewpoint. *Expert Review of Anti-infective Therapy, 12,* 117–129. doi:10.1586/14787210.2014.863148

Goltz, J.P., Janssen, H., Petritsch, B., & Kickuth, R. (2014). Femoral placement of totally implantable venous power ports as an alternative implantation site for patients with central vein occlusions. *Supportive Care in Cancer, 22,* 383–387. doi:10.1007/s00520-013-1984-3

Goltz, J.P., Noack, C., Petritsch, B., Kirchner, J., Hahn, D., & Kickuth, R. (2012). Totally implantable venous power ports of the forearm and the chest: Initial clinical experience with port devices approved for high-pressure injections. *British Journal of Radiology, 85,* e966–e972. doi:10.1259/bjr/33224341

Gonda, S.J., & Li, R. (2011). Principles of subcutaneous port placement. *Techniques in Vascular and Interventional Radiology, 14,* 198–203. doi:10.1053/j.tvir.2011.05.007

Goossens, G.A., Jerome, M., Janssens, C., Peetermans, W.E., Fieuws, S., Moons, P., ... Stas, M. (2013). Comparing normal saline versus diluted heparin to lock non-valved totally implantable venous access devices in cancer patients: A randomized, non-inferiority, open trial. *Annals of Oncology, 24,* 1892–1899. doi:10.1093/annonc/mdt114

Gorji, M.A.H., Rezaei, F., Jafari, H., & Cherati, Y. (2015). Comparison of the effects of heparin and 0.9% sodium chloride solutions in maintenance of patency of central venous catheters. *Anesthesiology and Pain Medicine, 5,* e22595. doi:10.5812/aapm.22595

Gossman, M.S., Seuntjens, J.P., Serban, M.M., Lawson, R.C., Robertson, M.A., Christian, K.J., ... Justice, T.E. (2009). Dosimetric effects near implanted vascular access ports: An examination of external

proton beam calculations. *Journal of Applied Clinical Medical Physics, 10,* 2886. doi:10.1120/jacmp.v10i3.2886

Granziera, E., Scarpa, M., Ciccarese, A., Filip, B., Cagol, M., Manfredi, V., ... Meroni, M. (2014). Totally implantable venous access devices: Retrospective analysis of different insertion techniques and predictors of complications in 796 devices implanted in a single institution. *BMC Surgery, 14,* 27. doi:10.1186/1471-2482-14-27

Guiffant, G., Durussel, J.J., Flaud, P., Vigier, J.P., & Merckx, J. (2012). Flushing ports of totally implantable venous access devices, and impact of the Huber point needle bevel orientation: Experimental tests and numerical computation. *Medical Devices, 5,* 31–37. doi:10.2147/MDER.S30029

Gyves, J., Ensminger, W., Niederhuber, J., Lipeman, M., Cozzi, E., Doan, K., ... Wheeler, R. (1982). Totally implanted system for intravenous chemotherapy in patients with cancer. *American Journal of Medicine, 73,* 841–845. doi:10.1016/0002-9343(82)90774-4

Ignatov, A., Hoffman, O., Smith, B., Fahlke, J., Peters, B., Bischoff, J., & Costa, S.-D. (2009). An 11-year retrospective study of totally implanted central venous access ports: Complications and patient satisfaction. *European Journal of Surgical Oncology, 35,* 241–246. doi:10.1016/j.ejso.2008.01.020

Indrajit, I.K., Sivasankar, R., D'Souza, J., Pant, R., Negi, R.S., Sahu, S., & Hashim, P. (2015). Pressure injectors for radiologists: A review and what is new. *Indian Journal of Radiology and Imaging, 25,* 2–10. doi:10.4103/0971-3026.150105

Iorio, O., & Cavallaro, G. (2015). External jugular vein approach for TIVAD implantation: First choice or only an alternative? A review of the literature. *Journal of Vascular Access, 16,* 1–4. doi:10.5301/jva.5000287

Justo, J.A., & Bookstaver, P.B. (2014). Antibiotic lock therapy: Review of technique and logistical challenges. *Journal of Infection and Drug Resistance, 12,* 343–363. doi:10.2147/IDR.S51388

Kefeli, U., Dane, F., Yumuk, P.F., Karamanoglu, A., Iyikesici, S., Basaran, G., & Turhal, N.S. (2009). Prolonged interval in prophylactic heparin flushing for maintenance of subcutaneous implanted port care in patients with cancer. *European Journal of Cancer Care, 18,* 191–194. doi:10.1111/j.1365-2354.2008.00973.x

Kim, J.T., Oh, T.Y., Chang, W.H., & Jeong, Y.K. (2012). Clinical review and analysis of complications of totally implantable venous access devices for chemotherapy. *Medical Oncology, 29,* 1361–1364. doi:10.1007/s12032-011-9887-y

Klösges, L., Meyer, C., Boschewitz, J., Andersson, M., Rudlowski, C., Schild, H.H., & Wilhelm, K. (2015). Long-term outcome of peripherally implanted venous access ports in the forearm in female cancer patients. *Cardiovascular and Interventional Radiology, 38,* 657–664. doi:10.1007/s00270-014-0975-1

Lamperti, M., Bodenham, A.R., Pittiruti, M., Blaivas, M., Augoustides, J.G., Elbarbary, M., ... Verghese, S.T. (2012). International evidence-based recommendations on ultrasound-guided vascular access. *Intensive Care Medicine, 38,* 1105–1117. doi:10.1007/s00134-012-2597-x

Linnemann, B. (2014). Management of complications related to central venous catheters in cancer patients: An update. *Seminars in Thrombosis and Hemostasis, 40,* 382–394. doi:10.1055/s-0034-1371005

López-Briz, E., Garcia, V.R., Cabello, J.B., Bort-Marti, S., Sanchis, R.C., & Burls, A. (2014). Heparin versus 0.9% sodium chloride intermittent flushing for prevention of occlusion in central venous catheters in adults. *Cochrane Database of Systemic Reviews, 2014*(10). doi:10.1002/14651858.CD008462.pub2

Moureau, N., Lamperti, M., Kelly, L.J., Dawson, R., Elbarbary, M., van Boxtel, A.J.H., & Pittiruti, M. (2013). Evidence-based consensus on the insertion of central venous access devices: Definition of minimal requirements for training. *British Journal of Anaesthesia, 110,* 347–356. doi:10.1093/bja/aes499

Odabas, H., Ozdemir, N.Y., Ziraman, I., Aksoy, S., Abali, H., Oksuzoglu, B., ... Zengin, N. (2014). Effect of port-care frequency on venous port catheter-related complications in cancer patients. *International Journal of Clinical Oncology, 19,* 761–766. doi:10.1007/s10147-013-0609-7

O'Grady, N.P., Alexander, M., Burns, L.A., Dellinger, E.P., Garland, J., Heard, S.O., ... Healthcare Infection Control Practices Advisory Committee. (2011). Guidelines for the prevention of intravascular catheter-related infections. *Clinical Infectious Diseases, 52,* E162–E193. doi:10.1093/cid/cir257

Raad, I., & Chaftari, A.-M. (2014). Advances in prevention and management of central line–associated bloodstream infections in patients with cancer. *Clinical Infectious Diseases, 59*(Suppl. 5), S340–S343. doi:10.1093/cid/ciu670

Rosenbluth, G., Tsang, L., Vittinghoff, E., Wilson, S., Wilson-Ganz, J., & Auerbach, A. (2014). Impact of decreased heparin dose for flush-lock of implanted venous access ports in pediatric oncology patients. *Pediatric Blood and Cancer, 61,* 855–858. doi:10.1002/pbc.24949

Rossetti, F., Pittiruti, M., Lamperti, M., Graziano, U., Celentano, D., & Capozzoli, G. (2015). The intracavitary ECG method for positioning the tip of central venous access devices in pediatric patients: Results of an Italian multicenter study. *Journal of Vascular Access, 16,* 137–143. doi:10.5301/jva.5000281

Schiffer, C.A., Mangu, P.B., Wade, J.C., Camp-Sorrell, D., Cope, D.G., El-Rayes, B.F., ... Levine, M. (2013). Central venous catheter care for the patient with cancer: American Society of Clinical Oncology clinical practice guideline. *Journal of Clinical Oncology, 31,* 1357–1370. doi:10.1200/JCO.2012.45.5733

Shin, H.-J., Kim, B.G., Na, H.S., Oh, A.-Y., Park, H.-P., & Jeon, Y.-T. (2015). Estimation of catheter insertion depth during ultrasound-guided subclavian venous catheterization. *Journal of Anesthesia, 29,* 724–727. doi:10.1007/s00540-015-2012-1

Sofue, K., Arai, Y., Takeuchi, Y., Tsurusaki, M., Sakamoto, N., & Sugimura, K. (2015). Ultrasonography-guided central venous port placement with subclavian vein access in pediatric oncology patients. *Journal of Pediatric Surgery, 50,* 1707–1710. doi:10.1016/j.jpedsurg.2015.05.013

Stroud, A., Zalieckas, J., Tan, C., Tracy, S., Zurakowski, D., & Mooney, D.P. (2014). Simple formulas to determine optimal subclavian central venous catheter tip placement in infants and children. *Journal of Pediatric Surgery, 49,* 1109–1112. doi:10.1016/j.jpedsurg.2013.12.024

Teichgräber, U.K.M., Kausche, S., Nagel, S.N., & Gebauer, B. (2011). Outcome analysis in 3,160 implantations of radiologically guided placements of totally implantable central venous port systems. *Eu-ropean Radiology, 21,* 1224–1232. doi:10.1007/s00330-010-2045-7

Thomopoulos, T., Meyer, J., Staszewicz, W., Bagetakos, I., Scheffler, M., Lomessy, A., ... Morel, P. (2014). Routine chest x-ray is not mandatory after fluoroscopy-guided totally implantable venous access device insertion. *Annals of Vascular Surgery, 28,* 345–350. doi:10.1016/j.avsg.2013.08.003

van de Wetering, M.D., van Woensel, J.B.M., & Lawrie, T.A. (2013). Prophylactic antibiotics for preventing gram positive infections associated with long-term central venous catheters in oncology patients. *Cochrane Database of Systematic Reviews, 2013*(11). doi:10.1002/14651858.CD003295.pub3

Walser, E.M. (2012). Venous access ports: Indications, implantation technique, follow-up, and complications. *Cardiovascular and Interventional Radiology, 35,* 751–764. doi:10.1007/s00270-011-0271-2

Wang, G., Guo, L., Jiang, B., Huang, M., Zhang, J., & Qin, Y. (2015). Factors influencing intracavitary electrocardiographic P-wave changes during central venous catheter placement. *PLOS ONE, 10,* e0124846. doi:10.1371/journal.pone.0124846

Webster, J., Gilllies, D., O'Riordan, E., Sherriff, K.L., & Rickard, C.M. (2011). Gauze and tape and transparent polyurethane dressings for central venous catheters. *Cochrane Database of Systematic Reviews, 2011*(11). doi:10.1002/14651858.CD003827.pub2

Wildgruber, M., Borgmeyer, S., Haller, B., Jansen, H., Gaa, J., Kiechle, M., ... Berger, H. (2015). Short-term and long-term outcome of radiological-guided insertion of central venous access port devices implanted at the forearm: A retrospective monocenter analysis in 1,704 patients. *European Radiology, 25,* 606–616. doi:10.1007/s00330-014-3417-1

Young, S.J., Young, L.J., Vogel, J., Sutkowski, R., & Venkataperumal, S. (2016). Accessing totally implantable venous access systems on the day of placement does not significantly increase the risk of infection. *Journal of Vascular Access, 17,* 261–264. doi:10.5301/jva.5000505

Zaghal, A., Khalife, M., Mukherji, D., El Majzoub, N., Shamseddine, A., Hoballah, J., ... Faraj, W. (2012). Update on totally implantable venous access devices. *Surgical Oncology, 21,* 207–215. doi:10.1016/j.suronc.2012.02.003

Zhang, L., Gowardman, J., Morrison, M., Runnegar, N., & Rickard, C.M. (2016). Microbial biofilms associated with intravascular catheter-related bloodstream infections in adult intensive care patients. *European Journal of Clinical Microbiology and Infectious Diseases, 35,* 201–205. doi:10.1007/s10096-015-2530-7

Chapter 8

Apheresis Catheters

Heather Thompson Mackey, RN, MSN, ANP-BC, AOCN®

I. History (Biffi, 2014; McLeod, 2010; Weinstein, 2014)
   A. Apheresis catheters were introduced with the first polyethylene IV catheters in 1945.
   B. The first type of tunneled central venous catheter, the Broviac® catheter, was introduced in 1973 for use in long-term hyperalimentation in children.
   C. A larger bore catheter, the Hickman® catheter, was introduced in 1976 to expand the applications of a tunneled catheter as well as the patient population (see Chapter 6).
   D. As improvements have been made in catheter technology (e.g., multilumen catheters, increased flow rates), clinical applications have expanded to areas such as hemodialysis and therapeutic apheresis.
II. Device characteristics (Dierickx & Macken, 2015; Golestaneh & Mokrzycki, 2013; Kalantari, 2012; O'Grady et al., 2011)
   A. A large-bore central venous catheter is designed with a high flow rate to allow for collection and reinfusion of blood products (i.e., red or white blood cells, platelets, plasma).
   B. Catheter designs are tunneled or nontunneled, depending on the intended duration of therapy.
      1. With proper care, tunneled catheters have a dwell time of several years.
      2. Nontunneled catheters are designed for temporary use, approximately seven days.
III. Device features (Delaney et al., 2014; Golestaneh & Mokrzycki, 2013; Hattori, 2014; Kalantari, 2012; Karakukcu & Unal, 2015; O'Grady et al., 2011; Schiffer et al., 2013)
   A. Typically shorter than other types of central venous access devices (VADs), with lengths ranging from 12–40 cm (4.7–15.8 inches)
   B. Designed with larger lumens compared with other types of central VADs, with sizes ranging from 10–18.5 Fr in adult patients and 6–8 Fr in pediatric patients
   C. Internal diameters range from 1.5–2 mm.
   D. Available in single- and double-lumen designs. Tunneled also are available in a triple-lumen design, with the third lumen consisting of a smaller diameter as compared to other lumens.
   E. A prime volume of 0.8–1.5 ml allows a flow rate of 300–400 ml/hour or greater.
   F. Typically stiffer as compared to other VADs to allow for higher blood flow rates and volumes. Stiff material makes the catheter more difficult to secure and preserve than other VADs.
   G. Catheters are made of polyurethane.
   H. Distal tips are open ended and require clamping during IV access for connection of IV tubing or syringes. Clamps typically are different colors to allow for identification of specific lumens.
   I. Tunneled are available with a cuff on the catheter.
      1. The cuff is positioned in the subcutaneous tunnel, 1–2 inches from the exit site for fixation of the catheter.
      2. The cuff potentially minimizes the risk of ascending infection from the exit site into the tunnel.
   J. Catheters have radiopaque markings.
IV. Device advantages and disadvantages (Golestaneh & Mokrzycki, 2013; Kalantari, 2012) (see Table 8-1)
V. Patient selection criteria (Delaney et al., 2014; Golestaneh & Mokrzycki, 2013; Kalantari, 2012; Karakukcu & Unal, 2015; O'Grady et al., 2011; Schwartz et al., 2013)
   A. Patient age, in general, does not restrict use of apheresis catheters.
   B. Indications
      1. Apheresis of blood components, including autologous stem cells, to be used with hematopoietic stem cell transplant. A temporary catheter may be used for stem cell collection from allogeneic donors who have poor peripheral venous access.
      2. Leukapheresis
      3. Plasmapheresis
      4. Tunneled catheters may be used for long-term IV access; however, other types of VADs usually are placed if this is the only indication for access.

Table 8-1. Advantages and Disadvantages of Apheresis Catheters		
Type of Catheter	**Advantages**	**Disadvantages**
Temporary apheresis catheter	Can be inserted at the bedside when immediate access is required Can be used immediately after placement	Designed for short-term use Increased incidence rate of catheter-related infection and sepsis Increased risk of catheter displacement because usually not sutured Often restricted to use for apheresis only
Tunneled apheresis catheter	Can be used immediately after placement Provide long-term access for apheresis Provide high flow rate because of large internal diameter of catheter Lower incidence rate of catheter-related infection than with temporary catheters	Insertion is a surgical procedure. Thrombosis: More likely with polyurethane catheter Poor flow may occur because of the technique used for catheter placement and the rigidity of catheter material.

C. Contraindications
1. Systemic infection or sepsis
2. Infection overlying the insertion site, presence of coagulopathies and platelet defects. Coagulopathies and thrombocytopenia should be corrected, when possible, prior to catheter insertion.
VI. Insertion techniques: Method is similar to nontunneled and tunneled VADs (Bowen, Mone, Nelson, & Scaife, 2014; Golestaneh & Mokrzycki, 2013; Kalantari, 2012) (see Chapters 4 and 6).
A. Inserted by a surgeon or interventional radiologist using ultrasound or fluoroscopy
B. Prior to placement, ensure that contraindications do not exist, informed consent is obtained, preplacement assessment is completed, laboratory studies are verified, and the medication/chemotherapy order is reviewed (see Appendix 4).
C. Vein selection
1. Selected according to the patient's anatomic structure, type and purpose of catheter, and vessel used. In children, vein selection also is dependent on age, activity level, and anatomy.

2. No definitive recommendation can be made regarding a preferred vein for insertion of tunneled VADs to minimize infection risk (Golestaneh & Mokrzycki, 2013; Kalantari, 2012; O'Grady et al., 2011).
3. Most common veins used for insertion
  a) Internal jugular vein
    (1) Preferred for tunneled apheresis catheters that will be used long term
    (2) Right internal jugular: Preferred due to ease of insertion into the junction of the superior vena cava and right atrium
  b) Subclavian vein: Due to the risk of venous stenosis, avoid if intended for apheresis.
  c) Femoral vein: Avoid in adult patients (O'Grady et al., 2011).
4. Verify catheter position prior to use. Verification of position is not required if placed by ultrasound or fluoroscopy (Bowen et al., 2014). The catheter tip is just above or in the lower third of the superior vena cava at the cavoatrial junction.
VII. Unique maintenance and care: No definitive recommendations can be made for flushing solution, volume, and frequency; frequency of dressing and needleless connector changes; or blood sampling technique (Delaney et al., 2014; Dierickx & Macken, 2015; Golestaneh & Mokrzycki, 2013; Infusion Nurses Society, 2016; O'Grady et al., 2011) (see Appendices 4, 5, and 9).
A. Replace all catheters inserted under emergency conditions as soon as possible when adherence to aseptic technique cannot be ensured.
B. Do not routinely replace apheresis catheters.
C. Apheresis catheter general care
1. Obtain specific manufacturer information for apheresis catheters prior to use.
2. Some institutions require a provider order if the catheter is to be used for reasons other than apheresis.
3. Clamps are used when accessing or deaccessing to prevent air embolisms or blood backflow.
4. Never use a hemostat or sharp-edged clamp, as these could damage or cut the catheter. Keep toothless plastic clamps available for emergency use. Scissors should never be used on or near the catheters.
5. If clamping is not possible, have the patient perform the Valsalva maneuver (forcefully exhale and hold breath) whenever the catheter is open to air.

6. A catheter becomes weakened with long-term use of alcohol and iodine-containing products.

D. Dressing changes
   1. Change dressing 24 hours after insertion. Change dressing if wet, soiled, contaminated, or nonocclusive. Apheresis catheter sites tend to bleed more easily due to the stiffness of the catheter, which may lead to increased dressing changes from bleeding or oozing around the exit site.
   2. Use an aseptic no-touch technique.
   3. No definitive recommendation can be made regarding the need for a dressing over a well-healed exit site of long-term, tunneled apheresis catheters (O'Grady et al., 2011).

E. Flushing
   1. Solution
      a) Use heparin 1,000 IU/ml after each use, 1–2 ml/day. Some settings support the use of concentrations of up to 5,000 IU/ml.
      b) If the heparinized saline is not aspirated and discarded, monitor coagulation levels (e.g., partial thromboplastin time), as this amount of heparin may lead to therapeutic serum levels.
      c) Data support the use of 3 ml of sodium citrate 4% in place of heparin for apheresis catheter locks in apheresis patients, although more research is needed for use with other catheters and patient populations (Passero et al., 2015).
      d) Acid citrate dextrose formula A (2 ml per lumen as locking solution) has been found to be as effective as heparin flush when evaluating for occlusion in short-term dwell times. Heparin was superior in long-term courses and long dwell times. No volume recommendation was given; further research is warranted (Osby, Barton, Lam, & Tran, 2014).
   2. Technique
      a) Flush vigorously using a pulsatile (push-pause motion) technique, maintaining pressure at the end of the flush to prevent reflux back into the catheter.
      b) Maintain a positive pressure technique while flushing an apheresis catheter by clamping the extension tubing while still flushing the line. This will help prevent the development of fibrin sheath, leading to withdrawal or infusion occlusions and contributing to the development of venous thrombosis.

F. Blood sampling techniques
   1. Clamp all lumens not being used for blood withdrawal on the apheresis catheter.
   2. Discard 3–5 ml of blood, obtain specimen, and flush vigorously using pulsatile technique with 10–20 ml of 0.9% normal saline after blood withdrawal.

VIII. Removal technique: Method is similar to nontunneled and tunneled VADs (see Chapters 4 and 6).

IX. Complications (Golestaneh & Mokrzycki, 2013; Osby et al., 2014) (see Chapter 9)

X. Education and documentation (see Chapter 17)

XI. Practicum on apheresis catheter care (see Appendix 9)

The author would like to acknowledge Susan A. Ezzone, MS, RN, CNP, AOCNP®, and Misty Lamprecht, MS, RN, CNS, AOCN®, for their contribution to this chapter that remains unchanged from the previous edition of this book.

References

Biffi, R. (2014). Introduction and overview of PICC history. In S. Sandrucci & B. Mussa (Eds.), *Peripherally inserted central venous catheters* (pp. 1–6). Milano, Italy: Springer.

Bowen, M.E., Mone, M.C., Nelson, E.W., & Scaife, C.L. (2014). Image-guided placement of long-term central venous catheters reduces complications and cost. *American Journal of Surgery, 208,* 937–941. doi:10.1016/j.amjsurg.2014.08.005

Delaney, M., Capocelli, K.E., Eder, A.F., Schneiderman, J., Schwartz, J., Sloan, S.R., ... Kim, H.C. (2014). An international survey of pediatric apheresis practice. *Journal of Clinical Apheresis, 29,* 120–126. doi:10.1002/jca.21301

Dierickx, D., & Macken, E. (2015). The ABC of apheresis. *Acta Clinica Belgica, 70,* 95–99. doi:10.1179/2295333714Y.0000000096

Golestaneh, L., & Mokrzycki, M.H. (2013). Vascular access in therapeutic apheresis: Update 2013. *Journal of Clinical Apheresis, 28*(1), 64–72. doi:10.1002/jca.21267

Hattori, M. (2014). Apheresis in children. In E. Noiri & N. Hanafusa (Eds.), *The concise manual of apheresis therapy* (pp. 403–411). Tokyo, Japan: Springer.

Infusion Nurses Society. (2016). *Infusion therapy standards of practice.* Norwood, MA: Author.

Kalantari, K. (2012). The choice of vascular access for therapeutic apheresis. *Journal of Clinical Apheresis, 27,* 153–159. doi:10.1002/jca.21225

Karakukcu, M., & Unal, E. (2015). Stem cell mobilization and collection from pediatric patients and healthy children. *Transfusion and Apheresis Science, 53,* 17–22. doi:10.106/j.transci.2015.05.010

McLeod, B.C. (2010). Therapeutic apheresis: History, clinical application, and lingering uncertainties. *Transfusion, 50,* 1413–1426. doi:10.1111/j.1537-2995.2009.02505.x

O'Grady, N.P., Alexander, M., Burns, L.A., Dellinger, E.P., Garland, J., Heard, S.O., ... Healthcare Infection Control Practices Advisory Committee. (2011). Guidelines for the prevention of intravascular catheter-related infections. *Clinical Infectious Diseases, 52,* E162–E193. doi:10.1093/cid/cir257

Osby, M., Barton, P., Lam, C.N., & Tran, M.-H. (2014). Acid-citrate-dextrose formula A versus heparin as primary catheter lock solutions for therapeutic apheresis. *Transfusion, 54,* 735–743. doi:10.1111/trf.12310

Passero, B.A., Zappone, P., Lee, H.E., Novak, C., Maceira, E.L., & Naber, M. (2015). Citrate versus heparin for apheresis catheter locks: An efficacy analysis. *Journal of Clinical Apheresis, 30,* 22–27. doi:10.1002/jca.21346

Schiffer, C.A., Mangu, P.B., Wade, J.C., Camp-Sorrell, D., Cope, D.G., El-Rayes, B.F., ... Levine, M. (2013). Central venous catheter care for the patient with cancer: American Society of Clinical Oncology clinical practice guideline. *Journal of Clinical Oncology, 31,* 1357–1370. doi:10.1200/JCO.2012.45.5733

Schwartz, J., Winters, J.L., Padmanabhan, A., Balogun, R.A., Delaney, M., Linenberger, M.L., ... Shaz, B.H. (2013). Guidelines on the use of therapeutic apheresis in clinical practice: Evidence-based approach from the Writing Committee of the American Society for Apheresis: The sixth special issue. *Journal of Clinical Apheresis, 28,* 145–284. doi:10.1002/jca.21276

Weinstein, S. (2014). History of infusion therapy. In S. Weinstein & M. Hagle (Eds.), *Plumer's principles and practice of infusion therapy* (9th ed., pp. 3–12). Philadelphia, PA: Wolters Kluwer Health/Lippincott Williams & Wilkins.

Chapter 9

Complications of Long-Term Venous Access Devices

Lisa Schulmeister, RN, MN, ACNS-BC, FAAN

I. Prevention of complications
   A. Staff education and training (Ferrer et al., 2014; Flodgren et al., 2013; Stone et al., 2014)
      1. Implementation of evidence-based measures helps prevent venous access device (VAD)-related complications, improves patient outcomes, and reduces healthcare costs.
      2. Higher levels of education and experience have been linked to a higher rate of successful VAD insertions and fewer complications.
      3. Training programs and dedicated staff (e.g., infection preventionists, vascular resource teams) decrease catheter-related bloodstream infection rates and increase patient satisfaction scores (Broadhurst, Moureau, & Ullman, 2016; Mermel & Parienti, 2015; Molas-Ferrer et al., 2015; O'Grady et al., 2011).
      4. Predictive simulation studies suggest that reduced nurse staffing resources are associated with higher catheter-related bloodstream infection rates; increasing the nurse workload is positively correlated to increased infection rates.
   B. Hand hygiene is critically important before patient contact, before performing an aseptic task, after patient contact and exposure to body fluids, and after contact with a patient's surroundings (O'Grady et al., 2011; World Health Organization, n.d.).
   C. Disinfection of catheter hubs, connectors, and injection ports is vital to VAD infection prevention (Berardi et al., 2015; Bustos, Aguinaga, Carmona-Torre, & Del Pozo, 2014; Chesshyre, Goff, Bowen, & Carapetis, 2015; Chopra, O'Horo, Rogers, Maki, & Safdar, 2013; García-Gabás et al., 2015; Kulkarni, Wu, Kasthuri, & Moss, 2014).
   D. Decisions about the need for a VAD should be individualized to the patient and based on patient factors (e.g., comorbidities, ability or willingness to participate in device care when applicable),

risks and benefits, and the overall cost to the patient, including ongoing maintenance costs such as dressing and flushing supplies.
   E. Considerations for the patient with cancer include the treatment regimen (e.g., irritants, vesicants), length of treatment (e.g., short- versus long-term infusion time, continuous infusion), overall duration of therapy (e.g., number of planned cycles), and need or potential need for parenteral nutrition.
   F. Select a device for insertion that minimally meets the patient's needs (e.g., minimum number of lumens, shortest dwell time).
   G. Central VADs must be considered at the initial treatment planning phase of care.
   H. Perform central venous catheterization only when potential benefits outweigh inherent risks.
   I. Central VAD tips are placed above or in the lower third of the superior vena cava at the cavoatrial junction; less commonly, the tip is placed in the inferior vena cava at the level of the diaphragm (Clemence & Maneval, 2014; York, 2012).
   J. VAD tips above the cavoatrial junction may result in subsequent malposition of the tip and catheter-related thrombosis, and VAD tips in the right atrium may trigger arrhythmias (Clemence & Maneval, 2014; York, 2012).
II. Insertion procedure–related complications (Calvache et al., 2014; Mermel & Parienti, 2015; Parienti et al., 2015) (see Table 9-1)
   A. Monitor the patient closely after placement of VAD for signs of complication, such as shortness of breath, edema, bleeding, or fever.
   B. Inform the patient and caregiver to notify the provider if symptoms occur after placement.
   C. Pediatric considerations: A case report cited that failure to place the catheter tip as close to the cavoatrial junction as possible can increase risk of vascular erosion into the pleural space (Blackwood, Farrow, Kim, & Hunter, 2015).

III. Postinsertion complications and management (see Table 9-1)
  A. Catheter migration: The catheter tip migrates spontaneously from the superior vena cava following initial placement (Ast & Ast, 2014; Beccaria et al., 2015; Brass, Hellmich, Kolodziej, Schick, & Smith, 2015; Jin et al., 2012; Prabaharan & Thomas, 2014).
    1. Etiologies: Change in intrathoracic pressure from coughing, sneezing, or vomiting; forceful flushing; vigorous upper extremity movements; changing body position, weight lifting, or by accidental pulling on an external catheter. Patient level of activity can be a contributor to late catheter migration.
    2. Signs and symptoms: Inability or difficulty infusing fluids or withdrawing blood, increased external VAD catheter length, reports of tingling sensation or gurgling in neck, arm or shoulder pain, vague back discomfort, swelling at exit site, pain during injection, or complaints of palpation or chest pain

		Table 9-1. Venous Access Device Insertion Complications	
Complication	**Etiology**	**Symptoms and Physical Exam Findings**	**Clinical Intervention**
Air embolism (Cook, 2013)	Occurs when intrathoracic pressure becomes less than atmospheric pressure at the open needle or catheter. Severity depends on the volume of air present, the rate of entry, and the patient's position at time of air embolus. Microbubbles join each other in the lung to create large bubbles, which are then trapped in pulmonary capillaries, causing a cascade of events, including tissue ischemia of the pulmonary walls and an inflammatory immune response.	Sudden dyspnea, tachypnea; cyanosis; shoulder and chest pain; anxiety, feeling of impending doom, feeling of air hunger, apnea; hypotension; cardiac arrest; aphasia; seizures; hemiplegia; pulmonary edema, coma; a churning sound heard over the pericardium on auscultation, which is produced by the presence of air and blood in the right ventricle (rare)	Symptoms may be subtle initially; requires immediate intervention. Treatment: Clamp catheter proximal to any breaks or leaks observed; place the patient on left side in Trendelenburg position; administer 100% oxygen; monitor and support vital signs; attempt to aspirate air from vascular access device (although rarely successful).
Arrhythmias (Hodzic et al., 2014; Khasawneh & Smalligan, 2011)	Insertion deep into the atrium can illicit extrasystoles, most often when more than two attempts at cannulation occur.	Tachycardia, heart sounds; most common arrhythmias are premature atrial or ventricular contractions; less commonly can cause right bundle branch block	Common complication of venous access device (VAD) insertion but is avoidable with careful placement; can be life-threatening, especially if ventricular overstimulation occurs; can typically resolve when guidewire tip is withdrawn so that endocardium is not touched; patients with preexisting bundle branch block can experience complete bundle branch block, requiring temporary pacing before resolution. Treatment: Reposition catheter tip
Brachial plexus injury (Kim et al., 2014)	Occurs when advancing catheter into jugular vein, causing direct needle trauma. Repeated attempts at subclavian vein cannulation can increase risk. This process can also injure the phrenic (diaphragmatic function, causing shortness of breath) and laryngeal nerves	Acute symptoms at time of catheter insertion: paresthesias, electric shock–like pain radiating distally, paralysis, which can be permanent	Prevention: skilled technique can minimize risk. Presence of paresthesias indicates catheter contact with brachial nerve. Treatment: Observe symptoms, which usually resolve in minutes to several hours after insertion; administer analgesics as necessary. Continued pain, paresthesia, weakness, or allodynia after cannulation requires immediate evaluation

(Continued on next page)

		Table 9-1. Venous Access Device Insertion Complications *(Continued)*	
Complication	**Etiology**	**Symptoms and Physical Exam Findings**	**Clinical Intervention**
Arterial puncture (Hodzic et al., 2014)	Occurs when artery is punctured during percutaneous catheterization; may affect carotid or subclavian arteries; can result in arterial embolism	Rapid hematoma formation; internal or external bleeding at insertion site; pallor; weak pulse; tachycardia; stroke; hypotension; upper airway impingement if trachea is compressed	Treatment: Remove needle or catheter; apply local pressure; obtain chest x-ray with order; observe site and patient closely for several hours.
Venous perforation (Khasawneh & Smalligan, 2011)	Occurs when excessive force is used when introducing the needle, guidewire, or dilator; can result in hemothorax	Shortness of breath, Internal bleeding, tachycardia; unexplained drop in hemoglobin, unilateral pleural effusion ipsilateral to a recently placed VAD	Can be catastrophic but avoidable with careful technique Treatment: Surgical intervention is required.
Cardiac tamponade (Khasawneh & Smalligan, 2011)	Results from cardiac compression of fluid accumulated within the pericardial sac, exerting increased pressure around the heart that restricts blood flow in and out of the ventricles. Occurs when catheter perforates cardium, typically the right atrium, followed by the right ventricle	May occur hours or days after insertion; anxiety; tachypnea; mild dyspnea to severe respiratory distress; light-headedness; restlessness; confusion; chest discomfort (fullness, heaviness); cyanosis; face and neck vein distention; decreased heart sounds; hypotension; tachycardia; syncope	Treatment: Requires immediate intervention. Immediate chest x-ray or echocardiogram is needed for diagnosis; pericardiocentesis may be life-saving. May require surgery to perform pericardial window and placement of drainage tubes.
Catheter fracture or embolism (Shah & Shah, 2014; Shimizu et al., 2014; Sundriya et al., 2014; Tamura et al., 2014)	May occur when catheter is pulled back and sheared off through inserting needle; catheter rupture; or pinch-off syndrome; the catheter fragment may embolize.	Chest pain, cardiac arrhythmias, hypotension, pallor, shortness of breath, tachycardia, confusion; can also be asymptomatic	Treatment: Requires immediate intervention. Place the patient in Trendelenburg; observe the patient for shortness of breath, tachycardia, confusion, and hypotension; obtain immediate consultation from interventional radiology, thoracic or vascular surgeon for removal. Percutaneous retrieval occurs under fluoroscopy or ultrasonography using goose-neck or conformational loop snare.
Catheter tip malposition (Cortellaro et al., 2014; Massmann et al., 2015; Salimi et al., 2015)	Occurs when catheter tip is misdirected on insertion Malposition of catheter can cause cardiac perforation, tamponade, venous thrombosis, or cardiac arrhythmias (especially ventricular). Inadvertent catheter placement into other veins (e.g., brachiocephalic, jugular) can occur.	Withdrawal occlusion; sluggish infusion; patient report of tingling sensation and gurgling sounds in neck; arm or shoulder pain; chest pain; cardiac dysrhythmias; cardiac arrest	Confirm placement. Treatment: Reposition catheter using imaging or guidewire exchange; remove catheter and replace. There is some conflicting evidence whether contrast-enhanced ultrasound versus traditional chest x-ray detects malposition most accurately; however, fluoroscopy, electrocardiogram, and increasingly ultrasound use during placement remains the standard of care for insertion.
Exit-site bleeding or hematoma (Hodzic et al., 2014)	Caused by introducer sheath larger than catheter left in place or traumatic insertion. May be significant if the patient has coagulopathies or thrombocytopenia or is taking anticoagulants	Oozing or frank bleeding from the exit site, sometimes persisting for several hours; discoloration or bruising; may result in compartment syndrome (large pooling of blood)	Treatment: Apply local pressure; change dressing, as needed; drain compartment; observe area frequently; remove catheter, if necessary. Apply hemostatic dressing to minimize bleeding.

(Continued on next page)

Table 9-1. Venous Access Device Insertion Complications *(Continued)*

Complication	Etiology	Symptoms and Physical Exam Findings	Clinical Intervention
Pneumothorax, hemothorax, chylothorax, or hydrothorax (Calvache et al., 2014; Tsotsolis et al., 2015)	Caused by air, blood, lymph, or infusion fluid into the pleural cavity due to pleura, vein, or thoracic duct injury during catheter insertion Risk increases significantly if three or more attempts to cannulate vein occur.	Chest pain; tachypnea; dyspnea; decreased breath sounds; shift in location of heart sounds; cyanosis; decreased cardiac output	Treatment: Obtain chest x-ray and discontinue infusions; administer oxygen; prepare for needle aspirations and chest tube drainage. Perform thoracotomy for drainage, if necessary. Remove device.
Left innominate vein stenosis (Song et al., 2015)	Can occur in some patients after placement via internal jugular vein; significantly more common in left-sided placement Incidence increased when the distance between sternum and left innominate vein was less than 16 mm.	Pain, swelling in affected arm and ipsilateral side of face and neck; headache; pressure	Prevention: Consider an ipsilateral approach in patients with right-sided cancer and a retrosternal space of < 16 mm. Treatment: Remove device.
Phlebitis (Cotogni & Pittiruti, 2014; Jumani et al., 2013; Schneider et al., 2015)	In peripherally inserted central catheters, can occur as a result of traumatic insertion or mechanical or chemical irritation	Pain, erythema, streak formation, palpable cord, edema	Prevention: Keep manipulation of the catheter to a minimum to prevent mechanical phlebitis and avoid stabilizing with sutures. Treatment: Apply warm compresses, elevate extremity, and administer pain medication.
Guidewire entanglement, kink, breakage, or loss (Khasawneh & Smalligan, 2011)	Kinking or looping of the guidewire, entanglement in existing intravascular equipment (e.g., pacer wires, superior vena cava filters), or loss of entire guidewire or breakage resulting from excessive force used to thread guidewire through introducer	May be dependent on location of defect; often causes inability to advance or withdraw guidewire; typically is observed as resistance during insertion or withdrawal of guidewire or complete loss of guidewire, which may result in arrhythmias, damage to vessels, or thrombosis	Prevention: Skilled technique can ensure avoidance of most guidewire complications. Treatment: Guidewire is retrieved by an interventional radiologist.

3. Diagnostic tests: Chest x-ray or dye study/cathetergram
   a) May be kinked, looped, coiled, or curled
   b) The tip may migrate from the cavoatrial junction to the internal jugular vein in the neck, contralateral brachiocephalic vein, or axillary vein.
4. Management: An appropriate repositioning method should be selected according to location of catheter tip, cause of malposition, length of malposition, and the patient's condition. Invasive and noninvasive procedures include the following:
   a) Percutaneous catheter repositioning using snares or wire-assisted long-loop snaring under fluoroscopic guidance

b) Catheter-exchange procedure using a guidewire (for nontunneled, percutaneous VADs)
c) Pulsatile (push-pause) flushing of device
d) Device removal and replacement
e) Repositioning can fail if the catheter length is insufficient to ensure proper placement; caution should be used to ensure that the catheter length is sufficient to allow for successful repositioning (Massmann, Jagoda, Kranzhoefer, & Buecker, 2015).
f) A catheter too deep into the atrium can be withdrawn to the correct placement at the time of insertion.
g) Consequences of uncorrected malposition: Delayed hydrothorax and sud-

den deaths have been reported (Jabeen, Murtaza, Hanif, Morabito, & Khalil, 2014).

B. Rotation of port (see Figure 9-1)
1. Etiologies
   a) Implanted portal bodies that are minimally secured during implantation may rotate or flip in the subcutaneous (SC) tissue upon rotation of the arm or shoulder, commonly referred to as "flipped port."
   b) Twiddler's syndrome occurs when a portal body is manipulated and rotated by the patient. It may result in malposition of the portal body or catheter fracture (Busch et al., 2012).
   c) Significant weight loss contributes to rotation of the portal body in the SC port pocket.
2. Signs and symptoms: Inability to palpate or access portal body
3. Diagnostic tests: Chest x-ray or chest computed tomography scan to visualize the portal body
4. Management: Depends on degree of rotation and coiling of catheter
   a) May be able to subcutaneously rotate into correct position
   b) May require surgical repositioning of device
   c) If catheter or portal device has become damaged during reposition, the device may need to be removed and replaced.

C. Portal body erosion: Erosion of portal body through the skin surface (Burris & Weis, 2014; Harish, 2014)
1. Etiologies
   a) Significant weight loss after port insertion
   b) Repeated improper access technique into port body
   c) Repeated use of ethyl chloride spray as topical anesthetic
   d) Wound dehiscence after port placement
   e) Poor wound healing of the insertion site after port placement
2. Signs and symptoms: Visualization of the portal body outline just below the skin surface (impending erosion) or visualization of the portal body (partial or complete explantation) (see Figure 9-2)
3. Diagnostic tests: Wound culture, as indicated
4. Management: Device removal

Figure 9-1. Rotation of Implanted Port

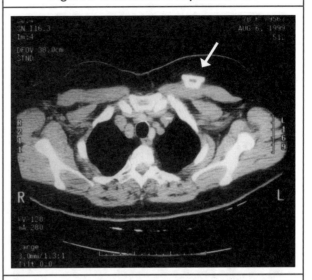

Note. From "Unusual Port Presentation," by D. Camp-Sorrell, 2001, *Clinical Journal of Oncology Nursing, 5,* p. 115. Copyright 2001 by Oncology Nursing Society. Reprinted with permission.

Figure 9-2. Skin Erosion of Implanted Port

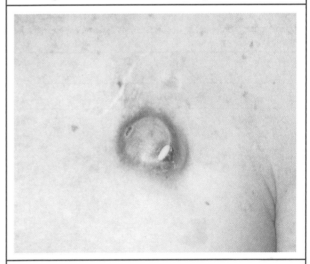

Note. From "Implanted Ports: Skin Erosion," by D. Camp-Sorrell, 2004, *Clinical Journal of Oncology Nursing, 8,* p. 309. Copyright 2004 by Oncology Nursing Society. Reprinted with permission.

D. Mechanical VAD catheter compression and fracture (El Hammoumi et al., 2014; Sugimoto, Nagata, Hayashi, & Kano, 2012; Sundriyal, Jain, & Manjunath, 2014; Tamura et al., 2014; Tazzioli et al., 2015): This also is called pinch-off syndrome or spontaneous catheter fracture (see Figures 9-3 and 9-4).
1. Etiology: The catheter is compressed between the clavicle and first rib in the cos-

Figure 9-3. Implanted Catheter Fracture

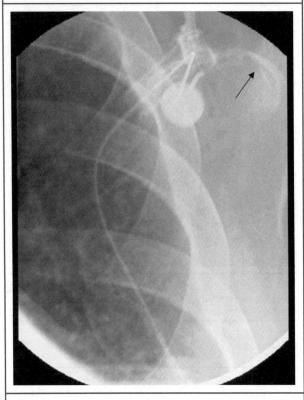

Note. Image courtesy of the Carole and Ray Neag Comprehensive Cancer Center, University of Connecticut Health Center. Used with permission.

Figure 9-4. Portal Body Fracture

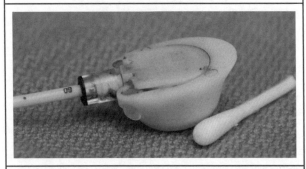

Note. Copyright 2009 by Seth Eisenberg. Used with permission.

toclavicular space. When a complete catheter fracture occurs, the distal portion of the catheter can travel to the jugular vein, superior vena cava, heart cavities, or lung.
2. Prevention: Research has shown that ultrasound-guided placement reduces the risk of catheter compression versus the use of the landmark technique (Brass et al., 2015).
3. Signs and symptoms

   a) Difficulty infusing fluids or withdrawing blood, despite patient repositioning
   b) Signs and symptoms of fracture depend on presence or location of embolized catheter fragment and may include palpitations, shortness of breath, and chest pain.
4. Diagnostic tests: Compression may be visualized on chest x-ray (with arms at the side and not rolled over) or dye study/ cathetergram.
5. Management
   a) If a complete fracture and embolization occurs, a catheter fragment may be retrievable.
   b) Remove any remaining device components.
   c) No definitive recommendation can be made regarding the frequency or type of imaging needed for surveillance to detect mechanical failure.
   d) Persistent withdrawal and flushing problems should be monitored closely, including imaging studies, as these findings in a catheter indicate compression.
E. Catheter occlusion: Partial to complete obstruction within the lumen or at the distal tip. Partial (incomplete) is defined as the ability to flush fluid yet unable to withdraw blood. Complete is defined as the inability to flush or withdraw blood (Anderson, Pesaturo, Casavant, & Ramsey, 2013; Baskin et al., 2012; Boddi et al., 2015; D'Ambrosio, Aglietta, & Grignani, 2014; Linnemann, 2014; Murray, Precious, & Alikhan, 2013).
   1. Etiologies
      a) Fibrin sheath: The fibrin adheres to the catheter tip and external surface forming a tail or sheath, which can extend the entire length of catheter. The sheath acts as a one-way valve that permits infusion but prevents withdrawal of blood. A fibrin sheath is one of the most common causes of thrombotic occlusion and is the most common cause of partial obstruction.
      b) Intraluminal clots: Form around the catheter surface, causing incomplete occlusion (see Figures 9-5 and 9-6)
      c) Mural thrombosis: Intraluminal clots adhere to the vessel wall, forming a venous thrombus and causing incomplete occlusion.

Figure 9-5. Intraluminal Surface of an Indwelling Vascular Catheter

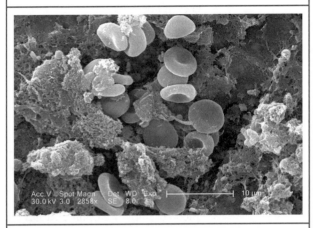

Note. Image courtesy of Janice Carr, Centers for Disease Control and Prevention.

Figure 9-6. Red Blood Cells Enmeshed in a Fibrinous Matrix on the Intraluminal Surface of an Indwelling Vascular Catheter

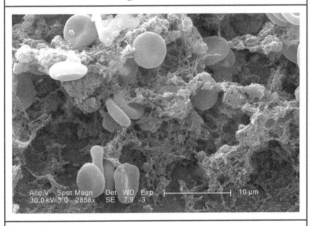

Note. Image courtesy of Janice Carr, Centers for Disease Control and Prevention.

  d) Deep vein thrombosis (DVT): Catheter-related thrombosis that occludes the vein; typically located in the upper extremity. It most commonly is found in the subclavian, followed by axillary, brachial, and brachiocephalic veins (Jasti & Streiff, 2014; Zwicker, Connolly, Carrier, Kamphuisen, & Lee, 2014).
  e) Infusion of incompatible solutions or inadequate flushing, causing precipitation, crystallization, or lipid deposits within the catheter or at the distal tip

2. Risk factors (Chopra et al., 2014, 2015; Clemence & Maneval, 2014; Dalton, Pheil, Lacy, & Dalton, 2014; Franchini, 2015; Geerts, 2014)
  a) Past medical history of venous thromboembolism; undergoing a surgery when a peripherally inserted central catheter (PICC) already is in place; hypercoagulable state
  b) Presence of sludge (sediment containing blood components, drug and mineral precipitates or residue, or lipid residue) adhering to the internal path of the port reservoir
  c) Use of larger gauge catheter or multiluminal catheter
  d) Improper positioning of the catheter tip
  e) Specific cancer tumor types (e.g., breast, lung, lymphoma)
  f) History of recent surgery, immobilization, chemotherapy, or targeted therapies (Elyamany, Alzahrani, & Bukhary, 2014)
3. Prevention (D'Ambrosio et al., 2014; Duffy, Rodgers, Shever, & Hockenberry, 2015; Hajjar, 2015; Odabas et al., 2014; O'Grady et al., 2011; Snarski et al., 2015; Stone et al., 2014)
  a) Early identification of at-risk patients helps guide practice.
  b) Adequate catheter flushing and heparinization (open-ended catheters). Data suggest that no difference exists in rate of occlusion when VADs are flushed with heparin or normal saline (Heidari Gorji, Rezaei, Jafari, & Yazdani Cherati, 2015), whereas some studies report statistical trends toward higher incidence of complications in saline-only cohorts (López-Briz et al., 2014). Manufacturers of open-ended VADs continue to advise the use of

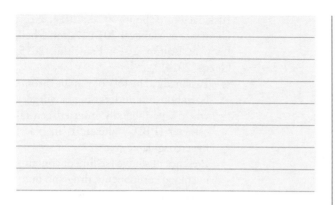

heparin flushes for "locking" after VAD use, and it continues as a common clinical practice (Heidari Gorji et al., 2015; López-Briz et al., 2014; Lyons & Phalen, 2014).

c) Pediatric: Weak evidence exists for daily flushing of noninfusing implanted ports to prevent fibrin accumulation; however, evidence does not support definitive heparin volumes and concentrations, as the study did not report heparin volumes and concentrations. No recommendations were made for PICC flushing in this population (Conway, McCollom, & Bannon, 2014).

d) Some studies suggest that systemic anticoagulation for thromboprophylaxis confers a benefit; use must be weighed against the potential harm associated with anticoagulant therapy. No recommendation can be made regarding prophylactic anticoagulation in pediatric and adult populations (Akl et al., 2014; Ast & Ast, 2014; Geerts, 2014; Jasti & Streiff, 2014; Park et al., 2014; Schiffer et al., 2013; Wiegering et al., 2014).

4. Signs and symptoms
   a) Partial occlusion allows fluid to be infused but not withdrawn.
   b) Total occlusion prevents infusion of fluids and withdrawal of blood.
   c) Mural thrombosis may cause pain or edema in neck or upper extremities.
   d) DVT reveals edema of extremity, warmth, and palpable cord.

5. Diagnostic tests
   a) Based on symptoms
   b) Based on medications administered prior to onset of symptoms
   c) A chest x-ray may be ordered to rule out mechanical causes of occlusion.

d) Perform a cathetergram/dye study to visualize catheter patency and the presence of fibrin tail, which may be causing backtracking along the catheter toward the venotomy site.

e) Ultrasound demonstrates high specificity and sensitivity as the initial diagnostic test if upper-extremity DVT is suspected (Fallouh, McGuirk, Flanders, & Chopra, 2015).

6. Management (see Figures 9-7 and 9-8)
   a) Treatment of occlusions caused by intraluminal blood or fibrin, precipitates, and lipid deposits (see Table 9-2)
   b) Blood or fibrin occlusion: Instill 2 mg tissue plasminogen activator, followed by a period of dwell time. Refer to the manufacturer's package insert for dosage and dwell time (Ragsdale, Oliver, Thompson, & Evans, 2014; Schiffer et al., 2013).
   c) Upper-extremity DVT: Initiate systemic anticoagulation therapy with low-molecular-weight heparin alone or low-molecular-weight heparin followed by warfarin for the life of the VAD. If the VAD is removed, continue anticoagulation therapy for three months. Consider VAD removal if symptoms persist, infection is suspected within the clot, or if the VAD is dysfunctional or no longer necessary (Debourdeau et al., 2013; National Comprehensive Cancer Network®, 2016).
   d) Removal: Although it is not always necessary to remove a catheter with a catheter-associated thrombosis, radiologically confirmed thrombi unresponsive to fibrinolytic treatment requires catheter removal (Schiffer et al., 2013).
   e) Removal alternative: Mechanical thrombolysis using a hair wire under fluoroscopy followed by aspiration of the fragments and remnant thrombus removal by saline flush has been reported to be successful (Oh, Choi, Chun, & Lee, 2015).

F. Infection (Berardi et al., 2015; Bustos et al., 2014; Chesshyre et al., 2015; Chopra et al., 2013; Ciocson, Hernandez, Atallah, & Amer, 2014; García-Gabás et al., 2015; Kulkarni et al., 2014; Mermel, 2015, Mermel & Parienti, 2015)
   1. Etiologies

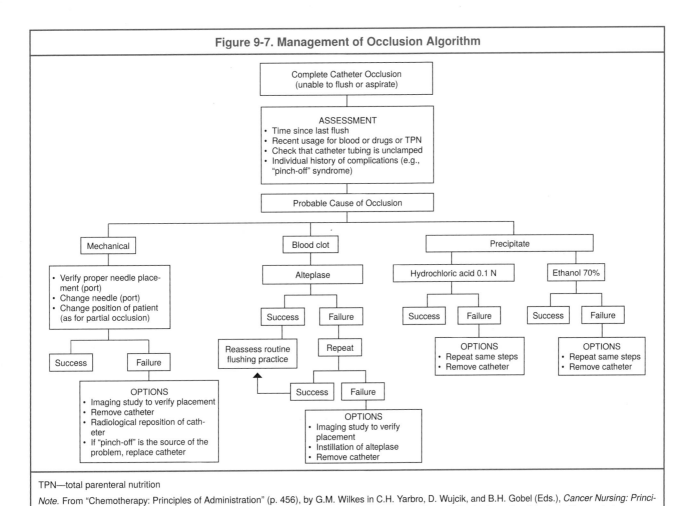

Figure 9-7. Management of Occlusion Algorithm

TPN—total parenteral nutrition

Note. From "Chemotherapy: Principles of Administration" (p. 456), by G.M. Wilkes in C.H. Yarbro, D. Wujcik, and B.H. Gobel (Eds.), *Cancer Nursing: Principles and Practice* (8th ed.), 2018, Burlington, MA: Jones & Bartlett Learning. Copyright 2018 by Jones & Bartlett Learning. Adapted with permission.

a) Most infections originate from the skin microbiota surrounding the catheter insertion site.

b) Catheter manipulation and repeated implanted port accessing are associated with development of intraluminal biofilm.

c) Biofilm development begins shortly after VAD insertion; however, clinical features of infection may not be apparent for days to weeks.

2. Risk factors (Bustos et al., 2014; Chesshyre et al., 2015; Chopra et al., 2013; Ciocson et al., 2014; Freire et al., 2013; Jia et al., 2015; Kaur, Gupta, Gombar, Chander, & Sahoo, 2015; Rhee, Heung, Chen, & Chenoweth, 2015)

a) Hematologic malignancies (particularly when immunosuppressed or if device is implanted when patient is neutropenic)

(1) Probability scoring using a modified Infection Probability Score has been shown to be a useful measure of probability of central line–associated bloodstream infection (CLABSI) development in patients with hematologic malignancies.

(2) Predictive factors: Number of days of catheter dwell, body temperature, heart and respiratory rates, white blood cell count, absolute neutrophil count, and C-reactive protein levels are scored using the modified scale.

(3) Scores from the Sequential Organ Failure Assessment tool are included in the final calculation. Final scores can effectively predict patients at high risk for CLABSI (Schalk, Hanus, Färber, Fischer, & Heidel, 2015).

b) Prolonged neutropenia

c) Older age

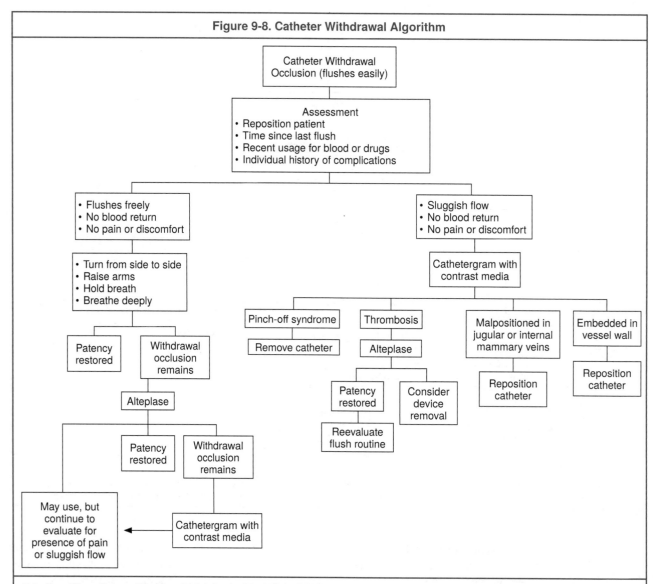

Figure 9-8. Catheter Withdrawal Algorithm

d) Use of catheter for nonchemotherapy indications

e) Comorbidities

f) Prolonged intensive care unit (ICU) hospitalization

g) Increased number of catheter days (e.g., dwell time)

h) PICCs are associated with a lower risk of CLABSI in outpatients; however, if a patient is admitted to the hospital with a PICC, the risk of CLABSI is equal to that of other VADs.

i) Research correlates central line infections in children with increased mortality, increased length of hospital and ICU stays, treatment interruptions, and increased complications (Chesshyre et al., 2015).

3. Prevention (Bustos et al., 2014; Duffy et al., 2015; Mermel, 2015; Mermel & Parienti, 2015; Morano et al., 2015; O'Grady et al., 2011; Schiffer et al., 2013; Snarski et al., 2015; Stone et al., 2014; Walz et al., 2015)

a) The goals are to diminish colonization of the catheter insertion site and hub, minimize the spread of microorganisms from the skin to the catheter hub, and reduce microbial spread through the catheter lumen to the bloodstream.

b) Incorporate central line bundle principles into daily maintenance and care, including hand hygiene, optimal catheter site selection, maximal barrier precautions during catheter insertion, chlorhexidine skin antisepsis during catheter insertion, and daily review line necessity, with prompt removal of unnecessary lines (Institute for Healthcare Improvement, 2016).

Table 9-2. Device Obstructions: Risks, Prevention, and Management			
Occlusion Type	At Risk	Prevention	Intervention
Mechanical obstruction	At catheter placement; inadequate securement of device	Astute assessment and early intervention of potential obstructions can prevent occurrence.	Dependent on etiology. May include catheter migration, port rotation, catheter compression (e.g., pinch-off syndrome), kinks in catheter or securement device, or catheter fracture
Blood/fibrin	Hypercoagulable state; type of malignancy; inadequate flushing	Meticulous catheter care and adequate flushing using a push-pause, pulsatile, or turbulent technique facilitates thorough rinsing of the intraluminal spaces and can prevent occurrence.	The goal is to dissolve the blood/fibrin: Instillation of 2 mg tissue plasminogen activator recommended, followed by a period of dwell time to restore patency and preserve catheter function occluded by intraluminal blood or fibrin. Refer to manufacturer's package insert for dosages and dwell times. Repeat if unsuccessful. Remove device if radiologically confirmed thrombosis is not responsive to fibrinolytic treatment or if fibrinolytic or anticoagulation therapy is contraindicated (Anderson et al., 2013; Ast & Ast, 2014; Ragsdale et al., 2014; Schiffer et al., 2013).
Deep vein thrombosis	Hypercoagulable state; type of malignancy; inadequate flushing	Evidence does not support routine administration of prophylactic systemic anticoagulation to decrease incidence of catheter-associated thrombosis. Routine and thorough flushing of the catheter in all lumens with normal saline with use and after blood sampling is recommended to prevent fibrin accumulation that can result in a thrombosis. Meticulous catheter care and adequate flushing using a push-pause, pulsatile, or turbulent technique facilitates thorough rinsing of the intraluminal spaces.	For an occluded clot of the upper extremity, three to six months of anticoagulant therapy with low-molecular-weight heparin (LMWH) or LMWH followed by warfarin is recommended for treatment of symptomatic thrombosis for the life of the catheter. Remove device if not functional, no longer needed, symptoms persist, if infection is suspected within the clot, if radiologically confirmed thrombosis is not responsive to fibrinolytic treatment, or if fibrinolytic or anticoagulation therapy is contraindicated (Ast & Ast, 2014; Jasti & Streiff, 2014; Ragsdale et al., 2014; Schiffer et al., 2013).
Mineral precipitate	Patients receiving concentrated levels of calcium and phosphate in total parenteral nutrition (TPN) at increased risk; inadequate flushing after incompatible medications or solutions	Be aware that 3-in-1 solutions can cause slow occlusions over time. Observe TPN for signs of precipitation prior to administration. Filtering is necessary to avoid occlusion; regular flushing with ethanol alcohol (EtOH) has been shown to decrease the incidence of TPN 3-in-1 precipitation. Change administration set used with TPN solution at least every 24 hours. Meticulous catheter care and adequate flushing using a push-pause, pulsatile, or turbulent technique facilitates thorough rinsing of the intraluminal spaces.	The goal is to increase the solubility of the identified precipitate by altering the pH in the catheter lumen. Sodium bicarbonate (8.4%) is used to dissolve alkaline precipitations. Sodium hydroxide (NaOH) (0.1 normality [N]) also may dissolve alkaline precipitations. Hydrochloric acid (HCl) (0.1 N) compounded specifically for this purpose is used to dissolve acidic precipitations. Extreme caution should be used when instilling HCl into the venous system, as fever, phlebitis, and sepsis can result. Cysteine HCl has been identified in the literature for use in neonates to decrease the pH of TPN solutions. Calcium-phosphate precipitation can be treated with an HCl (0.1 N) instillation (Ast & Ast, 2014; Baskin et al., 2012; Pai & Plogsted, 2014).

(Continued on next page)

Table 9-2. Device Obstructions: Risks, Prevention, and Management *(Continued)*			
Occlusion Type	At Risk	Prevention	Intervention
Drug precipitate	Patients who have received incompatible drugs, forming a precipitate often exhibited as an abrupt occlusion. Phenytoin and heparin are at high risk for precipitation; inadequate flushing between medications.	Proper saline flushing prior to and after drug administration can prevent precipitate formation. Assess for potential of drug incompatibility. Use separate lumens to infuse drugs, if possible. Meticulous catheter care and adequate flushing using a push-pause, pulsatile, or turbulent technique facilitates thorough rinsing of the intraluminal spaces. Ensure adequate flushing between medications. Examples of drugs prone to intraluminal precipitation include • Calcium gluconate • Phenytoin • Diazepam Examples of drugs incompatible with heparin include • Codeine • Cytarabine • Daunorubicin • Dobutamine • Erythromycin • Gentamycin • Hyaluronidase • Kanamycin • Levorphanol • Meperidine • Methadone • Morphine • Polymyxin B • Promethazine • Streptomycin	The goal is to dissolve precipitate. HCl 0.1 N instilled into occluded catheter lumen may dissolve low pH drug precipitates. Extreme caution should be used when instilling HCl into the venous system, as fever, phlebitis, and sepsis can result. Sodium bicarbonate instilled into occluded catheter lumen may dissolve high pH drug precipitates (Ast & Ast, 2014; Baskin et al., 2012).
Lipid residue	Patients receiving regular infusion containing lipids	Use TPN solutions in the first 28 hours after preparation to decrease risk of residue buildup in the catheter.	The goal is to dissolve lipid residue. Instillation of EtOH, NaOH, or ethanol into occluded catheter lumen may restore patency, especially if lipid emulsion buildup associated with TPN is suspected. Meticulous catheter care and adequate flushing using a push-pause, pulsatile, or turbulent technique facilitates thorough rinsing of the intraluminal spaces. A 70% EtOH solution is cited as successful in treatment for mainly lipid residue-based occlusion. Literature supports a combination treatment containing NaOH and EtOH if treatment with one of the agents is ineffective. Note: Alcohol solutions (ethanol or ethyl alcohol) may damage some catheter types; review manufacturer directions and warnings prior to instillation.
Unresolved controversies (see Chapter 1)	Ethanol locks may be associated with plasma protein precipitation	May be minimized or eliminated by limiting the concentration of the lock solution (Schilcher et al., 2013)	Most efficacious irrigation protocol (solution used, time between flushes) remains controversial (Palese et al., 2014; Ragsdale et al., 2014; Restrepo et al., 2015; Schiffer et al., 2013; Schilcher et al., 2013).

4. Research on infection prevention (O'Grady et al., 2011; Schiffer et al., 2013)
   a) Antibiotics: Do not administer antibiotics before the insertion of long-term VADs to prevent gram-positive catheter-related infections.
   b) Antimicrobial catheters: Limited evidence suggests that antimicrobial VADs reduce catheter colonization; however, benefits vary by setting and were only significant in studies conducted in ICUs. The use of antimicrobial-impregnated catheters (chlorhexidine and silver sulfadiazine, or minocycline/rifampin-coated) is recommended for short-term VADs; use remains controversial due to benefits weighed with increased costs. Limited evidence suggests that antimicrobial VADs do not appear to significantly reduce clinically diagnosed sepsis or mortality (Lai et al., 2016; Schiffer et al., 2013).
   c) One quasiexperimental study in ICU/burn/trauma patients found that a switch from uncoated catheters to chlorhexidine-silver-sulfadiazine-coated catheters resulted in a reduction in CLABSI incidence (Mermel, 2015).
   d) Further study is needed (Lai et al., 2016; Schiffer et al., 2013).
   e) No definitive recommendation can be made regarding routine use of antibiotic flushing or antibiotic lock solutions.
   f) Heparin-bonded catheters: Weak evidence exists that time to infection is longer in pediatric patients with heparin-bonded catheters, likely due to decreased fibrin accumulation. No definitive recommendation can be made based on available evidence (Shah & Shah, 2014).
   g) Use a chlorhexidine gluconate (CHG)-impregnated sponge dressing for all catheters, including specialty catheters in patients older than 2 months of age, unless sensitive to CHG (Karpanen et al., 2016; Kerwat et al., 2015; Safdar et al., 2014; Ullman et al., 2015; Wibaux et al., 2015).
   h) Analyses suggest increases in catheter-related bloodstream infections (CRBSIs) with polyurethane (transparent) dressing use; likewise, data also suggest no statistical differences between dressings (gauze versus transparent) in regard to infection incidence.
   i) Further research on gauze and tape versus polyurethane dressings for VAD sites is needed (Pedrolo, Danski, & Vayego, 2014; Webster, Gillies, O'Riordan, Sherriff, & Rickard, 2016).
   j) Catheter lock treatment: Meta-analysis in pediatric patients showed no significant difference between ethanol or urokinase lock treatments with concomitant systemic antibiotics and antibiotics alone regarding the number of catheter-related infections, days to first negative blood culture, number of ICU admissions or cases of sepsis, or number of catheters prematurely removed; however, study group sizes were small (Schoot, van Dalen, van Ommen, & van de Wetering, 2013).
   k) Use of topical antibiotic cream or ointment on insertion sites is not recommended because of the potential to promote fungal infections and antibiotic resistance (Schiffer et al., 2013).
5. Signs and symptoms (see Figure 9-9)
   a) Local infection signs and symptoms include swelling, tenderness, erythema, induration, cellulitis, drainage with positive culture, and tunnelitis (tunneled catheters).

Figure 9-9. Infected Implanted Port

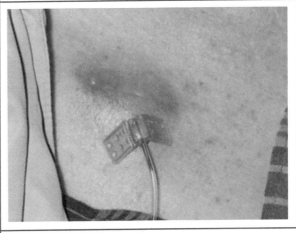

Note. From "Maintenance of Venous Access Devices in Patients With Neutropenia," by A.B. Moran and D. Camp-Sorrell, 2002, *Clinical Journal of Oncology Nursing, 6*, p. 128. Copyright 2002 by Oncology Nursing Society. Reprinted with permission.

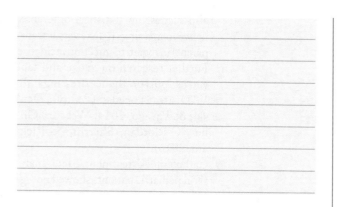

b) Signs of systemic infection include fever, chills, diaphoresis, fatigue, arthralgia, weakness, hypotension, tachycardia, hyperventilation, mental status changes, abdominal pain, vomiting, and diarrhea; may progress to infective endocarditis and septic shock.

6. Diagnostic tests (Bustos et al., 2014; Schiffer et al., 2013)

   a) VAD-related infection is diagnosed when no other detectable site of infection, except for the catheter, is identified.

   b) VAD-related infections can be grouped into three categories: localized insertion-site infections, tunnel or port pocket infections, and CRBSIs.

   c) Local infection is diagnosed by culture of insertion sites, tunnels, and local purulence.

   d) Diagnosis of CRBSIs is based on fever (> 38°C [100.4°F]), chills or hypotension, and positive blood cultures with isolation of the same microorganism from the catheter and bloodstream.

   e) Diagnosis requires that the same microorganism grows from at least one blood culture or from the culture of the catheter tip; with infections of less virulent microorganisms (e.g., *Micrococcus, Corynebacterium, Bacillus*), diagnosis requires that at least two positive results of blood cultures are obtained from samples from different sites. Research suggests that cultures of closed needleless connectors can be used to evaluate catheter tip colonization and are superior to hub cultures for identification of catheter colonization (Guembe, Pérez-Granda, Cruces, Martín-Rabadán, & Bouza, 2015).

   f) Draw blood cultures from each catheter lumen. A positive differential quantitative blood culture that is threefold greater than an identical bacterial colony count in a specimen from a peripheral vein is indicative of infection.

      (1) When it is not possible to obtain blood from a peripheral vein or if the patient has a multilumen catheter, guidelines suggest that diagnosis of catheter-related bacteremia can be made by isolating 100 or greater colony-forming units per milliliter of bacteria from a single quantitative blood culture drawn from one of the lumens of the catheter.

      (2) Recent evidence suggests that, in the event of inadequate sample size from any specific lumen, sampling each catheter lumen and pooling the blood into one culture bottle is as effective as individually cultured samples to substantiate colonization or CLABSI diagnosis. This option is considered a better choice than sampling only one lumen when sending multiple blood culture bottles (Herrera-Guerra, Garza-González, Martínez-Resendez, Llaca-Díaz, & Camacho-Ortiz, 2015).

   g) Diagnosing catheter-related bacteremia after catheter removal has traditionally required a culture of 4 cm of the catheter tip.

   h) Following removal, the portal bodies of implanted ports should be cultured by slicing the silicone septum and culturing the portal body reservoir. Microorganisms most commonly implicated in CRBSI are coagulase-negative *Staphylococcus, Staphylococcus aureus*, enteric gram-negative bacilli, *Pseudomonas* species, and *Candida* species.

7. Management (Bustos et al., 2014; Schiffer et al., 2013; Yacobovich et al., 2015)

   a) Most insertion-site infections can be successfully treated with appropriate antimicrobial therapy, with the catheter remaining in place.

b) Infected catheters are treated by initiating local and systemic antimicrobials. Choice of antimicrobial agent depends on culture results; empiric treatment is routinely started until culture results are available.

c) Vancomycin is considered the drug of choice for empiric treatment.

d) When the catheter remains in place, empiric antimicrobial treatment is administered systemically (IV) and locally (antibiotic lock technique) for 10–14 days and sometimes longer.

e) Use antibiotic lock therapy once catheter-related infection is diagnosed, or if the patient is at high risk of infection; however, the frequency, length of dwell time, and whether or not to discard or flush antibiotic dwell has not been determined. Sensitivities of the organism dictate antibiotic use (Chesshyre et al., 2015; Fernández-Hidalgo & Almirante, 2014; Justo & Bookstaver, 2014; Raad & Chaftari, 2014; van de Wetering, van Woensel, & Lawrie, 2013; Zhang, Gowardman, Morrison, Runnegar, & Rickard, 2016).

f) Flushing or locking long-term VADs with a combined antibiotic and heparin solution appears to reduce gram-positive catheter-related sepsis in people at risk of neutropenia from chemotherapy or bone marrow disease. However, the use of a combined antibiotic and heparin solution may increase microbial antibiotic resistance; therefore, it should be reserved for those at high risk or where baseline VAD infection rates are high (> 15%) (Centers for Disease Control and Prevention, 2016; Justo & Bookstaver, 2014; Raad & Chaftari, 2014; van de Wetering et al., 2013).

g) Antibiotic lock technique consists of infusing a concentrated antimicrobial solution in a small volume to fill the catheter lumen to penetrate biofilm and eradicate bacteria (Schiffer et al., 2013).

h) VAD removal is required for signs of SC tunnel infection (tunneled catheters); suppurative phlebitis; septic shock; peripheral or pulmonary embolization; infective endocarditis; persistent bacteremia; or recurrent infection despite adequate antimicrobial treatment.

i) Catheter retention is associated with a high risk of bacteremia recurrence as well as hospital readmission (Khong, Baggs, Kleinbaum, Cochran, & Jernigan, 2015).

G. Device damage (Balsorano et al., 2014; Busch et al., 2012; El Hammoumi et al., 2014; Ghaderian, Sabri, & Ahmadi, 2015; Gurkan et al., 2015)

1. Etiologies: Preinsertion damage or damage during insertion (e.g., nicking of catheter, guidewire puncture of catheter; suture occlusion of catheter); postinsertion damage of external catheters (e.g., nicking with scissors or clamping); forceful flushing that ruptures catheter; separation of catheter from portal body

2. Signs and symptoms: Visible leak, moist dressing, pain, edema, visible portal body, inability to withdraw blood; evidence of extravasation; note that the patient may be asymptomatic, despite catheter fracture with embolization of fragments (Shimizu et al., 2014).

3. Diagnostic tests: Observation of leak in external catheter during flushing; chest x-ray or dye study/cathetergram

4. Management

a) Over-the-guidewire exchange of ruptured external venous catheter

b) Repair of external portion of PICC or tunneled catheter using manufacturer's repair kit using maximum sterile barrier precautions

c) Device removal and replacement

H. Extravasation of vesicant or irritant chemotherapy and noncytotoxic drugs (Gonzalez, 2013; Le & Patel, 2014; Molas-Ferrer et al., 2015): Leakage or escape of infusate from the vessel into the surrounding tissue; severity depends on the drug used and its mechanism of action and/or properties (see Figure 9-10).

1. Etiology

a) Irritants may cause inflammation, pain, or burning, with rare subsequent tissue necrosis that is volume or high-concentration dependent.

b) Vesicants may cause local blisters, pain, or extensive damage of underlying layers of tissue, leading to tissue necrosis if left untreated.

Figure 9-10. Untreated Doxorubicin-Associated Extravasation

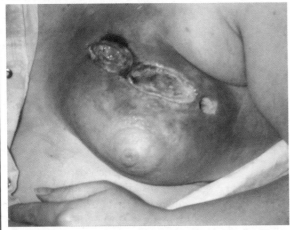

Photo A: Ulceration 8 weeks after doxorubicin administration

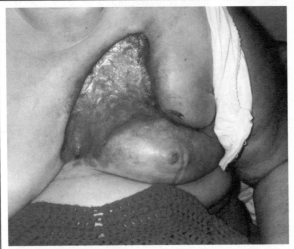

Photo B: Surgical debridement

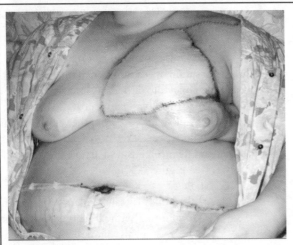

Photo C: Surgical resection 12 weeks post initial extravasation

Note. From "Chemotherapy Extravasation From Implanted Ports," by L. Schulmeister and D. Camp-Sorrell, 2000, *Oncology Nursing Forum, 27,* p. 535. Copyright 2000 by Oncology Nursing Society. Reprinted with permission.

---

    c) Irritants with vesicant properties can cause damage similar to vesicants.

    d) Antineoplastics that bind with DNA cause indolent and progressive tissue destruction; agents that do not bind with DNA remain contained locally.

2. Risk factors

    a) Patient movement that causes dislodgment of noncoring needle from implanted port

    b) Incomplete noncoring needle insertion into implanted port

    c) Separation of catheter from portal body

    d) Ruptured/damaged catheter

    e) VAD catheter tip migration into the SC tissue

    f) Backtracking of vesicant along extraluminal surface of catheter due to fibrin sheath

    g) Low pH and high osmolar solutions, diluents used in solutions, vasoactive properties of drug infused, presence of inactive ingredients that may cause vein irritation

    h) Treatment regimens with more than one vesicant or irritant drug

3. Prevention

    a) Use an appropriate size and length of noncoring needle and ensure needle stabilization.

    b) Ensure brisk blood return. Ensure consistent verification of blood return prior to, during, and after infusion.

    c) Use short-acting topical anesthetics prior to port access (if indicated) to ensure that the patient can sense early symptoms of extravasation.

    d) Use a transparent dressing to allow visualization of the site. Secure port needle. Consider tension loop or use of other securement device.

    e) Monitor IV site throughout the infusion.

    f) Instruct the patient to promptly report signs and symptoms of extravasation, such as burning, pain, or discomfort; discontinue vesicant administration at first sign of extravasation.

4. Signs and symptoms: Absence of blood return during or following infusion; redness; edema; pain; burning; difficulty infusing solution; leaking around the port noncoring needle, tunnel exit site, or PICC exit site or under dressing

5. Management (Polovich, Olsen, & LeFebvre, 2014)

a) Stop infusion.

b) Aspirate residual drug from the catheter or noncoring needle using a 5 ml syringe.

c) Remove noncoring needle from port septum, unless antidote is given through existing port needle; then remove.

d) Assess site of suspected extravasation; estimate amount of extravasated vesicant.

e) Administer antidote or extravasation treatment, as indicated.

f) Apply cold or heat, as indicated.

g) Determine the cause of extravasation, notify the physician, measure and photograph the site, document findings, provide patient education, and schedule follow-up appointments.

References

Akl, E.A., Ramly, E.P., Kahale, L.A., Yosuico, V.E.D., Barba, M., Sperati, F., … Schünemann, H. (2014). Anticoagulation for people with cancer and central venous catheters. *Cochrane Database of Systematic Reviews, 2014*(5). doi:10.1002/14651858.CD006468.pub5

Anderson, D.M., Pesaturo, K.A., Casavant, J., & Ramsey, E.Z. (2013). Alteplase for the treatment of catheter occlusion in pediatric patients. *Annals of Pharmacotherapy, 47*, 405–410. doi:10.1345/aph.1Q483

Ast, D., & Ast, T. (2014). Nonthrombotic complications related to central vascular access devices. *Journal of Infusion Nursing, 37*, 349–358. doi:10.1097/NAN.0000000000000063

Balsorano, P., Galducci, G., De Fanti, I., Evans, S.K., De Gaudio, A.R., & Pelagatti, C. (2014). Fractures of totally implantable central venous ports: More than fortuity. A three-year single center experience. *Journal of Vascular Access, 15*, 391–395. doi:10.5301/jva.5000261

Baskin, J.L., Reiss, U., Wilimas, J.A., Metzger, M.L., Ribeiro, R.C., Pui, C.-H., & Howard, S.C. (2012). Thrombolytic therapy for central venous catheter occlusion. *Haematologica, 97*, 641–650. doi:10.3324/haematol.2011.050492

Beccaria, P., Silvetti, S., Mucci, M., Battini, I., Brambilla, P., & Zangrillo, A. (2015). Contributing factors for a late spontaneous peripherally inserted central catheter migration: A case report and review of literature. *Journal of Vascular Access, 16*, 178–182. doi:10.5301/jva.5000337

Berardi, R., Rinaldi, S., Santini, D., Vincenzi, B., Giampieri, R., Maccaroni, E., … Cascinu, S. (2015). Increased rates of local complication of central venous catheters in the targeted anticancer therapy era: A 2-year retrospective analysis. *Supportive Care in Cancer, 23*, 1295–1302. doi:10.1007/s00520-014-2466-y

Blackwood, B.P., Farrow, K.N., Kim, S., & Hunter, C.J. (2015). Peripherally inserted central catheters complicated by vascular erosion in neonates. *Journal of Parenteral and Enteral Nutrition, 40*, 890–895. doi:10.1177/0148607115574000

Boddi, M., Villa, G., Chiostri, M., De Antoniis, F., De Fanti, I., Spinelli, A., … Pelagatti, C. (2015). Incidence of ultrasound-detected asymptomatic long-term central vein catheter-related thrombosis and fibrin sheath in cancer patients. *European Journal of Haematology, 95*, 472–479. doi:10.1111/ejh.12519

Brass, P., Hellmich, M., Kolodziej, L., Schick, G., & Smith, A.F. (2015). Ultrasound guidance versus anatomical landmarks for internal jugular vein catheterization. *Cochrane Database of Systematic Reviews, 2015*(2). doi:10.1002/14651858.CD006962.pub2

Broadhurst, D., Moureau, N., & Ullman, A.J. (2016). Central venous access devices site care practices: An international survey of 34 countries. *Journal of Vascular Access, 17*, 78–86. doi:10.5301/jva.5000450

Burris, J., & Weis, M.P. (2014). Reduction of erosion risk in adult patients with implanted venous access ports. *Clinical Journal of Oncology Nursing, 18*, 403–405. doi:10.1188/14.CJON.403-405

Busch, J.D., Herrmann, J., Heller, F., Derlin, T., Koops, A., Adam, G., & Habermann, C.R. (2012). Follow-up of radiologically totally implanted central venous access ports of the upper arm: Long-term complications in 127,750 catheter-days. *American Journal of Roentgenology, 199*, 447–452. doi:10.2214/AJR.11.7970

Bustos, C., Aguinaga, A., Carmona-Torre, F., & Del Pozo, J.L. (2014). Long-term catheterization: Current approaches in the diagnosis and treatment of port-related infections. *Infection and Drug Resistance, 4*(7), 25–35. doi:10.2147/IDR.S37773

Calvache, J.-A., Rodríguez, M.-V., Trochez, A., Klimek, M., Stolker, R.-J., & Lesaffre, E. (2014). Incidence of mechanical complications of central venous catheterization using landmark technique: Do not try more than 3 times. *Journal of Intensive Care Medicine, 31*, 447–452. doi:10.1177/0885066614541407

Centers for Disease Control and Prevention. (2016). Vital signs: Preventing antibiotic-resistant infections in hospitals: United States, 2014. *Morbidity and Mortality Weekly Report (MMWR)*. Retrieved from http://www.cdc.gov/mmwr/volumes/65/wr/mm6509e1.htm

Chesshyre, E., Goff, Z., Bowen, A., & Carapetis, J. (2015). Diagnosis and management of central venous line catheter infections in children. *Journal of Infection, 71*(Suppl. 1), S59–S75. doi:10.1016/j.jinf.2015.04.029

Chopra, V., Fallouh, N., McGuirk, H., Salata, B., Healy, C., Kabaeva, Z., … Flanders. S.A. (2015). Patterns, risk factors and treatment associated with PICC-DVT in hospitalized patients: A nested case-control study. *Thrombosis Research, 135*, 829–834. doi:10.1016/j.thromres.2015.02.012

Chopra, V., O'Horo, J.C., Rogers, M.A.M., Maki, D.G., & Safdar, N. (2013). The risk of bloodstream infection associated with peripherally inserted central venous catheters compared with central venous catheters in adults: A systematic review and meta-analysis. *Infection Control and Hospital Epidemiology, 34*, 908–918. doi:10.1086/671737

Chopra, V., Ratz, D., Kuhn, L., Lopus, T., Lee, A., & Krein, S. (2014). Peripherally inserted central catheter-related deep vein thrombosis: Contemporary patterns and predictors. *Journal of Thrombosis and Haemostasis, 12*, 847–854. doi:10.1111/jth.12549

Ciocson, M.A.F.R., Hernandez, M.G., Atallah, M., & Amer, Y.S. (2014). Central vascular access device: An adapted evidence-based clinical practice guideline. *Journal of the Association for Vascular Access, 19*, 221–237. doi:10.1016/j.java.2014.09.002

Clemence, B.J., & Maneval, R.E. (2014). Risk factors associated with catheter-related upper extremity deep vein thrombosis in patients with peripherally inserted central venous catheters: Literature review: Part I. *Journal of Infusion Nursing, 37*, 187–196. doi:10.1097/NAN.0000000000000037

Conway, M.A., McCollom, C., & Bannon, C. (2014). Central venous catheter flushing recommendations: A systematic evidence-based practice review. *Journal of Pediatric Oncology Nursing, 31*, 185–190. doi:10.1177/1043454214532028

Cook, L.S. (2013). Infusion-related air embolism. *Journal of Infusion Nursing, 36*, 26–36. doi:10.1097/NAN.0b013e318279a804

Cortellaro, F., Mellace, L., Paglia, S., Costantino, G., Sher, S., & Coen, D. (2014). Contrast enhanced ultrasound vs chest x-ray to determine correct central venous catheter position. *American Journal of Emergency Medicine, 32*, 78–81. doi:10.1016/j.ajem.2013.10.001

Cotogni, P., & Pittiruti, M. (2014). Focus on peripherally inserted central catheters in critically ill patients. *World Journal of Critical Care Medicine, 3*(4), 80–94. doi:10.5492/wjccm.v3.i4.80

Dalton, M., Pheil, N., Lacy, J., & Dalton, J. (2014). Does sludge/debris exist in today's vascular access ports? *Journal of the Association for Vascular Access, 19,* 23–26. doi:10.1016/j.java.2013.12.002

D'Ambrosio, L., Aglietta, M., & Grignani, G. (2014). Anticoagulation for central venous catheters in patients with cancer. *New England Journal of Medicine, 371,* 1362–1363. doi:10.1056/NEJMc1408861

Debourdeau, P., Farge, D., Beckers, M., Baglin, C., Bauersachs, R.M., Brenner, B., … Bounameaux, H. (2013). International clinical practice guidelines for the treatment and prophylaxis of thrombosis associated with central venous catheters in patients with cancer. *Journal of Thrombosis and Haemostasis, 11,* 71–80. doi:10.1111/jth.12071

Duffy, E.A., Rodgers, C.C., Shever, L.L., & Hockenberry, M.J. (2015). Implementing a daily maintenance care bundle to prevent central line–associated bloodstream infections in pediatric oncology patients. *Journal of Pediatric Oncology Nursing, 32,* 394–400. doi:10.1177/1043454214563756

El Hammoumi, M., El Ouazani, M., Arsalane, A., El Oueriachi, F., Mansouri, H., & Kabiri, E.H. (2014). Incidents and complications of permanent venous central access systems: A series of 1,460 cases. *Korean Journal of Thoracic and Cardiovascular Surgery, 47,* 117–123. doi:10.5090/kjtcs.2014.47.2.117

Elyamany, G., Alzahrani, A.M., & Bukhary, E. (2014). Cancer-associated thrombosis: An overview. *Clinical Medicine Insights: Oncology, 8,* 129–137. doi:10.4137/CMO.S18991

Fallouh, N., McGuirk, H.M., Flanders, S.A., & Chopra, V. (2015). Peripherally inserted central catheter-associated deep vein thrombosis: A narrative review. *American Journal of Medicine, 128,* 722–738. doi:10.1016/j.amjmed.2015.01.027

Fernández-Hidalgo, N., & Almirante, B. (2014). Antibiotic-lock therapy: A clinical viewpoint. *Expert Reviews of Anti-Infective Therapy, 12,* 117–129. doi:10.1586/14787210.2014.863148

Ferrer, J., Boelle, P.-Y., Salomon, J., Miliani, K., L'Hériteau, F., Astagneau, P., & Temime, L. (2014). Management of nurse shortage and its impact on pathogen dissemination in the intensive care unit. *Epidemics, 9,* 62–69. doi:10.1016/j.epidem.2014.07.002

Flodgren, G., Conterno, L.O., Mayhew, A., Omar, O., Pereira, C.R., & Shepperd, S. (2013). Interventions to improve professional adherence to guidelines for prevention of device-related infections. *Cochrane Database of Systematic Reviews, 2013*(2). doi:10.1002/14651858.CD006559.pub2

Franchini, M. (2015). Thromboembolic risk in hematological malignancies. *Clinical Chemistry and Laboratory Medicine, 53,* 1139–1147. doi:10.1515/cclm-2014-1010

Freire, M.P., Pierrotti, L.C., Zerati, A.E., Araújo, P.H.X.N., Motta-Leal-Filho, J.M., Duarte, L.P.G., … Abdala, E. (2013). Infection related to implantable central venous access devices in cancer patients: Epidemiology and risk factors. *Infection Control and Hospital Epidemiology, 34,* 671–677. doi:10.1086/671006

García-Gabás, C., Castillo-Ayala, A., Hinojo-Marín, B., Muriel-Abajo, M.A., Gómez-Gutiérrez, I., de Mena-Arenas, A.M., … Madroñero-Agreda, M.A. (2015). Complications associated to central venous catheters in hematology patients. *Enfermeria Clinica, 25,* 138–142. doi:10.1016/j.enfcli.2015.03.003

Geerts, W. (2014). Central venous catheter-related thrombosis. *Hematology: American Society of Hematology Education Program, 2014,* 306–311. doi:10.1182/asheducation-2014.1.306

Ghaderian, M., Sabri, M.R., & Ahmadi, A.R. (2015). Percutaneous retrieval of an intracardiac central venous port fragment using snare with triple loops. *Journal of Research in Medical Sciences, 20*(1), 97–99.

Gonzalez, T. (2013). Chemotherapy extravasations: Prevention, identification, management, and documentation. *Clinical Journal of Oncology Nursing, 17,* 61–66. doi:10.1188/13.CJON.61-66

Guembe, M., Pérez-Granda, M.J., Cruces, R., Martín-Rabadán, P., & Bouza, E. (2015). Cultures of needleless connectors are useful for ruling out central venous catheter colonization. *Journal of Clinical Microbiology, 53,* 2068–2071. doi:10.1128/JCM.00459-15

Gurkan, S., Seber, S., Gur, O., Yetisyigit, T., Okan Donbaloglu, M., & Ozkaramanli Gur, D. (2015). Retrospective evaluation of totally implantable venous access port devices: Early and late complications. *Journal of Balkan Union of Oncology, 20,* 338–345.

Hajjar, K.A. (2015). Central venous catheter thrombosis and the fibrin sleeve: Unraveling the mystery. *European Journal of Haematology.* Advance online publication. doi:10.1111/ejh.12642

Harish, K. (2014). Chemoport-skin erosion: Our experience. *International Journal of Angiology, 23,* 215–216. doi:10.1055/s-0033-1353734

Heidari Gorji, M.A., Rezaei, F., Jafari, H., & Yazdani Cherati, J. (2015). Comparison of the effects of heparin and 0.9% sodium chloride solutions in maintenance of patency of central venous catheters. *Anesthesiology and Pain Medicine, 5,* e22595. doi:10.5812/aapm.22595

Herrera-Guerra, A.S., Garza-González, E., Martínez-Resendez, M.F., Llaca-Díaz, J.M., & Camacho-Ortiz, A. (2015). Individual versus pooled multiple-lumen blood cultures for the diagnosis of intravascular catheter-related infections. *American Journal of Infection Control, 43,* 715–718. doi:10.1016/j.ajic.2015.02.028

Hodzic, S., Golic, D., Smajic, J., Sijercic, S., Umihanic, S., & Umihanic, S. (2014). Complications related to insertion and use of central venous catheters (CVC). *Medical Archives, 68,* 300–303.

Institute for Healthcare Improvement. (2016). Central line infection. Retrieved from http://www.ihi.org/topics/centrallineinfection/Pages/default.aspx

Jabeen, S., Murtaza, G., Hanif, M.Z., Morabito, A., & Khalil, B. (2014). Migration of indwelling central venous catheter and fatal hydrothorax. *European Journal of Pediatric Surgery Reports, 2*(1), 32–34. doi:10.1055/s-0033-1347130

Jasti, N., & Streiff, M.B. (2014). Prevention and treatment of thrombosis associated with central venous catheters in cancer patients. *Expert Review in Hematology, 7,* 599–616. doi:10.1586/17474086.2014.954541

Jia, L., Yu, H., Lu, J., Zhang, Y., Cai, Y., Liu, Y., & Ma, X. (2015). Epidemiological characteristics and risk factors for patients with catheter-related bloodstream infections in intensive care unit. *Zhonghua Yi Xue Za Zhi, 95,* 654–658. Retrieved from http://www.ivteam.com/intravenous-literature/epidemiological-characteristics-and-risk-factors-for-clabsi

Jin, J., Chen, C., Zhao, R., Li, A., Shentu, Y., & Jiang, N. (2012). Repositioning techniques of malpositioned peripherally inserted central catheters. *Journal of Clinical Nursing, 22,* 1791–1804. doi:10.1111/jocn.12004

Jumani, K., Advani, S., Reich, N.G., Gosey, L., & Milstone, A.M. (2013). Risk factors for peripherally inserted central venous catheter complications in children. *JAMA Pediatrics, 167,* 429–435. doi:10.1001/jamapediatrics.2013.775

Justo, J.A., & Bookstaver, P.B. (2014). Antibiotic lock therapy: Review of technique and logistical challenges. *Journal of Infection and Drug Resistance, 12,* 343–363. doi:10.2147/IDR.S51388

Karpanen, T.J., Casey, A.L., Whitehouse, T., Nightingale, P., Das, I., & Elliott, T.S.J. (2016). Clinical evaluation of a chlorhexidine intravascular catheter gel dressing on short-term central venous catheters. *American Journal of Infection Control, 44*(1), 54–60. doi:10.1016/j.ajic.2015.08.022

Kaur, M., Gupta, V., Gombar, S., Chander, J., & Sahoo, T. (2015). Incidence, risk factors, microbiology of venous catheter associated bloodstream infections: A prospective study from a tertiary care hospital. *Indian Journal of Medical Microbiology, 33,* 248–254. doi:10.4103/0255-0857.153572

Kerwat, K., Eberhart, L., Kerwat, M., Hörth, D., Wulf, H., Steinfeldt, T., & Wiesmann, T. (2015). Chlorhexidine gluconate dressings reduce bacterial colonization rates in epidural and peripheral regional catheters. *Biomed Research International, 2015,* 149785. doi:10.1155/2015/149785

Khasawneh, F.A., & Smalligan, R.D. (2011). Guidewire-related complications during central venous catheter placement: A case report and review of the literature. *Case Reports in Critical Care, 2011*, 287261. doi:10.1155/2011/287261

Khong, C.J., Baggs, J., Kleinbaum, D., Cochran, R., & Jernigan, J.A. (2015). The likelihood of hospital readmission among patients with hospital-onset central line–associated bloodstream infections. *Infection Control and Hospital Epidemiology, 36*, 886–892. doi:10.1017/ice.2015.115

Kim, H.J., Park, S.H., Shin, H.Y., & Choi, Y.S. (2014). Brachial plexus injury as a complication after nerve block or vessel puncture. *Korean Journal of Pain, 27*, 210–218. doi:10.3344/kjp.2014.27.3.210

Kulkarni, S., Wu, O., Kasthuri, R., & Moss, J.G. (2014). Centrally inserted external catheters and totally implantable ports for the delivery of chemotherapy: A systematic review and meta-analysis of device-related complications. *Cardiovascular and Interventional Radiology, 37*, 990–1008. doi:10.1007/s00270-013-0771-3

Lai, N.M., Chaiyakunapruk, N., Lai, N.A., O'Riordan, E., Pau, W.S.C., & Saint, S. (2016). Catheter impregnation, coating or bonding for reducing central venous catheter-related infections in adults. *Cochrane Database of Systematic Reviews, 2016*(3). doi:10.1002/14651858.CD007878.pub3

Le, A., & Patel, S. (2014). Extravasation of noncytotoxic drugs: A review of the literature. *Annals of Pharmacotherapy, 48*, 870–886. doi:10.1177/1060028014527820

Linnemann, B. (2014). Management of complications related to central venous catheters in cancer patients: An update. *Seminars in Thrombosis and Hemostasis, 40*, 382–394. doi:10.1055/s-0034-1371005

López-Briz, E., Garcia, V.R., Cabello, J.B., Bort-Marti, S., Sanchis, R.C., & Burls, A. (2014). Heparin versus 0.9% sodium chloride intermittent flushing for prevention of occlusion in central venous catheters in adults. *Cochrane Database of Systematic Reviews, 2014*(2). doi:10.1002/14651858.CD008462.pub2

Lyons, M.G., & Phalen, A.G. (2014). A randomized controlled comparison of flushing protocols in home care patients with peripherally inserted central catheters. *Journal of Infusion Nursing, 37*, 270–281. doi:10.1097/NAN.0000000000000050

Massmann, A., Jagoda, P., Kranzhoefer, N., & Buecker, A. (2015). Percutaneous re-positioning of dislocated portal-catheters in patients with dysfunctional central-vein port-systems. *Annals of Surgical Oncology, 22*, 4124–4129. doi:10.1245/s10434-015-4549-5

Mermel, L.A. (2015). Effectiveness of minocycline/rifampin vs. chlorhexidine/silver sulfadiazine-impregnated central venous catheters. *Journal of the American College of Surgeons, 221*, 891–892. doi:10.1001/jamainternmed.2015.36

Mermel, L.A., & Parienti, J.-J. (2015). Insertion site for central venous catheters. *JAMA Internal Medicine, 175*, 861–862. doi:10.1001/jamainternmed.2015.36

Molas-Ferrer, G., Farré-Ayuso, E., doPazo-Oubiña, F., deAndrés-Lázaro, A., Guell-Picazo, J., Borrás-Maixenchs, N., … Creus-Baró, N. (2015). Level of adherence to an extravasation protocol over 10 years in a tertiary care hospital [Online exclusive]. *Clinical Journal of Oncology Nursing, 19*, E25–E30. doi:10.1188/15.cjon.e25-e30

Morano, S.G., Latagliata, R., Girmenia, C., Massaro, F., Berneschi, P., Guerriero, A., … Foa, R. (2015). Catheter-associated bloodstream infections and thrombotic risk in hematologic patients with peripherally inserted central catheters (PICC). *Supportive Care in Cancer, 23*, 3289–3295. doi:10.1007/s00520-015-2740-7

Murray, J., Precious, E., & Alikhan, R. (2013). Catheter-related thrombosis in cancer patients. *British Journal of Haematology, 162*, 748–757. doi:10.1111/bjh.12474

National Comprehensive Cancer Network. (2016). *NCCN Clinical Practice Guidelines in Oncology (NCCN Guidelines®): Cancer-associated venous thromboembolic disease* [v.1.2016]. Retrieved from http://www.nccn.org/professionals/physician_gls/pdf/vte.pdf

Odabas, H., Ozdemir, N.Y., Ziraman, I., Aksoy, S., Abali, H., Oksuzoglu, B., … Zengin, N. (2014). Effect of port-care frequency on venous port catheter-related complications in cancer patients. *International Journal of Clinical Oncology, 19*, 761–766. doi:10.1007/s10147-013-0609-7

O'Grady, N.P., Alexander, M., Burns, L.A., Dellinger, E.P., Garland, J., Heard, S.O., … Healthcare Infection Control Practices Advisory Committee. (2011). Guidelines for the prevention of intravascular catheter-related infections. *Clinical Infectious Diseases, 52*, E162–E193. doi:10.1093/cid/cir257

Oh, J.S., Choi, B.G., Chun, H.J., & Lee, H.G. (2015). Mechanical thrombolysis of thrombosed central venous port. *Cardiovascular and Interventional Radiology, 37*, 1358–1362. doi:10.1007/s00270-014-0956-4

Pai, V.B., & Plogsted, S. (2014). Efficacy and safety of using L-cysteine as a catheter-clearing agent for nonthrombotic occlusions of central venous catheters in children. *Nutrition in Clinical Practice, 29*, 636–638. doi:10.1177/0884533614539177

Palese, A., Baldassar, D., Rupil, A., Bonanni, G., Capellari, M.T., Contessi, D., … Zanini, A. (2014). Maintaining patency in totally implantable venous access devices (TIVAD): A time-to-event analysis of different lock irrigation intervals. *European Journal of Oncology Nursing, 18*, 66–71. doi:10.1016/j.ejon.2013.09.002

Parienti, J.-J., Mongardon, N., Mégarbane, B., Mira, J.-P., Kalfon, P., Gros, A., …. du Cheyron, D. (2015). Intravascular complications of central venous catheterization by insertion site. *New England Journal of Medicine, 373*, 1220–1229. doi:10.1056/NEJMoa1500964

Park, C.K., Paes, B.A., Nagel, K., Chan, A.K., Murthy, P., & Thrombosis and Hemostasis in Newborns Group. (2014). Neonatal central venous catheter thrombosis: Diagnosis, management and outcome. *Blood Coagulation and Fibrinolysis, 25*, 97–106. doi:10.1097/MBC.0b013e328364f9b0

Pedrolo, E., Danski, M.T.R., & Vayego, S.A. (2014). Chlorhexidine and gauze and tape dressings for central venous catheters: A randomized clinical trial. *Revista Latino-Americana de Enfermagem, 22*, 764–771. doi:10.1590/0104-1169.3443.2478

Polovich, M., Olsen, M., & LeFebvre, K.B. (Eds.). (2014). *Chemotherapy and biotherapy guidelines and recommendations for practice*. Pittsburgh, PA: Oncology Nursing Society.

Prabaharan, B., & Thomas, S. (2014). Spontaneous migration of central venous catheter tip following extubation. *Saudi Journal of Anesthesia, 8*, 131–133. doi:10.4103/1658-354X.125975

Raad, I., & Chaftari, A.M. (2014). Advances in prevention and management of central line-associated bloodstream infections in patients with cancer. *Clinical Infectious Diseases, 59*(Suppl. 5), S340–S343. doi:10.1093/cid/ciu670

Ragsdale, C.E., Oliver, M.R., Thompson, A.J., & Evans, M.C. (2014). Alteplase infusion versus dwell for clearance of partially occluded central venous catheters in critically ill pediatric patients. *Pediatric Critical Care Medicine, 15*, e253–e260. doi:10.1097/PCC.0000000000000125

Restrepo, D., Laconi, N.S., Alcantar, N.A., West, L.A., Buttice, A.L., Patel, S., & Kayton, M.L. (2015). Inhibition of heparin precipitation, bacterial growth, and fungal growth with a combined isopropanol-ethanol locking solution for vascular access devices. *Journal of Pediatric Surgery, 50*, 472–477. doi:10.1016/j.jpedsurg.2014.07.003

Rhee, Y., Heung, M., Chen, B., & Chenoweth, C.E. (2015). Central line-associated bloodstream infections in non-ICU inpatient wards: A 2-year analysis. *Infection Control and Hospital Epidemiology, 36*, 424–430. doi:10.1017/ice.2014.86

Safdar, N., O'Horo, J.C., Ghufran, A., Bearden, A., Didier, M.E., Chateau, D., & Maki, D.G. (2014). Chlorhexidine-impregnated dressing for prevention of catheter-related bloodstream infection: A meta-analysis. *Critical Care Medicine, 42*, 1703–1713. doi:10.1097/CCM.0000000000000319

Salimi, F., Hekmatnia, A., Shahabi, J., Keshavarzian, A., Maracy, M.R., & Jazi, A.H.D. (2015). Evaluation of routine postoperative chest roentgenogram for determination of the correct position of permanent central venous catheters tip. *Journal of Research in Medical Sciences, 20*(1), 89–92.

Schalk, E., Hanus, L., Färber, J., Fischer, T., & Heidel, F.H. (2015). Prediction of central venous catheter-related bloodstream infections (CRBSIs) in patients with haematologic malignancies using a modified Infection Probability Score (miPS). *Annals of Hematology, 94*, 1451–1456. doi:10.1007/s00277-015-2387-y

Schiffer, C.A., Mangu, P.B., Wade, J.C., Camp-Sorrell, D., Cope, D.G., El-Rayes, B.F., … Levine, M. (2013). Central venous catheter care for the patient with cancer: American Society of Clinical Oncology clinical practice guideline. *Journal of Clinical Oncology, 31*, 1357–1370. doi:10.1200/JCO.2012.45.5733

Schilcher, G., Schlagenhauf, A., Schneditz, D., Scharnagl, H., Ribitsch, W., Krause, R., … Horina, J.H. (2013). Ethanol causes protein precipitation: New safety issues for catheter locking techniques. *PLOS ONE, 8*, e84869. doi:10.1371/journal.pone.0084869

Schneider, L., Duron, S., Arnaud, F.-X., Bousquet, A., Kervella, Y., Bouzad, C., … Potet, J. (2015). Evaluation of PICC complications in orthopedic inpatients with bone infection for long-term intravenous antibiotics therapy. *Journal of Vascular Access, 16*, 299–308. doi:10.5301/jva.5000389

Schoot, R.A., van Dalen, E.C., van Ommen, C.H., & van de Wetering, M.D. (2013). Antibiotic and other lock treatments for tunneled central venous catheter-related infections in children with cancer. *Cochrane Database of Systematic Reviews, 2013*(2). doi:10.1002/14651858.CD008975.pub2

Shah, P.S., & Shah, N. (2014). Heparin-bonded catheters for prolonging the patency of central venous catheters in children. *Cochrane Database of Systematic Reviews, 2014*(3). doi:10.1002/14651858.CD005983.pub3

Shimizu, A., Lefor, A., Nakata, M., Mitsuhashi, U., Tanaka, M., & Yasuda, Y. (2014). Embolization of a fractured central venous catheter placed using the internal jugular approach. *International Journal of Surgery Case Reports, 5*, 219–221. doi:10.1016/j.ijscr.2014.02.001

Snarski, E., Mank, A., Iacobelli, S., Hoek, J., Styczyński, J., Babic, A., … Johansson, E. (2015). Current practices used for the prevention of central venous catheter-associated infection in hematopoietic stem cell transplantation recipients: A survey from the Infectious Diseases Working Party and Nurses' Group of EBMT. *Transplant Infectious Disease, 17*, 558–565. doi:10.1111/tid.12399

Song, M.G., Seo, T.-S., Kang, E.Y., Yong, H.S., Seo, J.H., & Choi, Y.Y. (2015). Innominate vein stenosis in breast cancer patients after totally implantable venous access port placement. *Journal of Vascular Access, 16*, 315–320. doi:10.5301/jva.5000387

Stone, P.W., Pogorzelska-Maziarz, M., Herzig, C.T.A., Weiner, L.M., Furuya, E.Y., Dick, A., & Larson, E. (2014). State of infection prevention in US hospitals enrolled in the National Health and Safety Network. *American Journal of Infection Control, 42*, 94–99. doi:10.1016/j.ajic.2013.10.003

Sugimoto, T., Nagata, H., Hayashi, K., & Kano, N. (2012). Pinch-off syndrome: Transection of implantable central venous access device. *British Medical Journal Case Reports.* doi:10.1136/bcr-2012-006584

Sundriyal, D., Jain, S., & Manjunath, S. (2014). Difficult to flush chemoport: An important clinical sign. *Indian Journal of Surgical Oncology, 5*, 307–309. doi:10.1007/s13193-014-0354-z

Tamura, A., Sone, M., Ehara, S., Kato, K., Tanaka, R., Nakasato, T., & Itabashi, T. (2014). Is ultrasound-guided central venous port placement effective to avoid pinch-off syndrome? *Journal of Vascular Access, 15*, 311–316. doi:10.5301/jva.5000201

Tazzioli, G., Gargaglia, E., Vecchioni, I., Papi, S., DiBlasio, P., & Rossi, R. (2015). Retained embolized fragment of totally implantable central venous catheter in right ventricle: It is really necessary to remove? *Journal of Vascular Access, 16*, 431–433. doi:10.5301/jva.5000430

Tsotsolis, N., Tsirgogianni, K., Kioumis, I., Pitsiou, G., Baka, S., Papaiwannou, A., … Zarogoulidis, P. (2015). Pneumothorax as a complication of central venous catheter insertion. *Annals of Translational Medicine, 3*, 40. doi:10.3978/j.issn.2305-5839.2015.02.11

Ullman, A.J., Cooke, M.L., Mitchell, M., Lin, F., New, K., Long, D.A., … Rickard, C.M. (2015). Dressings and securement devices for central venous catheters (CVC). *Cochrane Database of Systematic Reviews, 2015*(2). doi:10.1002/14651858.CD010367.pub2

van de Wetering, M.D., van Woensel, J.B.M., & Lawrie, T.A. (2013). Prophylactic antibiotics for preventing gram positive infections associated with long-term central venous catheters in oncology patients. *Cochrane Database of Systematic Reviews, 2013*(3). doi:10.1002/14651858.CD003295.pub3

Walz, J.M., Ellison, R.T., Mack, D.A., Flaherty, H.M., McIlwaine, J.K., Whyte, K.G., … Heard, S.O. (2015). The bundle "plus": The effect of a multidisciplinary team approach to eradicate central line-associated bloodstream infections. *Anesthesia and Analgesia, 120*, 868–876. doi:10.1213/ANE.0b013e3182a8b01b

Webster, J., Gillies, D., O'Riordan, E., Sherriff, K.L., & Rickard, C.M. (2016). Gauze and tape and transparent polyurethane dressings for central venous catheters. *Cochrane Database of Systematic Reviews, 2016*(5). doi:10.1002/14651858.CD003827.pub3

Wibaux, A., Thota, P., Mastej, J., Prince, D.L., Carty, N., & Johnson, P. (2015). Antimicrobial activity of a novel vascular access film dressing containing chlorhexidine gluconate. *PLOS ONE, 10*, e0143035. doi:10.1371/journal.pone.0143035

Wiegering, V., Schmid, S., Andres, O., Wirth, C., Wiegering, A., Meyer, T., … Eyrich, M. (2014). Thrombosis as a complication of central venous access in pediatric patients with malignancies: A 5-year single-center experience. *BMC Hematology, 14*(1), 18. doi:10.1186/2052-1839-14-18

World Health Organization. (n.d.). The evidence for clean hands. Retrieved from http://www.who.int/gpsc/country_work/en

Yacobovich, J., Ben-Ami, T., Abdalla, T., Tamary, H., Goldstein, G., Weintraub, M., … Revel-Vilk, S. (2015). Patient and central venous catheter related risk factors for bloodstream infections in children receiving chemotherapy. *Pediatric Blood and Cancer, 62*, 471–476. doi:10.1002/pbc.25281

York, N. (2012). The importance of ideal central venous access device tip position. *British Journal of Nursing, 21*, S19–S20, S22, S24. doi:10.12968/bjon.2012.21.Sup21.S19

Zhang, L., Gowardman, J., Morrison, M., Runnegar, N., & Rickard, C.M. (2016). Microbial biofilms associated with intravascular catheter-related bloodstream infections in adult intensive care patients. *European Journal of Clinical Microbiology and Infectious Diseases, 35*, 201–205. doi:10.1007/s10096-015-2530-7

Zwicker, J.I., Connolly, G., Carrier, M., Kamphuisen, P.W., & Lee, A.Y.Y. (2014). Catheter-associated deep vein thrombosis of the upper extremity in cancer patients: Guidance from the SSC of the ISTH. *Journal of Thrombosis and Haemostasis, 12*, 796–800. doi:10.1111/jth.12527

Chapter 10

Subcutaneous (Hypodermoclysis) Infusion Devices

Andrea B. Moran, RN, APRN

I. History (Arthur, 2015; Bruno, 2015; Dychter, Gold, & Haller, 2012; Spandorfer, 2011)
  A. The term *hypodermoclysis* (originating from *hypo* + *derma* [skin] + *clysis* [to clean] [Greek]) is also used to describe subcutaneous (SC) infusions.
  B. The first reported use of hypodermoclysis was in 1913 for pediatric dehydration. By the 1950s, hypodermoclysis was out of favor because of reports of shock and deaths caused by severe osmotic shifts as a result of therapy. These complications subsequently were found to be the result of improper technique, inappropriate fluids, excessive fluid volumes, and rapid infusion rates.
  C. SC analgesia infusions were first introduced in England in 1979. Shortly after, this practice began in the United States.
  D. SC therapy has been recognized as a cost-effective means of delivering medication fluid. Although SC therapy is a viable choice for an access device, it often is not reimbursed.
II. Device characteristics (Bartz et al., 2014; Dychter et al., 2012)
  A. Provides continuous, prolonged, or short-term administration of parenteral drugs or fluids into the loose connective tissue underlying the dermis, which consists of large blood vessels, nerves, and adipose tissue (Arthur, 2015; Gabriel, 2013). A short-length catheter or needle is used for several days.
  B. Fluid is absorbed into the intravascular compartment by a combination of perfusion, diffusion, hydrostatic pressure, and osmotic pressure.
  C. SC infusions are particularly well suited for nonacute care settings because of the ease of maintenance, the low probability of systemic complications, the reduced pain on insertion, and the decreased number of needlesticks.
  D. Continuous SC infusion is shown to be as effective as and more cost-effective than IV ther-

apy; it is also a safe option for homecare delivery (Spandorfer, 2011).
III. Device features
  A. Several specific designs are available (Arthur, Goodloe, & Thomas, 2012; Gabriel, 2012, 2013, 2014a, 2014b).
    1. Products used for SC infusions are similar to peripheral IVs.
      a) Small-gauge, short-length, metal butterfly needles: Use only 24 or 27 gauge. Shielded needles are available.
      b) Small-gauge, short-length catheter
        (1) Over-the-needle design
        (2) Use only 24-gauge, ¾-inch catheter.
    2. Use a catheter instead of a butterfly needle to promote increased dwell time, improved patient comfort, and reduced risk of needlestick injury.
    3. Use smaller needles or cannulas to minimize discomfort during insertion.
    4. SC infusion sets are available with a 27-gauge, 90° needle situated on a clear, flexible anchoring disk. Various needle and tubing lengths are available. Sets are designed specifically for pediatric patients with a smaller half-inch disk and 27-gauge needle.
    5. Closed catheter systems are available in needle sizes from 18–24 gauge with an over-the-needle Vialon™ catheter. A telescoping needle shield device minimizes the risk of accidental needlestick (see Figure 10-1).
IV. Device advantages and disadvantages (see Figure 10-2)
V. Patient selection criteria (Arthur et al., 2012; Bartz et al., 2014; Humphrey, 2011; Neo, Khemlani, Sim, & Seah, 2016; Spandorfer, 2011)
  A. Patient age generally does not restrict use.
  B. Primarily used in geriatric and palliative medicine; suitable in acute care, home care, long-term facilities, or hospice settings

Figure 10-1. Closed Subcutaneous System

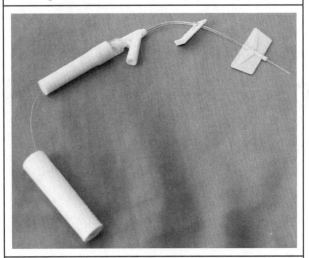

Note. Image courtesy of Andrea B. Moran. Used with permission.

Figure 10-2. Advantages and Disadvantages of Subcutaneous Infusions

Advantages	Disadvantages
• Simple insertion by RN • Can be used with patient-controlled analgesia ambulatory pumps • Limited supply requirements, minimizing costs • Alternative choice instead of a venous access device for pain management • Suitable for any patient-care setting • Less risk of systemic adverse effect (e.g., septicemia, respiratory distress, infection) • Caregiver can be taught to administer therapy. • No complication risk of thrombophlebitis or thrombosis	• Limited volume for rapid fluid replacement • Small volume available for continuous administration • Depending on infusion site, may cause mobility limitations • Limitations on types of fluids that can be administered • Local reactions can occur, with potential for insertion abscess or cellulitis formation. • Recommended to use volumetric controlled pump for infusions • Not an appropriate device for emergency use

C. Administered by a caregiver or nurse at home
D. Indications
   1. When an oral or transdermal route is inappropriate or ineffective (e.g., bowel obstruction, intractable nausea or vomiting, dysphagia, malabsorption, inadequate oral fluid intake secondary to confusion or infection)
   2. Poor peripheral veins (e.g., obese, older adults, very young patients, those whose veins have been overused)
   3. If a single-lumen, long-term venous access device is being used for other incompatible IV therapy

   4. Patients with delirium, confusion, stupor, or other mental status changes for which oral administration is contraindicated because of aspiration risk
   5. Pain management
     a) Acute pain management when vascular access is difficult (e.g., patients with sickle cell disease who are in pain crisis) (Sandoval, Coleman, Govani, Siddiqui, & Todd, 2013)
     b) Chronic pain management when oral or transdermal route is not available, transdermal route is not tolerated, or no other indications exist for IV therapy (Kawabata & Kaneishi, 2013)
     c) Short-term, self-limiting infusion with a local anesthetic directly into the incision site for operative and postoperative pain
   6. Reduction or alleviation of intractable nausea and vomiting
   7. Hypercalcemia treatment
   8. Iron chelation: For iron removal from transfusional iron overload or hemochromatosis
   9. Fluid replacement: For short-term, reversible fluid deficits when fluid replacement is not an emergency and is less than 3,000 ml/24 hours (Spandorfer, 2011)
  10. Infusion of amino acid solution (Lybarger, 2009)
  11. Infusion of immune gamma globulin
  12. Insulin infusion
E. Contraindications (Arthur, 2015; Spandorfer, 2011)
   1. Generalized edema, poor peripheral circulation, or minimal SC tissue. Cachexia is not an absolute contraindication for SC infusion.
   2. Severe pain when frequent boluses or changes are needed
   3. Bleeding or coagulation disorder
   4. Rapid infusion
   5. Emergency situations (e.g., circulatory failure, severe electrolyte imbalance, severe dehydration)
   6. Medications that are irritants to SC tissue which require IV administration (e.g., potassium, phenytoin)
VI. Insertion techniques (Bartz et al., 2014; Bruno, 2015; D'Arcy, 2010; Gabriel, 2012, 2013)
  A. Infusion sites: Anterior chest wall, upper abdomen, anterior or lateral aspects of thighs, between the scapula on the back, and outer upper arm
   1. For ambulatory patients, the upper chest area (subclavicular area) is recommended because it allows full range of movement.

2. The upper abdomen is best for patients with little peripheral SC tissue, such as with cachectic patients.
3. The access site must have intact skin and be located away from bony prominence and the patient's umbilical area (Scales, 2011).
4. Rotate sites when changing the needle; the needle may remain in the same region.
5. Interscapular or subscapular regions can be useful for confused patients who may attempt to remove the device.
B. Insertion procedure
   1. Explain the purpose of the infusion, the rationale for the type of infusion, and the procedure to the patient and family or significant others.
   2. Select the site. Maintain strict aseptic technique (see Appendix 4).
   3. Prepare the site with a cleansing agent and allow it to dry without fanning (see Appendix 2).
   4. Select the smallest gauge needle or catheter available.
   5. Attach the tubing and infusion bag with fluids or medication and prime the set.
   6. Put on gloves. Stabilize tissue with free hand, holding hand flat in a natural position, or pinching skin slightly. Local anesthetic may be used (see Appendix 7).
   7. Insert the needle with bevel down at about a 20°–30° angle almost up to the hub.
      a) A 45° insertion angle has been recommended as an alternate position (Gabriel, 2012; Spandorfer, 2011).
      b) The angle of the needle depends on the amount of SC tissue available and whether the tissue is held flat or pinched. When minimal SC tissue is available, use a smaller angle to ensure correct placement.
      c) Place needle bevel down so that the fluid is infused into the SC tissue and also to promote absorption.
   8. Secure wings or hub with a securement device.
   9. Check for blood return (i.e., lower unclamped solution bag or pull back on syringe). There should be no blood return, although an air bubble may be seen.
      a) If blood is seen in the tubing, clamp the tubing and remove the needle.
      b) Repeat this procedure using a new needle at an adjacent site.
      c) If no blood is seen, clamp the tubing.
   10. Attach the tubing to the pump, set the correct rate, unclamp the tubing, and turn the pump on. If infusion is not being used, attach a needleless connector.
   11. Cover with semipermeable, transparent dressing. Secure tubing to either dressing or skin.
VII. Unique maintenance and care (Arthur, 2015; D'Arcy, 2010; Gabriel, 2013, 2014a; Neo et al., 2016) (see Appendices 2 and 4)
   A. Observe the site every eight hours during infusions for local irritation or leakage, and assess the patient's comfort with placement and infusion rate.
   B. No definitive recommendation can be made regarding the frequency of catheter or needle placement. Intervals could include every three days, five days, weekly, or as clinically indicated.
   C. Change transparent dressings at one week and change with insertion of a new catheter or needle (O'Grady et al., 2011).
   D. Instruct patients and caregivers to report any leakage, erythema, edema, or pain at injection site as soon as possible.
   E. Use medications and fluids that are isotonic, nonirritating, nonviscous, and water soluble (Spandorfer, 2011).
      1. Medications for symptom management (Bruno, 2015)
         a) Analgesics: Any analgesic available for parenteral use is acceptable for SC infusion, except for meperidine hydrochloride, which causes tissue necrosis.
            (1) Morphine and hydromorphone are the preferred analgesics for home administration.
            (2) Hydromorphone is recommended as the most cost-effective analgesic because it is very potent, and high doses can be delivered in small amounts. Stability has been found to be 28 days. Hydromorphone is at least as effective as morphine using the SC infusion route (D'Arcy, 2010).
            (3) Morphine was found to be equianalgesic for IV and SC routes when administered as a continuous infusion (Arthur, 2015).
            (4) Other commonly used opioids include methadone, fentanyl, and ketorolac.
            (5) Methadone causes skin irritation with SC infusion (erythema and induration). Successful interventions to minimize this com-

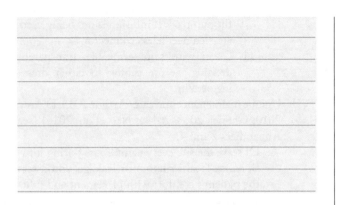

plication include the use of dexamethasone or hyaluronidase in the infusion and site rotation every 24 hours (Jabalameli & Kalantari, 2014).

    (6) Ambulatory pumps with a patient-controlled analgesia mode allow for rapid individual dose titration and provide a sense of control for the patient (see Chapter 16). This can be done in both the hospital and in the home.

b) Nonanalgesic medication examples (Kawabata & Kaneishi, 2013; Pérez, Farriols, Puente, Planas, & Ruiz, 2011)

    (1) Octreotide, scopolamine, lidocaine, and phenobarbital have been used for various symptom management needs.

    (2) Metoclopramide has been used for intractable nausea and vomiting in SC infusions.

2. Fluids

    a) Isotonic solutions can include 0.9% normal saline (NS) or a mixture of NS and 5% dextrose.

    b) The addition of the enzyme hyaluronidase to SC fluid infusion acts as a physical adjunct to increase absorption and dispersion of fluid (Wasserman, 2014). It facilitates fluid absorption, especially when fluid is infused rapidly or in large quantities.

        (1) The rate of perfusion is proportional to the amount of hyaluronidase present; the extent of diffusion is proportional to the volume of solution present.

        (2) Can cause systemic reaction; therefore, an intradermal test dose should be performed (0.02

of a 150 units/ml solution); see drug package insert for drug testing procedure. The usual dose is 150 units in a liter or more of fluid.

    c) Rate of infusions (Arthur, 2015)

        (1) Infusion rates for medications are 3–5 ml/hour. Faster infusion rates result in tissue irritation and sloughing, unless other measures are taken, such as using hyaluronidase in the infusate.

        (2) Concentrate the drug dose to ensure the maximum flow rate of 3–5 ml/hour or less, taking bolus dosing into consideration.

        (3) Rates for fluid replacement depend on how quickly the replacement must be achieved but range from 20–80 ml/hour. For patients who generally are active during the day, fluids can be administered at night (Scales, 2011).

    d) Rates as high as 400 ml/hour may be tolerated when administered with human recombinant hyaluronidase (Arthur, 2015; Arthur et al., 2012; Soremekun, Shear, Connolly, Stewart, & Thomas, 2012).

    e) An electronic infusion device should be used to deliver the infusion to lessen the likelihood of fluid overload or excess fluid into the SC tissue. Examples include an electronic syringe driver, elastomeric balloon pump, or peristaltic pump (see Chapter 16).

VIII. Removal technique

  A. Verify order or indication for removal when SC therapy is discontinued.

  B. Explain the procedure to the patient.

  C. Place the patient in a chair or bed for stabilization.

  D. Wash hands.

  E. Discontinue all infusions.

  F. Put on gloves, remove dressing, and observe site for edema, erythema, or discharge. Remove gloves. Wash hands and put on new gloves.

  G. Pull catheter/needle out in the same angle as insertion while stabilizing the skin with sterile gauze.

  H. Apply constant, firm pressure to the exit site if bleeding. Apply bandage.

  I. Instruct the patient and caregiver to report any discomfort or signs of bleeding, bruising, erythema, edema, or drainage.

J. Document observations, patient tolerance, catheter integrity, and actions.

IX. Complications (Dychter et al., 2012; Griffith, 2011; Mitchell, Pickard, Herbert, Lightfoot, & Roberts, 2012; Scales, 2011; Spandorfer, 2011)

A. Adverse effects are minimal and typically are local and associated with the type of solution, infusion rate, and volume. Instruct patients and caregivers to assess the SC site twice daily or every eight hours during infusions. Report any problems to the home health nurse or provider.

B. Local reactions at the insertion site include erythema, edema, or induration.
  1. Etiology: Prolonged duration of catheter or needle placement, rapid infusion, or irritation from solution
  2. Management: Remove needle and restart in another site.

C. Pain or discomfort at infusion site may develop.
  1. Etiology: Needle migration, prolonged duration of needle placement, inadvertent placement in muscle tissues, or rapid infusion
  2. Signs and symptoms: Edema; if present, try slowing infusion or restarting in another site.
  3. Management: Apply warm compress at the site after needle removal for comfort.

D. Leakage or pooling of fluid at infusion site also may occur.
  1. Etiology: Poor absorption or too-rapid infusion
  2. Signs and symptoms: Decreased infusion rate
  3. Management: If persistent leakage or pooling is noted despite rate reduction, stop infusion, remove catheter/needle, and restart in another site.

E. Management of edema
  1. If a small amount, slow infusion and monitor for absorption.
  2. If a large, generalized area, change the site for SC infusion.
  3. Gently massage the area and monitor for underlying tissue damage. Excessive or deep massage can cause tissue damage.
  4. Add hyaluronidase to the infusate to improve absorption.

F. Management of insertion site abscess or cellulitis formation
  1. Remove the device and culture the insertion site.
  2. Administer systemic antibiotics as indicated per culture results.
  3. Apply warm compresses to the site for comfort.

G. Rare complications: Sloughing of tissue, infection, and puncture of vessels with bleeding and bruising. Prevention includes frequently assessing the site and avoiding SC infusion in patients with coagulation or bleeding disorders to minimize possibility of occurrence.

X. Education and documentation (see Chapter 17)

References

Arthur, A.O. (2015). Innovations in subcutaneous infusions. *Infusion Nursing Society, 38,* 179–187. doi:10.1097/NAN.0000000000000099

Arthur, A.O., Goodloe, J.M., & Thomas, S.H. (2012). Subcutaneous fluid administration: A potentially useful tool in prehospital care. *Emergency Medicine International, 2012,* 904521. doi:10.1155/2012/904521

Bartz, L., Klein, C., Seifert, A., Herget, I., Ostgathe, C., & Stiel, S. (2014). Subcutaneous administration of drugs in palliative care: Results of a systematic observational study. *Journal of Pain and Symptom Management, 48,* 540–547. doi:10.1016/j.jpainsymman.2013.10.018

Bruno, V.G. (2015). Hypodermoclysis: A literature review to assist in clinical practice. *Einstein (São Paulo), 13*(1), 122–128. doi:10.1590/S1679-45082015RW2572

D'Arcy, Y. (2010). Is continuous subcutaneous infusion a good route for pain medication? *Nursing, 40,* 59–60. doi:10.1097/01.NURSE.0000388322.36758

Dychter, S.S., Gold, D.A., & Haller, M.F. (2012). Subcutaneous drug delivery: A route to increased safety, patient satisfaction, and reduced costs. *Journal of Infusion Nursing, 35,* 154–160. doi:10.1097/NAN.0b013e31824d2271

Gabriel, J. (2012). Subcutaneous infusion in palliative care: The neria soft infusion set. *International Journal of Palliative Nursing, 18,* 526, 528–530. doi:10.12968/ijpn.2014.20.11.536

Gabriel, J. (2013). The use of subcutaneous infusion in medication administration. *British Journal of Nursing, 22*(Suppl. 14), S6–S12. doi:10.12968/bjon.2013.22.Sup14.S10

Gabriel, J. (2014a). Subcutaneous fluid administration and the hydration of older people. *British Journal of Nursing, 23*(Suppl. 14), S10–S14. doi:10.12968/bjon.2014.23.Sup14.S10

Gabriel, J. (2014b). The role of subcutaneous infusion in integrated, patient-centered palliative care. *International Journal of Palliative Nursing, 20,* 216. doi:10.12968/ijpn.2014.20.5.216

Griffith, S. (2011). Improving practice using action research: Resolving the problem of kinking with non-metal cannulae. *International Journal of Palliative Nursing, 17,* 531–536. doi:10.12968/ijpn.2011.17.11.531

Humphrey, P. (2011). Hypodermoclysis: An alternative to I.V. infusion therapy. *Nursing, 41,* 16–17. doi:10.1097/01.NURSE.0000405126.91849.e3

Jabalameli, M., & Kalantari, F. (2014). Evaluation of the analgesic effect of subcutaneous methadone after cesarean section. *Advanced Biomedical Research, 3,* 197. doi:10.4103/2277-9175.140679

Kawabata, M., & Kaneishi, K. (2013). Continuous subcutaneous infusion of compound oxycodone for the relief of dyspnea in patients with terminally ill cancer: A retrospective study. *American Journal of Hospice and Palliative Medicine, 30,* 305–311. doi:10.1177/1049909112448924

Lybarger, E.H. (2009). Hypodermoclysis in the home and long-term care settings. *Journal of Infusion Nursing, 32,* 40–44. doi:10.1097/NAN.0b013e3181922552

Mitchell, K., Pickard, J., Herbert, A., Lightfoot, J., & Roberts, D. (2012). Incidence and causes for syringe driver site reactions in palliative care: A prospective hospice-based study. *Palliative Medicine, 26,* 979–985. doi:10.1177/0269216311428096

Neo, S.H., Khemlani, M.H., Sim, L.K., & Seah, A.S. (2016). Winged metal needles versus plastic winged and nonwinged cannulae for subcutaneous infusions in palliative care: A quality improvement project to enhance patient care and medical staff safety in a Singaporean hospital. *Journal of Palliative Medicine, 19,* 318–322. doi:10.1089/jpm.2015.0085

O'Grady, N.P., Alexander, M., Burns, L.A., Dellinger, E.P., Garland, J., Heard, S.O., … Healthcare Infection Control Practices Advisory Committee. (2011). Guidelines for the prevention of intravascular catheter-related infections. *Clinical Infectious Diseases, 52,* E162–E193. doi:10.1093/cid/cir257

Pérez, L.M., Farriols, C., Puente, V., Planas, J., & Ruiz, I. (2011). The use of subcutaneous scopolamine as a palliative treatment in Parkinson's disease. *Palliative Medicine, 25,* 92–93. doi:10.1177/0269216310381662

Sandoval, M., Coleman, P., Govani, R., Siddiqui, S., & Todd, K.H. (2013). Pilot study of human recombinant hyaluronidase-enhanced subcutaneous hydration and opioid administration for sickle cell disease acute pain episodes. *Journal of Pain and Palliative Care Pharmacotherapy, 27,* 10–18. doi:10.3109/15360288.2012.758683

Scales, K. (2011). Use of hypodermoclysis to manage dehydration. *Nursing Older People, 23,* 16–22. doi:10.7748/nop2011.06.23.5.16.c8528

Soremekun, O., Shear, M.L., Connolly, J., Stewart, C.E., & Thomas, S.H. (2012). Basic-level emergency medical technician administration of fluids and glucose via enzyme-assisted subcutaneous infusion access. *Prehospital and Disaster Medicine, 27,* 220–225. doi:10.1017/S1049023X12000829

Spandorfer, P. (2011). Subcutaneous rehydration: Updating a traditional technique. *Pediatric Emergency Care, 27,* 230–236. doi:10.1097/PEC.0b013e31820e1405

Wasserman, R. (2014). Overview of recombinant human hyaluronidase-facilitated subcutaneous infusion of IgG in primary immunodeficiencies. *Immunotherapy, 6,* 553–567. doi:10.2217/imt.14.34

Chapter 11

Arterial Access Devices

Lisa Hartkopf Smith, MS, RN, AOCN®, CNS

I. History (Inoue & Kusunoki, 2014; Karanicolas et al., 2014; Leal & Kingham, 2015; Parks & Routt, 2015; Petre, Sofocleous, & Solomon, 2015; Shields et al., 2014)
   A. The first use of intra-arterial devices to administer chemotherapy appeared in the literature in the 1950s with the administration of nitrogen mustard to treat melanoma.
   B. The percutaneous catheter placement technique for hepatic arterial infusion with chemotherapy initially was developed in the 1980s in Japan. It was fully established in the United States by 2000 (Arai et al., 2015).
   C. Other early reports included the treatment of gliomas and sarcomas (Joshi, Ellis, & Emala, 2014).
   D. The technology to deliver intra-arterial infusions into the hepatic artery has evolved since its inception.
      1. Initially, temporary external catheters were used; treatment advanced to using tunneled catheters and intra-arterial ports connected to ambulatory infusion pumps.
      2. The first subcutaneous (SC) implanted hepatic intra-arterial infusion pump was placed in 1977 for the treatment of hepatic metastases from colon cancer.
      3. More recently, hepatic chemoembolization using chemotherapy, followed by embolization of the hepatic artery, has become a recommended treatment for a subgroup of patients with unresectable hepatocellular carcinoma and neuroendocrine tumors involving the liver using a temporary arterial catheter (National Comprehensive Cancer Network® [NCCN®], 2016).
      4. Intra-arterial chemotherapy also is used in combination with systemic chemotherapy (Kemeny et al., 2011).
II. Device characteristics (De Baere & Mariani, 2014; Deschamps et al., 2010; Inoue & Kusunoki, 2014; Leal & Kingham, 2015; Petre et al., 2015; Shi et al., 2015)
   A. Temporary percutaneous catheters, ports, and implanted pumps are most frequently used to deliver intra-arterial therapies. Arterial pressure lines are outside the scope of these standards.
   B. Delivers high concentrations of drug directly to the tumor, with decreased systemic exposure (Royal, 2013)
   C. Intra-arterial therapies are considered regional forms of treatment. For all types of intra-arterial devices, the catheter is threaded directly to the artery that feeds the tumor.
   D. Temporary devices remain in place for minutes to hours and are removed immediately after drug administration; long-term devices may remain in place a year or longer (Perez et al., 2014).
III. Device features
   A. Compared to venous catheters, arterial catheters have smaller internal diameters and thicker catheter walls to withstand higher arterial pressures.
   B. Temporary percutaneous catheters
      1. Type, French size (e.g., 2.7–5 Fr), and length of catheter used is dependent on the procedure to be performed, the artery that is being cannulated, and provider preference.
      2. Open ended and commonly made of polyurethane
      3. A tapered tip design is available.
   C. Arterial ports (De Baere & Mariani, 2014; Ganeshan, Upponi, Hon, Warakaulle, & Uberoi, 2008; Shi et al., 2015): At the time of publication, intra-arterial ports are not being manufactured specifically for this use in the United States.
      1. Design is similar to venous ports, consisting of a portal body with a self-sealing silicone septum connected to a catheter.
      2. Portal body is plastic or titanium and typically is not preattached to a catheter made of polyurethane or silicone.
      3. Catheter is designed with a fixed tip versus nonfixed tip with side hole. Metallic coils are an available design to secure the catheter fixed tip within the artery. Catheter design can be tapered or nontapered.

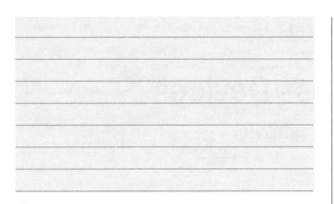

D. Hepatic artery infusion pumps (Leal & King-ham, 2015; Liu, Cui, Guo, Li, & Zeng, 2014; Parks & Routt, 2015): At the time of publication, one implanted pump is approved for intra-arterial drug delivery. The following details relate to the Codman pump (Codman & Shurtleff, Inc., 2016). It is a fully implanted drug delivery system. The pump is connected to an arterial catheter that is placed into the hepatic artery.
   1. The pump typically delivers a constant infusion rate, ranging from 1–2.5 ml/day.
   2. Reservoir volumes range from 16 ml, 20 ml, and 50 ml.
   3. Side bolus port and center septum for access to reservoir
   4. Titanium disk pump is 7 cm in diameter, ¾–1 inch thick, and weighs 4–6 oz.
   5. Pump typically consists of two chambers.
      a) The inner chamber contains drug to be infused.
      b) The outer chamber contains charging fluid (a volatile liquid/vapor mixture) used as the chemical power source.
      c) Once inserted in the body, the pump is regulated to the temperature of the body, leading to expansion of the charging fluid, which pressurizes the medication chamber to push the drug through the chamber.
      d) The pump does not need to be recharged and does not require batteries.
IV. Device advantages and disadvantages (see Table 11-1)
V. Patient selection criteria (Allard & Malka, 2014; Basile, Carrafiello, Ierardi, Tsetis, & Brountzos, 2012; Ganeshan et al., 2008; Grigorovski et al., 2014; Guillaume et al., 2010; Inoue & Kusunoki, 2014; Karanicolas et al., 2014; Ko & Karanicolas, 2014; Koganemaru et al., 2012; Leal & Kingham, 2015; Liu et al., 2014; Parks & Routt, 2015; Petre et al., 2015; Shi et al., 2015)
   A. Use arterial devices in the following types of therapies and treatments.
      1. Transhepatic chemoembolization
      2. Isolated limb perfusion and infusions such as for melanoma, sarcoma, or cancerous ulcers in extremities
      3. Intra-arterial chemotherapy with osmotic blood–brain barrier disruption
      4. Intra-arterial therapy for retinoblastoma
      5. Local regional unresectable liver metastases
      6. Palliative treatment for unresectable disease
   B. Appropriate arterial anatomy providing adequate blood supply to tumor bed documented by arteriogram
   C. Expertise in administration of therapies through arterial devices
VI. Insertion techniques (Allard & Malka, 2014; Basile et al., 2012; De Baere & Mariani, 2014; Deschamps et al., 2010; Ganeshan et al., 2008; Gottlieb & Bailitz, 2016; Parks & Routt, 2015; Shi et al., 2015)
   A. Prior to placement, ensure that contraindications do not exist, informed consent is obtained, a preplacement assessment is completed, and laboratory studies are verified (see Appendix 4). An angiogram or similar study is done preplacement and/or postplacement to confirm location, confirm arterial blood flow, and to assess for complications.
   B. Temporary percutaneous catheter placement
      1. Placed by interventional radiologist. Ultrasound guidance is used.
      2. Maximum sterile barrier precautions are used during artery catheter insertion (O'Grady et al., 2011).
      3. Location of the catheter and tip are dependent on the area to be infused. The most common sites for insertion are the femoral or brachial artery, and then threaded into the artery that perfuses the tumor (Abdalla et al., 2013; Basile et al., 2012).
      4. Postprocedure care
         a) Monitor the patient's vital signs postprocedure every 15 minutes for at least 2 hours. Monitoring varies among institutions.
         b) Assess the involved limb for peripheral pulses, color, temperature, capillary refill, numbness or tingling, edema or signs of bleeding, or hematoma formation with each set of vital signs.
         c) Certain activities are restricted depending on location of catheter.
   C. Arterial port: Placed by surgeon or interventional radiologist
      1. With side-hole technology, the catheter tip is fixed within the artery (Deschamps et al., 2010; Ishikawa et al., 2012; NCCN, 2016; Shi et al., 2015).

Device	Advantages	Disadvantages
Percutaneous temporary arterial catheters (those removed at the end of each infusion cycle)	Can be used for multiple drug infusions at one setting Can be used in palliative or neoadjuvant setting No device in place after the procedure	Potential activity restriction until catheter removal depending on location Hospitalization is required. Short-term infusions of eight hours or less can be done during a 23-hour observation instead of a full hospitalization admission. Insertion of the catheter typically performed in interventional radiology by trained personnel Tip of catheter stability is less than with implanted devices. Possible complications secondary to repeated insertions into artery Required monitoring of site during infusion
Arterial ports	Allows repeated access to arterial system Allows for long-term use Can be used for multiple drug infusions at one setting Tip of catheter stability increased compared to percutaneous temporary catheter Depending on insertion site, the patient may be able to ambulate during infusion. More cost-effective if long-term use is planned Can be used in an outpatient or inpatient setting if properly trained personnel are available	Patient discomfort with needlesticks Special noncoring, single-use needle required Required monitoring of site during infusion Specially trained personnel required for all care
Arterial implanted pumps	Allows prolonged access to arterial system Allows repeated access to arterial system No immobility required Tip of catheter stability increased compared to percutaneous temporary catheter Has lower rate of malfunction than arterial ports	Cost of initial insertion Specially trained personnel are required for all care. Patient discomfort with needlesticks Special noncoring straight needle required for access Limited indication for liver perfusion

Table 11-1. Advantages and Disadvantages of Arterial Catheters, Ports, and Pumps

2. The portal body is placed in a SC pocket, frequently over a bone to stabilize. The catheter is threaded into the appropriate artery to be infused.

D. Implanted arterial pump: Used for hepatic artery placement for liver cancer involvement (Abdalla et al., 2013; Karanicolas et al., 2014; Leal & Kingham, 2015).

1. Implanted by surgeon or interventional radiologist

2. Pump insertion into the gastroduodenal artery and threaded to the hepatic artery is preferred. The catheter is attached to the pump placed in a SC pocket. The pocket is created superficial to the abdominal wall fascia for ease of pump refill (Kanat, Gewirtz, & Kemeny, 2012; Ko & Karanicolas, 2014).

3. To prevent possible drug-induced cholecystitis, the gallbladder is removed at the time of surgical resection or pump placement.

4. Blood vessels from the distal stomach and proximal duodenum are embolized to pre-

vent extrahepatic perfusion. A methylene blue dye study and/or a nuclear hepatobiliary scan (i.e., TC-99m) verifies pump placement (Kanat et al., 2012; Perez et al., 2014).

VII. Unique maintenance and care: Prior to accessing arterial catheters, ports, and pumps, scope of practice must be verified with the individual state board of nursing and institutional guidelines. RNs managing arterial devices must be knowledgeable of the principles of drug administration and care of patients with these devices (see Appendices 2, 4, 7, 11, and 12). Use strict sterile technique at all times (i.e., sterile gloves, face mask, sterile field).

A. Avoid blood pressure monitoring on the involved extremity.

B. Ensure that all tubing connections are Luer lock. Label all lines as close to the patient as feasible. Secure catheter to prevent kinks and tension, which may lead to malposition. Consider tension loop.

C. Use specialized tubing without injection ports, as indicated, to prevent accidental injection of unintended medication.

D. Trace tubing or catheter from the patient to point of origin each time the catheter is accessed, at hand-off, and at transitions to a new setting or service.

E. Temporary percutaneous catheters (Ashton, 2012; Robertson-Malt, Malt, Farquhar, & Greer, 2014; Scales, 2010)
   1. Frequently assess the involved extremity for peripheral pulses, skin color and temperature, capillary refill, swelling, numbness, tingling, dysesthesias, bleeding, and hematoma formation. Frequently observe dressing for drainage and bleeding.
   2. Place infusions on pumps (see Chapter 16).
   3. Because of the circulatory risk associated with flushing and potential for dislodgment of clots and creation of air bubbles, no definitive recommendation can be made regarding the frequency or volume of flushing. During periods where chemotherapy is not infusing, heparinized solution may be ordered as a continuous infusion to maintain patency. Volume, concentration, and frequency varies; no evidence exists to support a particular volume or concentration. The literature reports use of heparin solution 1,000–5,000 IU/ml, 1–3 ml every eight hours (daily) to maintain patency.
   4. No definitive recommendation can be made regarding blood sampling from temporary percutaneous arterial catheters.
   5. Access location
      a) Femoral access (Ashton, 2012; Barosh et al., 2011)
         (1) Place the patient on bed rest to prevent catheter dislodgment.
         (2) Consider placing a loose restraint on the involved extremity as a reminder to keep leg straight and to not get out of bed. If a restraint is used, follow the institutional policy and procedure for restraints.
         (3) Implement strategies for deep vein thrombosis prophylaxis.
      b) Brachial or subclavian access
         (1) Secure arm in a sling or other immobilization device.
         (2) Assist the patient with ambulation until the patient's understanding of restrictions regarding arm use is validated (e.g., do not use arm to support weight).
   6. Dressing changes: A chlorhexidine dressing/sponge has been found to decrease infection in temporary arterial lines (Saf-

dar et al., 2014). The dressing may be left intact to prevent dislodgment or may be changed 24 hours after insertion.

F. Arterial ports (Arai et al., 2015; De Baere & Mariani, 2014; Deschamps et al., 2010; Matsumoto et al., 2014; Shi et al., 2015): No definitive recommendations regarding blood sampling through long-term catheters can be made.
   1. No definitive recommendation can be made regarding the frequency, volume, or concentration of flush. Flushing protocols include 2–5 ml of heparinized saline (100–1,000 IU/ml) every week. If 1,000 IU/ml is used, aspirate and discard prior to infusions and monitor coagulation values as warranted (i.e., every 12 hours, daily).
   2. After infusions, flush with 10 ml of 0.9% normal saline followed by heparinized saline lock.
   3. Safety considerations
      a) Ensure that all tubing connections are Luer lock.
      b) Label all arterial lines as close to the patient as feasible.
      c) Use specialized tubing without injection ports, as indicated, to prevent accidental injection of unintended medication.
      d) Secure tubing to prevent kinks, tension, and possible needle dislodgment. Consider tension loop.
      e) Place infusions on pumps (see Chapter 16).
      f) Refer to Chapter 7 for instructions on port access with a noncoring needle and for dressing recommendations.
      g) Educate the patient regarding signs and symptoms of infiltration, occlusion, tubing disconnection, infection, pump malfunction, and interventions to prevent and manage complications.
      h) No definitive recommendation can be made regarding blood sampling from arterial ports. Typically, blood sampling is avoided due to the high pressure in arterial systems.

G. Implanted arterial pumps (Leal & Kingham, 2015; Parks & Routt, 2015): Prior to pump care, obtain the specific pump model and maintenance procedures from the manufacturer for further details. Use a noncoring needle to prevent damage to the pump's septum (see Appendix 11).
   1. The current pump approved for intra-arterial use delivers at a constant infusion rate and cannot be programmed to change rates. The medication delivered per hour is

changed by modifying the concentration of the medication; the rate and total volume of the medication remains the same.

2. Locate the septum(s) to refill pump: The pump may be designed with a side port to provide bolus dosing and a center port to refill the center chamber where medication infuses.

3. Reservoir volume: Verify reservoir volume to ensure that the amount and volume of medication ordered can be instilled into the pump.

4. Refill pump reservoir with chemotherapy or heparinized saline to maintain patency every two weeks. If the pump will not be used for an extended period of time, glycerin has been used to decrease the frequency of pump refill. The refill interval varies with the pump reservoir volume (e.g., 16 ml, 20 ml, 50 ml) and the percentage of glycerin used (Parks & Routt, 2015). Refill schedules should accommodate office closures and holidays. Detailed instructions are available from the manufacturer.

5. Pump refill kits are available from the pump manufacturer.

   a) Kits contain 22-gauge straight noncoring needles, an extension tubing with clamp or stopcock, an empty syringe, antiseptic for cleansing the site, sterile gloves, sterile drape, and adhesive dressing.

   b) One type of noncoring needle is used for the bolus side port and another type of noncoring needle is for the mid-septum reservoir. These needles are not interchangeable. Do not use the bolus needle to fill the reservoir; the bolus needle has a slot opening midway on the needle shaft.

   c) In contrast to the noncoring needles used to access venous implanted ports, noncoring needles for pumps are straight (i.e., not bent at 90 degrees).

   d) To verify correct needle placement prior to pump refill and to determine dose of medication delivered (total volume infused at previous fill minus amount removed), empty the pump completely prior to refilling.

   e) Pumps are not designed for blood sampling.

VIII. Removal technique (Barosh et al., 2011; Deschamps et al., 2010)

   A. Whether a trained RN or an advanced practice nurse can remove arterial temporary percutaneous catheters depends on the individual state board of nursing. For states that do permit RNs to remove arterial catheters, training and competency records must be maintained.

   B. Temporary percutaneous catheters can be removed at the bedside or in interventional radiology, depending on location of catheter, mechanism of catheterization securement, and institutional policy or preference.

   1. Remove securement mechanism (e.g., sutures) and remove line in one uninterrupted motion.

   2. Apply prolonged digital pressure. The amount and duration of pressure is specific to the institution and the patient. No definitive recommendation supports the use of sandbags.

      a) Vascular closure devices are sometimes used for femoral arterial catheters. Delivery mechanisms use a suture, a bovine collagen plug, and a polymer (polylactic and polyglycolic acid) to form a mechanical plug that is fully bioabsorbable over time.

      b) Other bioabsorbable devices use a polyethylene glycol polymer to adhere to the contours of the vessel lumen. These devices decrease the time required for hemostasis, with more rapid insertion site healing and earlier patient mobility (Alshehri & Elsharawy, 2015; Hon et al., 2010; Lucatelli et al., 2013).

   3. Assess circulation in the involved extremity after catheter removal (e.g., pulse, temperature, color, swelling).

   4. Activity restrictions following temporary catheter removal are dependent on the location of the catheter. Femoral sites traditionally involve bed rest for up to eight hours following removal; however, vascular closure devices can decrease this time (Alshehri & Elsharawy, 2015; Hon et al., 2010; Lucatelli et al., 2013). One study with a small number of patients with short-term femoral artery catheters used for hemody-

namic monitoring suggested that mobility and walking are safe with no catheter-related complications (Perme, Lettvin, Throckmorton, Mitchell, & Masud, 2011).

C. Arterial ports are removed by a surgeon or an interventional radiologist in a method similar to venous implanted port removal (see Chapter 7).

D. Implanted arterial pumps are removed by a surgeon or an interventional radiologist.

IX. Complications (Basile et al., 2012; Deschamps et al., 2010; Ganeshan et al., 2008; Karanicolas et al.,

2014; Leal & Kingham, 2015; Perez et al., 2014) (see Table 11-2)

A. Temporary percutaneous catheters: Complications are related to the type of procedure, the length of time the catheter remains in place, and the catheter location.

B. Arterial ports: Extravasation can occur if the needle is dislodged from the portal body or if the catheter migrates, resulting in the infusion of chemotherapy into the SC tissue (Seo et al., 2015).

Table 11-2. Major Complications Associated With Arterial Access Devices

Complication	Prevention	Signs and Symptoms	Intervention
Infection	Sterile barrier precautions. Sterile, occlusive dressings over ports when accessed and over percutaneous catheters until removed. Remove temporary catheters as soon as possible. Within four days is optimal, after which the risk of infection increases	Tenderness, erythema, or drainage at site; fever; skin necrosis over port or pump; dehiscence; pump or port extrusion	If chemotherapy is infusing, notify provider, as infusion may need to be stopped. Culture site and catheter exit tip, as ordered. Administer port or pump pocket washout with local antibiotics, or give systemic antibiotics, as ordered. Have the surgeon or interventional radiologist assess if the device requires removal. If removed, send the catheter for culture, if ordered.
Catheter migration/ dislodgment	The catheter is sutured in place during placement. Braided or beaded catheter can assist to secure placement. Routine assessment of placement with imaging study	Hepatic artery infusion: Epigastric pain, nausea, vomiting, or diarrhea. Extrahepatic infusion: Pain over site or in surrounding area of infusion; edema or erythema over site. For any arterial infusion: Weak or absent peripheral pulse. Inability to infuse infusate; patient discomfort during infusion. Temporary percutaneous catheter: Patient discomfort, wet dressing, leakage, and increase length of external catheter	Stop infusion and notify the provider or interventional radiologist. Flush the catheter, as ordered, with normal saline or other solution compatible with chemotherapy that was infusing. Obtain imaging study, as ordered. The device may require removal.
Occlusion/ thrombosis	Apply positive pressure when deaccessing the catheter or port. Flush with saline or compatible solution between drugs. Use heparinized solution for flushing the catheter between use.	Unable to flush or withdraw fluid (If catheter has a one-way valve, withdrawal of fluid is not possible.) If a temporary percutaneous catheter is in place, a change occurs in color, pulse, and temperature of the involved extremity. If catheter tip is in hepatic artery, any abdominal pain needs to be assessed immediately.	Do not force flushing, as it could cause a rupture of the catheter or diaphragm. Notify the provider. After assessment by a trained provider, tissue plasminogen activator may be used. Evaluate the need to remove the device. A replacement will be based on the clinical situation, as such replacement may not be able to be done at the same time as removal.
Bleeding at exit site	Baseline and frequent observation of exit site	For temporary percutaneous catheter placement, more drainage than would be expected after placement should be considered a problem.	Apply a pressure dressing. Notify the provider. Educate the patient to immediately report any swelling, erythema, or pain.

Note. Based on information from De Baere & Mariani, 2014; Deschamps et al., 2010; Karanicolas et al., 2014; Leal & Kingham, 2015.

C. The arterial port or pump may rotate in the SC pocket (i.e., "flip"), requiring surgical manipulation.

D. The pump can cause abdominal herniation from the pump weight. An abdominal binder may be worn to stabilize the pump.

X. Education and documentation (see Chapter 17)

The author would like to acknowledge Donna L. Gerber, PhD, RN, AOCN®, for her contribution to this chapter that remains unchanged from the previous edition of this book.

References

Abdalla, E.K., Bauer, T.W., Chun, Y.S., D'Angelica, M., Kooby, D.A., & Jarnagin, W.R. (2013). Locoregional surgical and interventional therapies for advanced colorectal cancer liver metastases: Expert consensus statements. *HPB (Oxford), 15,* 199–130. doi:10.1111/j.1477-2574.2012.00597.x

Allard, M.A., & Malka, D. (2014). Place of hepatic intra-arterial chemotherapy in the treatment of colorectal liver metastases. *Journal of Visceral Surgery, 151*(Suppl. 1), S21–S24. doi:10.1016/j.jviscsurg.2013.12.003

Alshehri, A.M., & Elsharawy, M. (2015). Comparison of angioseal and manual compression in patients undergoing transfemoral coronary and peripheral vascular interventional procedures. *International Journal of Angiology, 24,* 133–136. doi:10.1055/s-0035-1547449

Arai, Y., Aoyama, T., Inaba, Y., Okabe, H., Ihaya, T., Kichikawa, K., … Saji, S. (2015). Phase II study on hepatic arterial infusion chemotherapy using percutaneous catheter placement techniques for liver metastases from colorectal cancer (JFMC28 study). *Asia-Pacific Journal of Clinical Oncology, 11,* 41–48. doi:10.1111/ajco.12324

Ashton, K.S. (2012). Nursing care of patients undergoing isolated limb procedures for recurrent melanoma of the extremity. *Journal of Perianesthesia Nursing, 27,* 94–109. doi:10.1016/j.jopan.2012.01.005

Barosh, B.A., Holmes, C., Keerikattu, L.M., Manappurathu, M.S., Segovia, J.H., Hasen, P.C., … Kurzrock, R. (2011). Advancing the scope of nursing practice: Hepatic arterial catheter removal. *Clinical Journal of Oncology Nursing, 15,* 465–468. doi:10.1188.11.CJON.465-468

Basile, A., Carrafiello, G., Ierardi, A.M., Tsetis, D., & Brountzos, E. (2012). Quality-improvement guidelines for hepatic transarterial chemoembolization. *Cardiovascular and Interventional Radiology, 35,* 765–774. doi:10.1007/s00270-012-0423-z

Codman & Shurtleff, Inc. (2016). Retrieved from http://www.codmanpumps.com/index.asp

De Baere, T., & Mariani, P. (2014). Surgical or percutaneous hepatic artery cannulation for chemotherapy. *Journal of Visceral Surgery, 151*(Suppl. 1), S17–S20. doi:10.1016/j.jvissurg.2013.12.004

Deschamps, F., Rao, P., Teriitehau, C., Hakime, A., Malka, D., Boige, V., … De Baere, T. (2010). Percutaneous femoral implantation of an arterial port catheter for intraarterial chemotherapy: Feasibility and predictive factors of long-term functionality. *Journal of Vascular and Interventional Radiology, 21,* 1681–1688. doi:10.1016/j.jvir.2010.08.003

Ganeshan, A., Upponi, S., Hon, L.Q., Warakaulle, D., & Uberoi, R. (2008). Hepatic arterial infusion of chemotherapy: The role of diagnostic and interventional radiology. *Annals of Oncology, 19,* 847–851. doi:10.1093/annonc/mdm528

Gottlieb, M., & Bailitz, J. (2016). Is ultrasonographic guidance more successful than direct palpation for arterial line placement? *Annals of Emergency Medicine, 68,* 227–229. doi:10.1016/j.annemergmed.2016.03.024

Grigorovski, N., Lucena, E., Mattosinho, C., Parareda, A., Ferman, S., Catalá, J., & Chantada, G. (2014). Use of intra-arterial chemotherapy for retinoblastoma: Results of a survey. *International Journal of Ophthalmology, 7,* 726–730. doi:10.3980/j.issn.2222-3959.2014.04.26

Guillaume, D.J., Doolittle, N.D., Gahramanov, S., Hedrick, N.A., Delashaw, J.B., & Neuwelt, E.A. (2010). Intra-arterial chemotherapy with osmotic blood-brain barrier disruption for aggressive oligodendroglial tumors: Results of a phase I study. *Neurosurgery, 66*(1), 48–58.

Hon, L.Q., Ganeshan, A., Thomas, S.M., Warakaulle, D., Jagdish, J., & Uberoi, R. (2010). An overview of vascular closure devices: What every radiologist should know. *European Journal of Radiology, 73,* 181–190. doi:10.1016/j.ejrad.2008.09.023

Inoue, Y., & Kusunoki, M. (2014). Advances and directions in chemotherapy using implantable port systems for colorectal cancer: A historical review. *Surgery Today, 44,* 1406–1414. doi:10.1007/s00595-013-0672-8

Ishikawa, M., Kakizawa, H., Hieda, M., Toyota, N., Katamura, Y., Aikata, H., … Awai, K. (2012). Long-term outcomes of hepatic arterial port implantation using a coaxial microcatheter system in 176 patients with hepatocellular carcinoma. *Hiroshima Journal of Medical Sciences, 61,* 7–13. Retrieved from http://www.ncbi.nlm.nih.gov/pubmed/22702214

Joshi, S., Ellis, J.A., & Emala, C.W. (2014). Revisiting intra-arterial drug delivery for treating brain disease or is it "déjà-vu, all over again"? *Journal of Neuroanesthesiology and Critical Care, 1,* 108–115. doi:10.4103/2348-0548.130386

Kanat, O., Gewirtz, A., & Kemeny, N. (2012). What is the potential role of hepatic arterial infusion chemotherapy in the current armamentorium against colorectal cancer? *Journal of Gastrointestinal Oncology, 3,* 130–138. doi:10.3978/j.issn.2078-6891.2011.025

Karanicolas, P.J., Metrakos, P., Chan, K., Asmis, T., Chen, E., Kingham, T.P., … Ko, Y.J. (2014). Hepatic arterial infusion pump chemotherapy in the management of colorectal liver metastases: Expert consensus statement. *Current Oncology, 21,* e129–e136. doi:10.374/co.21.1577

Kemeny, N.E., Jarnagin, W.R., Capanu, M., Fong, Y., Gewirtz, A.N., Dematteo, R.P., & D'Angelica, M.I. (2011). Randomized phase II trial of adjuvant hepatic arterial infusion and systemic chemotherapy with or without bevacizumab in patients with resected hepatic metastases from colorectal cancer. *Journal of Clinical Oncology, 29,* 884–889. doi:10.1200/JCO.2010.32.5977

Ko, Y.J., & Karanicolas, P.J. (2014). Hepatic arterial infusion pump chemotherapy for colorectal liver metastases: An old technology in a new era. *Current Oncology, 21,* e116–e121. doi:10.3747/co.21.1592

Koganemaru, M., Abe, T., Iwamoto, R., Nonoshita, M., Yoshida, S., Uchiyama, D., & Hayabuchi, N. (2012). Hepatic arterial infusion chemotherapy with a coaxial reservoir system using a non-braided spiral tip microcatheter. *Japanese Journal of Radiology, 30,* 10–17. doi:10.1007/s11604-011-0001-3

Leal, J.N., & Kingham, T.P. (2015). Hepatic artery infusion chemotherapy for liver malignancy. *Surgical Oncology Clinics of North America, 24,* 121–148. doi:10.1016/j.soc.2014.09.005

Liu, C., Cui, Q., Guo, J., Li, D., & Zeng, Y. (2014). Intra-arterial intervention chemotherapy for sarcoma and cancerous ulcer via an implanted pump. *Pathology and Oncology Research, 20,* 229–234. doi:10.1007/s12253-013-9673-6

Lucatelli, P., Fanelli, F., Cannavale, A., Corona, M., Cirelli, C., D'adamo, A., … Catalano, C. (2013). Angioseal VIP® vs. Starclose SE® closure devices: A comparative analysis in non-cardiological procedures. *Journal of Cardiovascular Surgery.* Advance online publication.

Matsumoto, T., Yamagami, T., Yoshimatsu, R., Morishita, H., Kitamura, N., Sato, O., & Hasebe, T. (2014). Hepatic arterial infusion chemotherapy by the fixed-catheter-tip method: Retrospective comparison of percutaneous left subclavian and femoral port-catheter system implantation. *American Journal of Roentgenology, 202,* 211–215. doi:10.2214/AJR.12.10502

National Comprehensive Cancer Network. (2016). *NCCN Clinical Practice Guidelines in Oncology (NCCN Guidelines®): Colon cancer* [v.2.2016]. Retrieved from http://www.nccn.org/professionals/physician_gls/pdf/colon.pdf

O'Grady, N.P., Alexander, M., Burns, L.A., Dellinger, E.P., Garland, J., Heard, S.O., … Healthcare Infection Control Practices Advisory Committee. (2011). Guidelines for the prevention of intravascular catheter-related infections. *Clinical Infectious Diseases, 52,* E162–E193. doi:10.1093/cid/cir257

Parks, L., & Routt, M. (2015). Hepatic artery infusion pump in the treatment of liver metastases. *Clinical Journal of Oncology Nursing, 19,* 316–320. doi:10.1188/15.CJON.316-320

Perez, D.R., Kemeny, N.E., Brown, K.T., Gewirtz, A.N., Paty, P.B., Jarnagin, W.R., & D'Angelica, M.I. (2014). Angiographic identification of extrahepatic perfusion after hepatic arterial pump placement: Implications for surgical prevention. *HPB (Oxford), 16,* 744–748. doi:10.1111/hpb.12208

Perme, C., Lettvin, C., Throckmorton, T.A., Mitchell, K., & Masud, F. (2011). Early mobility and walking for patients with femoral arterial catheters in intensive care unit: A case series. *Journal of Acute Care Physical Therapy, 2,* 30–34. doi:10.1097/01592394-201102010-00004

Petre, E.N., Sofocleous, C.T., & Solomon, S.B. (2015). Ablative and catheter-directed therapies for colorectal liver and lung metastases. *Hematology/Oncology Clinics of North America, 29,* 117–133. doi:10.1016/j.hoc.2014.09.007

Robertson-Malt, S., Malt, G.N., Farquhar, V., & Greer, W. (2014). Heparin versus normal saline for patency of arterial lines. *Cochrane Database of Systematic Reviews, 2014*(5). doi:10.1002/14651858.CD007364.pub2

Royal, R.E. (2013). Principles of isolated regional limb perfusion. In S.T. Kee, D.C. Madoff, & R. Murthy (Eds.), *Clinical interventional oncology* (pp. 26–38). St. Louis, MO: Elsevier Saunders.

Safdar, N., O'Horo, J.C., Ghufran, A., Bearden, A., Didier, M.E., Chateau, D., & Maki, D.G. (2014). Chlorhexidine-impregnated dressing for prevention of catheter-related bloodstream infection: A meta-analysis. *Critical Care Medicine, 42,* 1703–1713. doi:10.1097/CCM.0000000000000319

Scales, K. (2010). Arterial catheters: Indications, insertion and use in critical care. *British Journal of Nursing, 19,* S16–S21. doi:10.12968/bjon.2010.19.Sup9.79306

Seo, B.F., Jung, H., Han, H.H., Moon, S.H., Oh, D.Y., Ahn, S.T., & Rhie, J.W. (2015). Extravasation of a percutaneous femoral hepatic infusion device. *Archives of Plastic Surgery, 42,* 93–95. doi:10.5999/aps.2015.42.1.93

Shi, L., Zhao, J., Lu, Q., Chen, X., Wang, H., Jiang, Y., … Wu, C. (2015). Initial hepatic artery infusion and systemic chemotherapy for asymptomatic colorectal cancer with un-resectable liver metastasis. *International Journal of Clinical and Experimental Medicine, 8,* 1000–1008.

Shields, C.L., Manjandavida, F.P., Lally, S.E., Pieretti, G., Arepalli, S.A., Caywood, E.H., … Shields, J.A. (2014). Intra-arterial chemotherapy for retinoblastoma in 70 eyes: Outcomes based on the international classification of retinoblastoma. *Ophthalmology, 121,* 1453–1460. doi:10.1016/j.ophtha.2014.01.026

Chapter 12

Intraventricular Access Devices

Carole Marie Elledge, RN, MSN, AOCN®

I. History: In 1963, Dr. Ayub K. Ommaya developed the Ommaya® subcutaneous (SC) reservoir for sterile access to the ventricular system as an alternative to repeated lumbar punctures in patients with cryptococcal meningitis (Kramer, Smith, & Souweidane, 2014; Ommaya, 1963; Szvalb et al., 2014; Weiner et al., 2015).

II. Device characteristics: Intraventricular catheter connected to an SC drug delivery reservoir to give medications directly to the intraventricular system

III. Device features (Mascitelli, De Los Reyes, Steinberger, & Zou, 2013; Szvalb et al., 2014) (see Figure 12-1)
   A. A dome-shaped, self-sealing silicone reservoir is attached to an intraventricular catheter.
   B. The reservoir volume is 1.5–2.5 ml.
   C. The dome size is 1.5–3.5 cm in diameter.
   D. Catheter length is measured and cut intraoperatively to fit within the ipsilateral frontal horn of the lateral ventricle.
   E. The reservoir is radiopaque.
   F. The device also may include a ventriculoperitoneal shunt with an on/off valve.

IV. Device advantages and disadvantages (see Figure 12-2)

V. Patient selection criteria (Aiello-Laws & Rutledge, 2008; Gabay, Thakkar, Stachnik, Woelich, & Villano, 2012; Graber & Omuro, 2011; Kramer et al., 2014; Lee et al., 2014; Roguski et al., 2015; Van Horn & Chamberlain, 2012)
   A. Leptomeningeal disease or primary central nervous system (CNS) tumors
   B. Need for intermittent administration of chemotherapy or antibiotics into the cerebrospinal fluid (CSF)
   C. Intractable headaches: Limited publications exist referencing the use of intraventricular access devices to instill opioid medications for individuals with refractory headaches.
   D. Alternative device for anticipated repeated lumbar punctures for CSF access
   E. Pediatric patients receiving radioimmunotherapy for CNS malignancies

VI. Insertion techniques (Mascitelli et al., 2013; Ozerov, Mel'nikov, Ibragimova, Tereshchenko, & Rachkov, 2014) (see Figure 12-3)
   A. Prior to placement, ensure that contraindications do not exist, informed consent is obtained, a preplacement assessment is completed, and laboratory studies and medication/chemotherapy orders are verified (see Appendix 4).
   B. While the patient is under general anesthesia, the device is inserted by a surgeon with maximum sterile barrier precautions.
      1. The patient is placed in a supine position, and the insertion site is cleaned and draped.

Figure 12-1. Intraventricular Reservoir

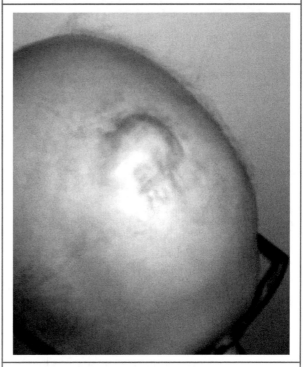

Figure 12-2. Advantages and Disadvantages of Intraventricular Reservoirs

Advantages
- Provide repeated access to the cerebrospinal fluid (CSF)
- Obviate the need for repeated lumbar punctures
- Permit consistent and predictable drug delivery through the CSF
- Can be used for multiple therapies, such as chemotherapy, antibiotics, and antifungals
- Allow for sampling of CSF
- Low infection risk

Disadvantages
- Require surgical insertion and removal
- Possible catheter migration
- Require specialized training for access and care

Figure 12-3. Use of an Intraventricular Reservoir

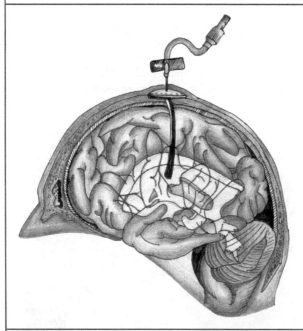

Note. From "Vascular Access Devices" (p. 64), by J.S. Webster in M.M. Gullatte (Ed.), *Clinical Guide to Antineoplastic Therapy: A Chemotherapy Handbook*, 2001, Pittsburgh, PA: Oncology Nursing Society. Copyright 2001 by Oncology Nursing Society. Reprinted with permission.

---

2. A flap is created by cutting a U-shaped incision in the scalp, and a burr hole is made through the cranial bone.
3. A reservoir is implanted subcutaneously under the scalp above the frontal lobe and secured to the pericranium, while the catheter is threaded through the burr hole into the ventricle. The catheter tip typically is placed in the frontal horn of the lateral ventricle.

4. The reservoir is covered by the flap of scalp tissue, which is then sutured closed. Patency is verified by withdrawal of CSF through the reservoir, and a sterile dressing is applied.
5. The use of stereotactic placement with a neuronavigation system improves placement success in patients with narrow and slit-like ventricles.
6. A postoperative imaging is required to confirm placement prior to use.

C. Postoperative care
   1. Maintain original sterile dressing for at least 24 hours. Follow with gauze and tape dressing for several days. After, no dressing is needed. Keep sutures dry until removal (approximately 7–10 days).
   2. Monitor site for bleeding, leakage of CSF, and excessive edema.
   3. Monitor for and notify the provider of changes in neurologic status (e.g., headache, vomiting, cognitive changes, vision changes, progressive lethargy, dysarthria, seizures) and signs of infection (e.g., fever, neck stiffness, headache, changes in level of consciousness).
   4. Ensure that radiologic imaging and flow studies verify patency and CSF flow tracts prior to use.
   5. Caution the patient regarding protection of the insertion site to prevent damage to the reservoir or dehiscence of the surgical wound.

VII. Unique maintenance and care (Aiello-Laws & Rutledge, 2008; Kramer et al., 2014; Peyrl et al., 2014) (see Appendices 2, 4, and 12)
   A. Prior to accessing or caring for an intraventricular device, verify scope of practice with the individual state board of nursing and institutional guidelines. RNs and advanced practice nurses managing these devices must be knowledgeable of the principles of drug administration and the care of patients with these devices.
   B. No definitive recommendation can be made regarding time interval between placement and first access of an intraventricular device; intervals range from day of surgery to multiple days after placement.
   C. Use strict sterile technique at all times (i.e., sterile gloves, face mask, sterile field). Use maximum sterile barrier precautions.
   D. Use only preservative-free drugs and diluents to prevent meningeal irritation.
   E. Use a 25-gauge or smaller needle to preserve dome integrity.

F. Ensure CSF patency prior to intraventricular drug administration.
G. Accessing technique (Gabay et al., 2012)
    1. Assess the patient's vital signs and neurologic status prior to procedure.
    2. Clip (do not shave) hair, if needed. The syringe containing the medication is not sterile. Once retrieved, the hand is no longer sterile and should touch only the nonsterile syringe throughout the remainder of the procedure.
    3. Cleanse reservoir. Ensure antiseptic is air-dried prior to access.
    4. Palpate the reservoir and assess for signs of infection. Pump the reservoir three to four times to fill with CSF from the ventricle.
    5. Insert a butterfly needle with extension tubing at a 45°–90° angle into the reservoir (see Figure 12-2). A release of resistance will be felt when the reservoir is penetrated. The presence of blood in the tubing indicates needle tunneling between the scalp and dome of the reservoir; if present, withdraw the needle and insert a new sterile needle at a 90° angle.
        a) Withdraw CSF volume equal to the amount of drug to be infused, plus an additional volume to use as flush following the procedure, according to institutional policy.
        b) If CSF is bloody or cloudy, preserve the specimen, notify the provider, and stop the procedure. An order may be given to send the sample for culture, sensitivity, Gram stain, protein, glucose, and cell count with differential.
        c) Infuse the medication into the reservoir, followed by reserved CSF flush or preservative-free normal saline, according to institutional policy.
    6. Remove the needle and apply gentle pressure with a sterile gauze.
    7. Gently pump the reservoir three to five times to distribute the drug. Apply sterile dressing.
H. Postprocedure care
    1. Obtain vital signs and assess neurologic status following the procedure.
    2. Keep the patient supine or in a semirecumbent position for at least 30 minutes following medication administration. Monitor for drug-related side effects and potential complications of the reservoir.
    3. Instruct the patient to report headache, nausea, dizziness, neck or back pain, stiffness, or other neurologic symptoms (e.g., change in level of consciousness).
VIII. Removal technique
    A. Rarely removed once implanted, except for unresolvable device malfunction or infection
    B. Intraventricular reservoirs removed by surgeon
    C. May be removed if implanted for the purpose of delivering prophylactic therapy
IX. Complications (Kramer et al., 2014; Peyrl et al., 2014; Weiner et al., 2015; Zairi et al., 2015)
    A. Infection
        1. Etiology (Bin Nafisah & Ahmad, 2015; Mead, Safdieh, Nizza, Tuma, & Sepkowitz, 2013; Ng, Mabasa, Chow, & Ensom, 2014; Szvalb et al., 2014)
            a) Improper access technique
            b) Surgical contamination
            c) Systemic complication of immunosuppressed patient
            d) Noniatrogenic trauma to site
        2. Prevention
            a) Maintain sterile barrier precautions when accessing the system.
            b) Ensure that only specially trained personnel access the device.
            c) Protect the device from trauma and damage.
        3. Signs and symptoms
            a) Site tenderness, warmth, erythema, or drainage
            b) Fever
            c) Headache with or without vomiting, neck stiffness, seizures, altered level of consciousness
            d) Bloody or purulent CSF
            e) Wound dehiscence with device exposure
        4. Diagnostic tests
            a) Complete blood count: Elevated white blood cell count
            b) CSF specimen: Obtain sample for culture and sensitivity, Gram stain,

protein, glucose, and cell count with differential. Typical findings indicative of infection in CSF include elevated protein, low glucose, and microbial growth (gram-positive organisms commonly found).

  c) Infection may be present without abnormal laboratory findings.

 5. Management

  a) Systemic antimicrobials or direct instillation of antimicrobials into the reservoir

  b) Persistent infection requires device removal.

B. Malposition or migration of catheter (Bot, Constantini, & Roth, 2013; Kramer et al., 2014)

 1. Etiology

  a) Kinking of catheter

  b) Migration of catheter out of ventricle

 2. Signs and symptoms

  a) Poor or absent refilling of the reservoir when depressed

  b) Inability to gently aspirate CSF

  c) Inability to instill fluid into the reservoir

  d) CSF leakage around the reservoir

  e) Change in neurologic status (i.e., dizziness, headache, lethargy, altered level of consciousness)

 3. Diagnostic tests: Radiologic imaging (e.g., computed tomography [CT] or magnetic resonance imaging [MRI] scan of brain).

 4. Management: Referral to a neurosurgeon to evaluate the need for revision or removal

C. Blood in CSF

 1. Etiology

  a) Intraventricular hemorrhage

  b) Subdural hematoma

  c) Subarachnoid hematoma

  d) Improper positioning of butterfly needle during access, causing SC bleeding

 2. Signs and symptoms

  a) Change in neurologic status (e.g., vision changes, headaches, confusion)

  b) Sensory or motor deficits (e.g., ataxia, slurred speech)

 3. Diagnostic tests: CT or MRI of brain

 4. Management: May require surgical intervention

X. Education and documentation (see Chapter 17)

XI. Patient education special considerations

A. Care of device

 1. Avoid getting incision wet while sutures are present.

 2. No special care is required once sutures are removed.

 3. Hair may grow back, except for a small 2–3 cm area over the device.

 4. Protect the site from trauma.

B. Signs and symptoms of infection or malfunction (e.g., fever, headache, neck stiffness, vision changes, nausea/vomiting, neurologic changes, altered level of consciousness)

XII. Special considerations

A. Pediatric

 1. The use of ventriculoperitoneal shunts with programmable valves for administration of chemotherapy has been described in pediatric patients with hematologic malignancies, intracerebral hemorrhage, or hydrocephalus (Kramer et al., 2014; Palejwala et al., 2014). The device allows for intraventricular chemotherapy and subsequent concomitant CSF diversion through the shunt.

 2. Pericatheter cyst formation has been reported in one series of pediatric patients following placement of an intraventricular reservoir or ventriculoperitoneal shunt (Kramer et al., 2014).

B. Older adults: Underlying dementia may complicate assessment and diagnosis of medication-induced mental status changes in patients receiving intrathecal chemotherapy.

The author would like to acknowledge Julie G. Walker, MSN, RN, FNP-C, for her contribution to this chapter that remains unchanged from the previous edition of this book.

References

Aiello-Laws, L., & Rutledge, D.N. (2008). Management of adult patients receiving intraventricular chemotherapy for the treatment of leptomeningeal metastasis. *Clinical Journal of Oncology Nursing, 12,* 429–435. doi:10.1188/08.CJON.429-435

Bin Nafisah, N., & Ahmad, M. (2015). Ommaya reservoir infection rate: A 6-year retrospective cohort study of Ommaya reservoir in pediatrics. *Child's Nervous System, 31,* 29–36. doi:10.1007/s00381-014-2561-x

Bot, G., Constantini, S., & Roth, J. (2013). Intraventricular migration of ventricular access device. *Child's Nervous System, 29,* 1975–1976. doi:10.1007/s00381-013-2292-4

Gabay, M.P., Thakkar, J.P., Stachnik, J.M., Woelich, S.K., & Villano, J.L. (2012). Intra-CSF administration of chemotherapy medications. *Cancer Chemotherapy and Pharmacology, 70,* 1–15. doi:10.1007/s00280-012-1893-z

Graber, J.J., & Omuro, A. (2011). Pharmacotherapy for primary CNS lymphoma: Progress beyond methotrexate? *CNS Drugs, 25,* 447–457. doi:10.2165/11589030-000000000-00000

Kramer, K., Smith, M., & Souweidane, M.M. (2014). Safety profile of long-term intraventricular access devices in pediatric patients receiving radioimmunotherapy for central nervous system malignancies. *Pediatric Blood and Cancer, 61,* 1590–1592. doi:10.1002/pbc.25080

Lee, D.J., Gurkoff, G.G., Goodarzi, A., Muizelaar, J.P., Boggan, J.E., & Shahlaie, K. (2014). Intracerebroventricular opiate infusion for refractory head and facial pain. *World Journal of Clinical Cases, 2,* 351–356. doi:10.12998/wjcc.v2.i8.351

Mascitelli, J., De Los Reyes, K., Steinberger, J., & Zou, H. (2013). Lack of functionality and need for revision of an Ommaya reservoir placed into a cavum septum pellucidum: Case report. *Journal of Neurosurgery, 118,* 502–504. doi:10.3171/2012.10.JNS12818

Mead, P.A., Safdieh, J.E., Nizza, P., Tuma, S., & Sepkowitz, K.A. (2013). Ommaya reservoir infections: A 16-year retrospective analysis. *Journal of Infection, 68,* 225–230. doi:10.1016/j.jinf.2013.11.014

Ng, K., Mabasa, V.H., Chow, I., & Ensom, M.H. (2014). Systematic review of efficacy, pharmacokinetics, and administration of intraventricular vancomycin in adults. *Neurocritical Care, 29,* 158–171. doi:10.1007/s12028-012-9784-z

Ommaya, A.K. (1963). Subcutaneous reservoir and pump for sterile access to ventricular cerebrospinal fluid. *Lancet, 282,* 983–984. doi:10.1016/S0140-6736(63)90681-0

Ozerov, S.S., Mel'nikov, A.V., Ibragimova, D.I., Tereshchenko, G.V., & Rachkov, V.E. (2014). Placement of the Ommaya reservoir in narrow and slit-like ventricles using a neuronavigation system. Author's own experience and literature review. *Zhurnal Voprosy Neĭrokhirurgii Imeni N.N. Burdenko, 78*(3), 38–43.

Palejwala, S.K., Stidd, D.A., Skoch, J.M., Gupta, P., Lemole, G.M., & Weinand, M.E. (2014). Use of a stop-flow programmable shunt valve to maximize CNS chemotherapy delivery in a pediatric patient with acute lymphoblastic leukemia. *Surgical Neurology International, 5*(Suppl. 4), S273–S277.

Peyrl, A., Chocholous, M., Azizi, A.A., Czech, T., Dorfer, C., Mitteregger, D., … Slavc, I. (2014). Safety of Ommaya reservoirs in children with brain tumors: A 20-year experience with 5472 intraventricular drug administrations in 98 patients. *Journal of Neuro-Oncology, 120,* 139–145. doi:10.1007/s11060-014-1531-1

Roguski, M., Rughani, A., Lin, C.-T., Cushing, D.A., Florman, J.E., & Wu, J.K. (2015). Survival following Ommaya reservoir placement for neoplastic meningitis. *Journal of Clinical Neuroscience, 22,* 1467–1472. doi:10.1016/j.jocn.2015.04.003

Szvalb, A.D., Raad, I.I., Weinberg, J.S., Suki, D., Mayer, R., & Viola, G.M. (2014). Ommaya reservoir-related infections: Clinical manifestations and treatment outcomes. *Journal of Infection, 68,* 216–244. doi:10.1016/j.jinf.2013.12.002

Van Horn, A., & Chamberlain, M.C. (2012). Neoplastic meningitis. *Journal of Supportive Oncology, 10,* 45–53. doi:10.1016/j.suponc.2011.06.002

Weiner, G.M., Chivukula, S., Chen, C.-J., Ding, D., Engh, J.A., & Amankulor, N. (2015). Ommaya reservoir with ventricular catheter placement for chemotherapy with frameless and pinless electromagnetic surgical neuronavigation. *Clinical Neurology and Neurosurgery, 130,* 61–66. doi:10.1016/j.clineuro.2014.12.018

Zairi, F., Le Rhun, E., Bertrand, N., Boulanger, T., Taillibert, S., Aboukais, R., … Chamberlain, M.C. (2015). Complications related to the placement of intraventricular chemotherapy device for the treatment of leptomeningeal metastases from solid tumor: A single centre experience in 112 patients. *Journal of Neuro-Oncology, 124,* 317–323. doi:10.1007/s11060-015-1842-x

Chapter 13

Epidural and Intrathecal Access Devices

Carole Marie Elledge, RN, MSN, AOCN®, and Mady Stovall, RN, MSN, ANP-BC

I. History (Bauer, George, Seif, & Farag, 2012; Bottros & Christo, 2014; Calthorpe, 2004; Toledano & Tsen, 2014)
   A. In 1885, Dr. J. Leonard Corning accidentally discovered epidural anesthesia when he introduced cocaine between the lumbar vertebral processes to treat habitual masturbation.
   B. In 1901, French physicians Jean-Anthanase Sicard and Fernand Cathelin independently introduced single-shot epidural blocks via the caudal approach for neurologic and genitourinary procedures, respectively (Toledano & Tsen, 2014).
   C. By 1910, caudal block use for gynecologic and obstetric procedures was found beneficial (Toledano & Tsen, 2014).
   D. Intrathecal injections of alcohol for palliation of pain associated with malignant and nonmalignant disease was first described in the 1930s.
   E. In 1940, Dr. William Lemmon developed a malleable spinal needle made of German silver to provide continuous spinal anesthesia.
   F. By 1942, continuous caudal analgesia techniques were developed for obstetrical patients using a modified Lemmon needle (Toledano & Tsen, 2014).
   G. In 1944, Dr. Edward Tuohy developed a nylon ureteric catheter for continuous spinal analgesia, thereby eliminating some of the drawbacks associated with the malleable needle.
   H. By the early 1950s, intraspinal segmental alcohol blocks used the Tuohy catheter to treat intractable pain associated with malignancy.
   I. Broad commercial availability of epidural catheters, the first report of intrathecal opioid efficacy, and the formation of pain services began in the 1970s (Toledano & Tsen, 2014).
   J. Implantable drug delivery systems were trialed in the early 1980s for treatment of cancer-related pain and chemotherapy administration (Wilkes, 2014).
II. Anatomy and physiology (Bauer et al., 2012; Farquhar-Smith & Chapman, 2012; McHugh, Miller-

Saultz, Wuhrman, & Kosharskyy, 2012; National Cancer Institute, n.d.)
   A. Vertebral column (see Figure 13-1)
      1. 33 vertebrae
         a) Cervical: 7 (C1–C7)
         b) Thoracic: 12 (T1–T12)
         c) Lumbar: 5 (L1–L5)
         d) Fused sacral: 5 (S1–S5)
         e) Coccyx, formed by four fused vertebrae; small, triangle-shaped bone attached to the bottom of the sacrum
      2. The spinal cord typically ends between the last thoracic and first lumbar vertebrae; subsequently, lumbar punctures are performed below the second lumbar vertebra (L2).

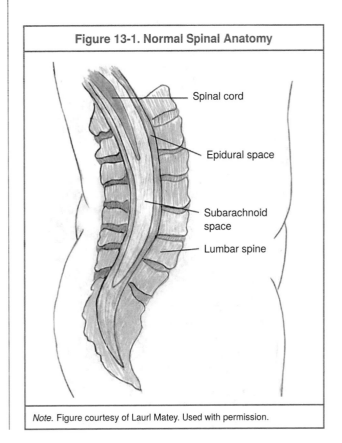

Figure 13-1. Normal Spinal Anatomy

Spinal cord

Epidural space

Subarachnoid space

Lumbar spine

Note. Figure courtesy of Laurl Matey. Used with permission.

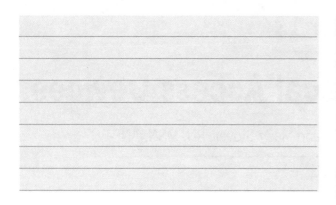

3. Cerebrospinal fluid (CSF) flows throughout the vertebral column.
  B. Intraspinal spaces
    1. Epidural space
      a) Lies between periosteum (the inner portion of the vertebrae) and dura mater of the vertebral column
      b) Extends from the foramen magnum (base of the skull) to the sacrococcygeal ligament (sacrum)
      c) Contains adipose tissue, blood vessels, lymphatic vessels, and spinal nerves
    2. Intrathecal space (subdural space)
      a) A potential space is located between the dura mater and arachnoid membrane.
      b) The small volume space is filled with CSF.
      c) Drug delivery catheters are usually placed in this space to provide site-specific delivery of pain medications, antibiotics, or antineoplastic therapy (e.g., morphine).
III. Device characteristics (Bottros & Christo, 2014; Calthorpe, 2004; Farquhar-Smith & Chapman, 2012; Heo et al., 2014; Kim, Jung, & Cho, 2013; McHugh et al., 2012; Smyth, Jarvis, & Poulin, 2014)
  A. Epidural
    1. Medications injected into the epidural space are slowly spread throughout the thoracic, lumbar, and sacral areas.
    2. Catheters inserted into the epidural space are used to deliver opioids with or without anesthetics or steroids.
  B. Intrathecal
    1. Medications are delivered directly into CSF fluid surrounding the spinal column.
    2. Catheters inserted into the intrathecal space are used to deliver medications with or without anesthetics or steroids.
IV. Device features (Bottros & Christo, 2014; Calthorpe, 2004; Farquhar-Smith & Chapman, 2012; Kim et al., 2013; McHugh et al., 2012)
  A. External epidural or intrathecal catheters

1. Percutaneous or short tunneled catheters
  a) Short-term use only (hours to days) due to increased risk of infection, dislodgment, and skin irritation
  b) Made of radiopaque polyamide, polyurethane, Teflon™, or nylon
  c) Available with open- or closed-end tips with three-eyed multiport configuration
  d) Sizes from 19 to 20 gauge, 40-inch length; pediatric sizes 20 and 24 gauge
  e) Exit site: Lower back
  f) Drug delivery: Intermittent injection or an external pump
2. Long-term tunneled catheters
  a) Made of radiopaque polyamide, polyurethane, or nylon
  b) Exit site: Usually the abdomen
  B. Implanted epidural or intrathecal ports (Heo et al., 2014; Kim et al., 2013; Smyth et al., 2014)
    1. Similar in structure to venous ports (e.g., comprising a portal body, reservoir, septum, catheter) (see Chapter 7)
    2. Reservoirs contain a filter (e.g., 20 or 60 micron filter) to prevent infusion of large particulate matter into the catheter.
    3. Reservoir volume approximately 0.3–0.5 ml
    4. Completely implanted, similar to venous port in a subcutaneous (SC) pocket
    5. Indicated for long-term therapy
    6. At the time of publication, not being manufactured in the United States
  C. Implanted pump with attached intrathecal or epidural catheter (Bottros & Christo, 2014; Farquhar-Smith & Chapman, 2012; Smyth et al., 2014; Wesemann et al., 2014)
    1. Contains an intrinsic power source and refillable drug reservoir
    2. Totally implanted in an SC pocket
    3. Pump: Small and disc-shaped septum(s), reservoir, and catheter
    4. Catheter: Radiopaque silicone, attached at time of surgery or available preattached
    5. Pump reservoir: 20 ml or 40 ml with a diameter of 6.5 mm, weighing 30 g and up to 212.6 g (7.5 oz) when full
    6. Indicated for long-term therapy
    7. Available with side port for bolus injection
    8. Available with filter to prevent infusion of large particulate matter into the catheter
    9. Pump types (Bottros & Christo, 2014; McHugh et al., 2012; Rosen et al., 2013; Wilkes, 2014)
      a) Battery powered

(1) Drug delivery is achieved with a battery-powered peristaltic pump.

(2) Within the pump, pressurized gas exerts pressure on the reservoir to assist in drug delivery.

(3) Because of the pressurized gas, the pump will deliver different drug amounts in high pressure atmospheres (e.g., high altitudes) or high temperatures (e.g., hot tubs).

(4) The pump is available with an external device to allow bolus infusion and is programmed similarly to ambulatory pumps, where bolus dose, lockout time, and total number of doses are programmed.

b) Non–battery powered

(1) The pump is divided into inner and outer chambers by accordion-like bellows.

(2) The inner chamber contains the drug to be infused.

(3) The outer chamber contains propellant permanently sealed inside.

(4) Body temperature warms the propellant, exerting constant pressure on the bellows and infusing the drug through the inner chambers filter and through the catheter.

(5) Dosages are changed by adjusting drug concentration during the pump refill process.

c) Externally operated programmable pump

(1) A drug reservoir automatically delivers a controlled amount of the drug through a filter and then through the catheter.

(2) Constant pressure on the reservoir mechanically pushes the medication forward.

(3) An external, handheld, battery-operated programmer is used to control flow rate by electronically controlled valves in the pump.

10. Pumps are magnetic resonance imaging (MRI) compatible; however, a pump may have to be emptied prior to MRI imaging. The magnetic field can increase pump infu-

sion rate. Refer to the manufacturer's operational manual prior to imaging.

V. Device advantages and disadvantages (see Table 13-1)

VI. Patient selection criteria (Bhatnagar & Gupta, 2015; Farquhar-Smith & Chapman, 2012; Heo et al., 2014; Kim et al., 2013; Lin et al., 2012; Saulino, Kim, & Shaw, 2014; Smyth et al., 2014; Wesemann et al., 2014; Wilkes, 2014)

A. Indications for epidural or intrathecal access devices

1. Chronic localized intractable cancer pain

2. Noncancer pain (e.g., chronic, intractable back or pelvic pain)

3. Postsurgical pain needing temporary epidural anesthesia or patient-controlled anesthesia

4. Spasticity requiring an intrathecal baclofen pump

5. Leptomeningeal or primary neurologic cancers requiring frequent administration of intrathecal chemotherapy

6. Frequent intrathecal access, such as acute lymphoblastic leukemia

B. Contraindications for epidural or intrathecal access device

1. Local or systemic infection

2. Uncorrected coagulopathy (international normalized ratio > 1.5; platelet count < 50,000)

3. Epidural metastasis or suspected spinal cord compression

4. Patients with opioid addiction or drug-seeking behavior

5. Patients with multiple sites or various types of pain

6. Large volume infusion required

7. Increased intracranial pressure

8. Some institutions will not place in the presence of unstable neurologic findings and brain metastases due to risk of herniation and hemorrhage.

9. Cancer of the spine (depending on the spinal level and degree of stenosis)

VII. Insertion techniques (Bauer et al., 2012; Bottros & Christo, 2014; Farquhar-Smith & Chapman, 2012; Heo et al., 2014; Smyth et al., 2014; Wilkes, 2014)

A. Before insertion procedure, verify scope of practice with the individual state board of nursing and institutional guidelines. Credentialing and ongoing competency validation is required. Advanced practice nurses in many states have the ability to insert temporary catheters within scope of practice (see Appendix 4).

B. Patient preparation: Prior to placement, review the provider order for catheter placement and recent imaging studies and laboratory studies,

	Table 13-1. Advantages and Disadvantages of Epidural or Intrathecal Access Devices	
Type	**Advantages**	**Disadvantages**
Overall (compared to other routes)	Less sedation with narcotics Less effect on cardiovascular or respiratory status	Require skilled personnel to manage catheter, which may be problematic in some rural areas Preservative-free medications used with epidural and intraspinal may be difficult to obtain.
Temporary catheters	Indicated postoperatively for short-term pain control (e.g., trauma pain, postoperative pain) Indicated for infrequent access for medications Ease and speed of insertion Used for pain control when life expectancy is weeks Can give intrathecal chemotherapy Test efficacy of epidural or intrathecal opioid therapy prior to placement of long-term device	Leak around insertion site Require frequent, meticulous site care
Permanent catheters	Facilitate ambulation and activities of daily living with adequate pain control Less risk of catheter dislodgment Can be used long term	Require surgical placement and removal Involve expensive placement costs when compared to temporary catheters Cost of maintenance supplies Greater risk of infection
Implantable ports	Less chance of infection Facilitate ambulation and activities of daily living with adequate pain control Less risk of catheter dislodgment Can be used long term	Require surgical procedure for placement and removal Involve expensive placement costs compared to temporary catheters Require access with a noncoring needle
Implantable pumps	Less chance of infection Infusion rates can be changed by a computerized programmer, depending on pump type. Less risk of catheter dislodgment Catheter can be placed epidurally or intrathecally. Because of the pump reservoir's capacity, refills are required every one to six months. Increase freedom to perform daily activities Reduce systemic side effects Continuous and bolus therapy available	The complexity of the technology requires healthcare professionals who are trained in computer technology, internal pump access, and pump maintenance. Costly to insert Fever increases pump mechanism. May require emptying if magnetic resonance imaging is needed, depending on pump type

including coagulation tests, current medications, and the most recent doses and clinical notes.

C. Procedure
1. Typically performed under fluoroscopy. Ultrasound is preferred for intraoperative and bedside insertion and is beneficial as a radiation-free technique (Bauer et al., 2012; Bottros & Christo, 2014).
2. Use sterile technique and maximum sterile barrier precautions for insertion and handling of devices.
   a) Epidural insertion: Percutaneously into epidural space and advanced approximately 4 cm, usually at L2–L3, L3–L4, or L4–L5
   b) Intrathecal insertion: Advanced below the dura where the CSF circulates, usually at L2–L3, L3–L4, or L4–L5
3. Percutaneous temporary catheters (epidural or intrathecal)
   a) May be placed at the bedside or in a procedural area using local anesthesia
   b) The external portion is secured using tape along the patient's back to the anterior chest wall or around the flank and secured using a transparent dressing and securement device.
   c) Label the transparent dressing with date of insertion and placement site.
   d) Label the device as either epidural or intrathecal.
4. Tunneled catheters (epidural or intrathecal)
   a) Placed by a surgeon or interventional radiologist. The procedure is similar to venous tunneled catheter placement (see Chapter 6).
   b) The distal tip is placed in the epidural or intrathecal space, and the proximal tip is tunneled under SC tissue, exiting at the waist or abdomen.

c) The exit site is secured using a transparent dressing and securement device.

d) Label the transparent dressing with date of insertion and placement site (e.g., epidural, intrathecal).

e) Label the tubing as either intrathecal or epidural.

5. Implanted port (epidural or intrathecal)

a) Placed by a surgeon or interventional radiologist

b) The proximal end of the catheter is subcutaneously tunneled around the flank to the abdomen or anterior chest wall and connected to the portal body.

c) The port is attached to the catheter that is inserted percutaneously approximately 4 cm into the epidural space.

d) The portal body is sutured to the fascia over a bony prominence, such as the lower rib.

e) Cover the portal body insertion site with a transparent dressing.

f) Label the transparent dressing with date of insertion and placement site (e.g., epidural or intrathecal).

6. Implantable pump (intrathecal)

a) Inserted in the operating room or interventional radiology using local anesthesia with fluoroscopic guidance

b) Pumps should be placed away from bony landmarks, such as the lower thoracic ribs or iliac crest, to avoid irritation.

c) The pump is implanted into an SC pocket in the lower quadrant of the left or right abdomen or gluteal region approximately 2.5 cm deep to accommodate refilling of the pump. The catheter is tunneled and threaded into the epidural or intrathecal space (Bottros & Christo, 2014).

d) The pump reservoir is filled and catheter access port is flushed after connecting the catheter to the pump.

D. Immediate postoperative care (McHugh et al., 2012)

1. Check dressing for bleeding or drainage.
2. Assess site for hematoma or excessive postoperative edema.
3. Perform frequent neurologic assessments.
4. Monitor vital signs per postoperative routine and then every four hours until stable. Monitor blood pressure frequently for hypotension.
5. Analgesics may take one hour to take effect.

6. Assess for pain.
7. Assess respiratory rate after placement, then frequently if device is being used for pain medication.

VIII. Unique maintenance and care (Bottros & Christo, 2014; McHugh et al., 2012)

A. Prior to accessing or caring for epidural or intrathecal catheters or pumps, verify scope of practice with the individual state board of nursing and institutional guidelines. RNs managing epidural and intrathecal devices must be knowledgeable of the principles of epidural and intrathecal drug administration and the care of patients with these devices.

B. Maintain maximum sterile barrier precautions with mask and sterile gloves with any access or maintenance procedure (O'Grady et al., 2011).

C. Use preservative-free medications and preservative-free solutions. Attach a 0.2 micron filter to eliminate debris entering into the epidural or intrathecal space.

D. Do not use alcohol for cleaning these devices; alcohol is neurotoxic. Use chlorhexidine gluconate and let dry (see Appendix 2).

E. Flushing: Routine flushing is not indicated.
1. Catheter (temporary and tunneled): 1–2 ml of preservative-free 0.9% normal saline (NS) after each use
2. Epidural or intrathecal port: 3 ml of preservative-free NS after each use
3. Infusion pump: No flushing is required.

F. Tubing
1. Ensure that all tubing connections are Luer lock. Label all lines closest to the patient as feasible. Secure the catheter to prevent kinks and tension, which may lead to malposition. Consider a tension loop.
2. Attach a 0.2 micron filter to all epidural and intrathecal infusions and change if damaged, leaking, and when tubing is changed. A filter may not be needed if the drug is filtered prior to administration or if the portal body or pump contains a filter.

3. Use specialized tubing without injection ports, as indicated, to prevent accidental injection of unintended medication into epidural or intrathecal space (Institute for Safe Medication Practices, 2008) (see Chapter 17).
4. Label any injection tubing for epidural or intrathecal use only (see Figure 13-2).
5. Trace the tubing or catheter from the patient to point of origin each time the catheter is accessed, at handoff, and at transitions to a new setting or service.

G. A chlorhexidine-impregnated dressing or sponge has been found to significantly reduce the rate of epidural catheter infections (Kerwat et al., 2015).

H. Medication administration considerations (Bottros & Christo, 2014; Saulino et al., 2014)
1. Only preservative-free NS may be used as diluent for medications administered via an epidural or intrathecal catheter, with the exception of methotrexate and cytarabine administration; Elliotts B® Solution should be used as the diluent.
2. Be aware that opioid dosing for epidural drug administration may be up to 10 times higher than intrathecal administration.
3. Ensure placement prior to drug administration by gently aspirating. If clear fluid volume is greater than 0.5 ml or if blood is obtained, notify the provider and do not administer the drug. The presence of CSF indicates that the catheter has punctured the dura and migrated into the intrathecal space.
4. Continuous infusions of epidural or intrathecal medication: Secure with a tension loop or other securement device to prevent accidental dislodgment.

I. Routine monitoring for opioid administration (Bottros & Christo, 2014; Saulino et al., 2014)
1. Monitor carefully during initial dose of opiate and with each subsequent increase in dose. Assess pain levels before, during, and after opioid administration.
2. The patient may be weaned off other systemic opioids while receiving epidural analgesia.
3. Monitor for signs of respiratory and central nervous system depression based on individual risk factors, treatment-related risks, and type of drug regimen administered (Jarzyna et al., 2011).
   a) Patients are at highest risk for opioid-induced respiratory depression within the first 24 hours of epidural or intrathecal opioid administration.
   b) Delayed respiratory depression usually occurs 3–12 hours after administration, but may occur as late as 24 hours following opioid administration.
   c) Ensure that resuscitation equipment is available.
   d) Ensure presence of IV access for at least 24 hours after initiation of epidural or intrathecal opioids for rescue drug, if needed.
   e) Use evidence-based recommendations for monitoring patients at risk for opioid-induced sedation (e.g., American Society for Pain Management Nursing, National Comprehensive Cancer Network®).

J. Implanted pump (Bottros & Christo, 2014; Saulino & Gofeld, 2014)
1. Ensure familiarity with the device and its complications.
2. Document the pump model number, reservoir size, and flow rate in the patient's medical record. Prior to pump care, obtain the specific pump model and maintenance procedures from the manufacturer for further details.
3. Use maximum sterile barrier precautions when accessing the pump septum. A kit is provided by the pump manufacturer, which includes an access needle and pump template to locate the septum. Ultrasound has successfully been used to access the pump septum (Gofeld & McQueen, 2011; Saulino & Gofeld, 2014).
4. The pump must be refilled on a schedule. The refill interval depends on drug concentration, drug stability, pump reservoir vol-

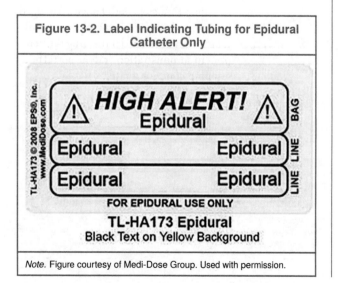

Figure 13-2. Label Indicating Tubing for Epidural Catheter Only

⚠ HIGH ALERT! ⚠
Epidural

| Epidural | Epidural |
| Epidural | Epidural |

BAG / LINE / LINE

TL-HA173 © 2008 EPS®, Inc.
www.MediDose.com

FOR EPIDURAL USE ONLY
TL-HA173 Epidural
Black Text on Yellow Background

Note. Figure courtesy of Medi-Dose Group. Used with permission.

ume, and daily dose. Never allow the pump to become completely empty.

5. Pump refills typically occur every two to eight weeks; however, they can occur up to six months. Refill schedules should accommodate office closures and holidays.

6. The U.S. Food and Drug Administration requires pumps to be refilled every six months, even if the pump is not completely empty.

7. Do not overfill pump, which can result in overpressurization and subsequent overinfusion of medication.

8. Drug dose calculations
   a) Use manufacturer guidelines for calculating the amount of drug needed to refill the pump.
   b) Evaluate the actual (measured) volume (the volume initially placed in the pump) minus the volume of drug withdrawn from reservoir.

9. Document refill.
   a) Date and time of refill and the number of days since last refill
   b) Return volume from pump after access
   c) Infused volume (previous refill volume minus return volume)
   d) Pump flow rate (infused volume divided by number of days since last refill)
   e) Pump drug, concentration, and drug refill volume
   f) Patient's response to the procedure

IX. Removal technique
A. Whether a trained RN or advanced practice nurse can remove temporary catheters depends on the individual state board of nursing and institutional guidelines. Training and competency records must be maintained.
B. Temporary catheters are pulled directly out of the epidural or intrathecal system using maximum sterile barrier precautions. The catheter is assessed for integrity.
C. Pumps and ports are removed by a surgeon or interventional radiologist. Devices may be left in place except in the occurrence of catheter migration, infection, CSF leak, hematoma, meningitis, sciatic nerve damage, catheter occlusion, or persistent or severe spinal headaches.

X. Complications (Bauer et al., 2012; Bottros & Christo, 2014; Deer & Provenzano, 2013; Farquhar-Smith & Chapman, 2012; Gevirtz, 2010; Heo et al., 2014; Smyth et al., 2014)
A. Infection
   1. Etiology
      a) Surgical contamination
      b) Improper technique when accessing the system
      c) Systemic complication of an immunosuppressed patient
      d) Non-iatrogenic trauma to the site
   2. Potential sites of infection
      a) Catheter exit site
      b) Tunnel
      c) Port pocket
      d) Pump pocket
      e) Epidural space
      f) Surgical wound or wound dehiscence
   3. Signs and symptoms
      a) Site tenderness, warmth, erythema, or drainage
      b) Hypo- or hyperthermia
      c) Headache with or without vomiting
      d) Bloody or purulent CSF from reservoir
      e) Pain during injection
      f) Decreased analgesic effects following pain medication administration
      g) Changes in sensory or motor function
      h) Nuchal rigidity
      i) Mental status changes
      j) Port or pump pocket erythema
      k) Seizures
      l) Photophobia
   4. Diagnostic testing
      a) Complete blood count: Elevated white blood cell count
      b) CSF: Elevated protein and microbial growth
      c) Wound culture: Culture of CSF
   5. Prevention
      a) Evidence-based recommendations for preventing infections in epidural and intrathecal devices are limited in the literature.
         (1) For implanted drug delivery devices, preoperative prophylactic antibiotic therapy has been recommended (Deer & Provenzano, 2013; Gevirtz, 2010).
         (2) A randomized, prospective trial by Kerwat et al. (2015) of 337 patients with epidural and peripheral regional catheters used for pain medication administration demonstrated that chlorhexidine gluconate dressings significantly reduced bacterial colonization of the tip and insertion site of epidural and peripheral regional catheters compared to

conventional dressings with no difference in local infections between the two groups. Subsequently, the use of chlorhexidine-impregnated dressings may decrease infection rate.

    (3) Recommendations

        (a) Use maximum sterile barrier precautions during insertion, routine maintenance, and medication administration.

        (b) Maintain integrity of dressing for percutaneous catheters and all others until insertion site has healed.

        (c) Ensure that only specially trained personnel access the device.

        (d) Protect the exit site from injury and the device from damage.

        (e) Use a microporous filter to decrease introduction of pathogens.

6. Management

   a) Administer antibiotics systemically.

   b) Persistent infection may require device removal. If the device is removed, a culture of the catheter tip may be obtained if ordered.

B. Epidural hematoma (Margo et al., 2011)

   1. Etiology: Blood filling the brain area and compressing the brain tissue, resulting in intracranial hypertension; considered an emergency situation

   2. Signs and symptoms: Headache, neurologic changes, behavior changes, aphasia, dizziness, nausea and vomiting, lethargy, and confusion

   3. Diagnostic tests: computed tomography (CT) or MRI of brain

   4. Management: Surgical drainage of hematoma by a surgeon

C. Post–dural puncture headache syndrome (Neuman, Eldrige, Qu, Freeman, & Hoelzer, 2013; Zencirci, 2010)

   1. Etiology: Leakage of CSF through the dura mater puncture, causing reduced CSF levels in the brain and spinal cord; more common with intrathecal devices

   2. Signs and symptoms: Headache, neck pain, shoulder pain, paresthesia, nausea and vomiting, photophobia, and vision changes

   3. Prevention: Keep the patient supine after procedure; encourage fluids.

   4. Management

      a) Epidural blood patch

      b) Postprocedure: Hydration and oral intake of caffeine

D. Fibrin formation at catheter tip (Jhas & Tuli, 2008)

   1. Etiology: Fibrin sheath forms around catheter distal tip, applying pressure to the dorsal nerve, nerve roots, and spinal cord. Backtracking of the drug can occur outside the catheter, with deposition of drug into the SC tissue.

   2. Signs and symptoms

      a) Inadequate pain management

      b) Neurologic deficits

      c) Paralysis

      d) Bowel or bladder retention or incontinence

      e) Pain with injection: Radicular pain is more frequent with intrathecal catheters.

   3. Diagnostic test: Imaging of catheter tip

   4. Management

      a) Evaluate the location of the catheter tip by imaging procedure.

      b) Removal of the device may be necessary.

E. Bleeding (Bauer et al., 2012)

   1. Etiology: Epidural or subarachnoid bleeding, exit-site bleeding; considered a potential emergency

   2. Signs and symptoms

      a) Neurologic changes

      b) Severe back pain

      c) Sensory or motor deficits

      d) Bleeding noted at exit site

   3. Management

      a) Notify the provider; a CT or MRI may be ordered.

      b) Establish IV access.

      c) Elevate the head of the bed 30°.

      d) Monitor neurologic status and vital signs.

e) If neurologic status is deteriorating, obtain a neurosurgery consult.

f) If bleeding persists, the provider may need to remove the device.

F. Displacement or migration of catheter (Jeon, Lee, Yoon, Kim, & Lee, 2013; Strandness, Wiktor, Varadarajan, & Weisman, 2015; Tandon & Pandey, 2015)

1. Etiology
   a) Kinking or blockage of catheter
   b) Catheter migration out of epidural space
   c) Inadvertent dural puncture during epidural placement
   d) Spinal cord puncture either by migration of the intrathecal catheter or during insertion

2. Signs and symptoms: Associated with a variety of effects from the displacement
   a) Ineffective pain control
   b) Traumatic syrinx (fluid filled cavity inside the spinal cord or brain stem)
   c) Epigastric arterial erosion
   d) Cerebral hypotension
   e) Herniation associated with excessive CSF leakage

3. Assessment parameters
   a) Change in neurologic status
   b) Spinal headache
   c) CSF leakage around the exit site, port, or pump pocket
   d) Slow or resistant filling of pump reservoir or port
   e) Easy mobility of the port under the skin
   f) Outward migration of the catheter judged by catheter marks outside the patient's body

4. Prevention: Avoid trauma to the implant site or device. Patients who weigh less than 40 kg (88 lbs) are at increased risk for epidural catheters that move inward and fall out as compared to patients who weigh more (Strandness et al., 2015).

5. Management
   a) Attempt to gently irrigate with preservative-free NS.
   b) Notify the provider if blood or greater than 0.5 ml of CSF is aspirated, and do not administer drug.
   c) Imaging studies may be ordered to assess placement of the catheter.
   d) Radiation therapy may be considered to decrease size of the tumor if growth blocks the catheter.
   e) Administer pain medication, as needed.
   f) The device may be removed.

G. Dislodgment of the needle from port or pump
1. Etiology: Needle dislodged from septum
2. Signs and symptoms: Edema at insertion site, possible erythema, pain
3. Prevention: Secure needle within the septum with securement device and place occlusive dressing.
4. Management: Reaccess device.

H. Implantable pump complications (see Table 13-2)
1. "Pocket fill" (Gofeld & McQueen, 2011; Saulino & Gofeld, 2014; Wesemann et al., 2014; Wilkes, 2014)
   a) Etiology: Medication is improperly administered into the SC tissue pump pocket.
   b) Signs and symptoms: Depend on drug administered and concentration
   c) Prevention
      (1) Use ultrasound guidance to locate septum for access.
      (2) Use the template provided by the manufacturer to locate the septum prior to access. Management includes supportive care and possible reversal agents.

2. Radiation effects on implanted pump functioning (Gebhardt, Ludwig, Kirsner, Kisling, & Kosturakis, 2013)
   a) Gebhardt et al. (2013) studied 39 patients (12 of whom received external beam radiation therapy with either the pump or the catheter in the treatment field) with cumulative device doses ranging from 5–36 Gy and 15–45 Gy, respectively. At the completion of radiation, no evidence was found of pump malfunction for any of the 39 patients. Median follow-up was 4.5 months.
   b) Guidelines from manufacturers have recommended a cumulative dose of 5 Gy; however, no definitive recommendation can be made.
   c) Check device functioning following completion of radiation or sooner if analgesic requirements change.

3. Silicone septum leakage (Perruchoud, Bovy, Rutschmann, Durrer, & Buschser, 2013)
   a) Etiology: Multiple access within septum, needles constantly rubbing against metallic pump body, inability to access septum
   b) Signs and symptoms: Depend on drug administered

Table 13-2. Implantable Intrathecal Pump Complications

Complication	Prevention	Presentation	Interventions
Seroma, hematoma	Instruct the patient to avoid sports and other activities that may cause injury.	Tenderness, edema, fluid leakage, and erythema occurring within 72 hours after surgery	Apply pressure dressing or abdominal binder daily for 1–2 months, if needed. Avoid trauma to the pump.
Catheter occlusion: Thrombus, catheter kinking/dislodgment	Instruct the patient to keep refill appointments. Do not let the pump become completely empty.	Excess fluid remaining in pump, abdominal pain, medication withdrawal symptoms Lower extremity weakness Groin pain Uncontrolled pain	Imaging or catheter contrast study to confirm placement Prepare the patient for pump removal (rare) if occlusion cannot be cleared.
Equipment problems, program problems, incorrect setup, improper rate	Confer with company technical support staff. Provide competency-based education.	Excess or less fluid remains in the pump, and systemic toxicity from incorrect drug dose infusion	Preprogram pump or remove fluid/drug from reservoir and refill with proper concentration. Avoid extreme temperature or altitudes.
Infection: Subcutaneous pocket, sepsis	Use sterile technique. Examine fluid for discoloration. Maintain closed system.	Tenderness, warmth, erythema, swelling, drainage at pump site Fever/chills Headache Neck pain	Culture site or fluid. Administer antibiotics, as prescribed. Assess for signs of sepsis. Pump removal may be necessary.
Pump inversion in subcutaneous pocket	Instruct the patient to avoid sports and other activities that may cause injury. Encourage patient to maintain weight.	Unable to access pump	Imaging to evaluate pump Surgical intervention to reposition pump
Skin necrosis over pump	Implant with sufficient tissue over pump. Encourage patient to maintain weight. Routinely inspect skin over pump.	Erythema, pain, and skin breakdown	Apply semipermeable transparent dressing over skin to avoid friction with clothing. Remove pump and consider a new pump site.

Note. Based on information from Bottros & Christo, 2014; Farquhar-Smith & Chapman, 2012; Rosen et al., 2013; Saulino et al., 2014; Wesemann et al., 2014.

c) Prevention: Use ultrasound guidance to access; only trained personnel should access the pump.
d) Diagnostic tests: CT of abdomen
e) Management: Remove pump and replace.
XI. Education and documentation (see Chapter 17)

The authors would like to acknowledge Julie G. Walker, MSN, RN, FNP-C, for her contribution to this chapter that remains unchanged from the previous edition of this book.

References

Bauer, M., George, J.E., III., Seif, J., & Farag, E. (2012). Recent advances in epidural analgesia. *Anesthesiology Research and Practice, 2012,* 309219. doi:10.1155/2012/309219

Bhatnagar, S., & Gupta, M. (2015). Evidence-based clinical practice guidelines for interventional pain management in cancer pain. *Indian Journal of Palliative Care, 21,* 137–147. doi:10.4103/0973-1075.156466

Bottros, M.M., & Christo, P.J. (2014). Current perspectives on intrathecal drug delivery. *Journal of Pain Research, 7,* 615–626. doi:10.2147/JPR.S37591

Calthorpe, N. (2004). The history of spinal needles: Getting to the point. *Anaesthesia, 59,* 1231–1241. doi:10.1111/j.1365-2044.2004.03976.x

Deer, T.R., & Provenzano, D.A. (2013). Recommendations for reducing infection in the practice of implanting spinal cord stimulation and intrathecal drug delivery devices: A physician's playbook. *Pain Physician, 16,* E125–E128.

Farquhar-Smith, P., & Chapman, S. (2012). Neuraxial (epidural and intrathecal) opioids for intractable pain. *British Journal of Pain, 6,* 25–35. doi:10.1177/2049463712439256

Gebhardt, R., Ludwig, M., Kirsner, S., Kisling, K., & Kosturakis, A.K. (2013). Implanted intrathecal drug delivery systems and radiation treatment. *Pain Medicine, 14,* 398–402. doi:10.1111/pme.12037

Gevirtz, C. (2010). Infection control for patients with implanted pain management devices. *Nursing, 40*(2), 62–63. doi:10.1097/01.nurse.0000376304.90970.24

Gofeld, M., & McQueen, C.K., (2011). Ultrasound-guided intrathecal pump access and prevention of the pocket fill. *Pain Medicine, 12,* 607–611. doi:10.1111/j.1526-4637.2011.01090.x

Heo, B.H., Pyeon, T.H., Lee, H.G., Kim, W.M., Choi, J.I., & Yoon, M.H. (2014). Epidural infusion of morphine and levobupivacaine through a subcutaneous port for cancer pain management. *Korean Journal of Pain, 27,* 139–144. doi:10.3311/jkp.2014.27.2.139

Institute for Safe Medication Practices. (2008). Epidural-IV route mix-ups: Reducing the risk of deadly errors. *Acute care ISMP medication safety alert!* Retrieved from https://www.ismp.org/newsletters/acutecare/articles/20080703.asp

Jarzyna, D., Jungquist, C.R., Pasero, C., Willens, J.S., Nisbet, A., Oakes, L., ... Polomano, R.C. (2011). American Society for Pain Management Nursing guidelines on monitoring for opioid-induced sedation and respiratory depression. *Pain Management Nursing, 12,* 118–145. doi:10.1016/j.pmn.2011.06.008

Jeon, J., Lee, I.H., Yoon, H.-J., Kim, M.-G., & Lee, P.-M. (2013). Intravascular migration of a previously functioning epidural catheter. *Korean Journal of Anesthesiology, 64,* 556–557. doi:10.4097/kjae.2013.64.6.556

Jhas, S., & Tuli, S. (2008). Intrathecal catheter-tip inflammatory masses: An intraparenchymal granuloma. *Journal of Neurosurgery Spine, 9,* 196–199. doi:10.3171/SPI/2008/9/8/196

Kerwat, K., Eberhart, L., Kerwat, M., Hörth, D., Wulf, H., Steinfeldt, T., & Weismann, T. (2015). Chlorhexidine gluconate dressings reduce bacterial colonization rates in epidural and peripheral regional catheters. *Biomed Research International, 2015,* 149785. doi:10.1155/2015/149785

Kim, J.H., Jung, J.Y., & Cho, M.S. (2013). Continuous intrathecal morphine administration for cancer pain management using an intrathecal catheter connected to a subcutaneous injection port: A retrospective analysis of 22 terminal cancer patients in Korean population. *Korean Journal of Pain, 26,* 32–38. doi:10.3344/kjp.2013.26.1.32

Lin, C.P., Lin, W.Y., Lin, F.S., Lee, Y.S., Jeng, C.S., & Sun, W.Z. (2012). Efficacy of intrathecal drug delivery system for refractory cancer pain patients: A single tertiary medical center experience. *Journal of the Formosan Medical Association, 111,* 253–257. doi:10.1016/j.jfma.2011.03.005

Margo, E., Remy-Neris, O., Seizeur, R., Allano, V., Quinio, B., & Dam-Hieu, P. (2011). Bilateral subdural hematoma following implantation of intrathecal drug delivery device. *Neuromodulation, 14,* 179–182. doi:10.1111/j.1525-1403.2011.00335.x

McHugh, M.E., Miller-Saultz, D., Wuhrman, E., & Kosharskyy, B. (2012). Interventional pain management in the palliative care patient. *International Journal of Palliative Nursing, 18,* 426–428, 430–433. doi:10.12968/ijpn.2012.18.9.426

National Cancer Institute: SEER Training Modules. (n.d.). Anatomy and physiology. Retrieved from http://training.seer.cancer.gov/anatomy

Neuman, S.A., Eldrige, J.S., Qu, W., Freeman, E.D., & Hoelzer, B.C. (2013). Post dural puncture headache following intrathecal drug delivery system placement. *Pain Physician, 16,* 101–107.

O'Grady, N.P., Alexander, M., Burns, L.A., Dellinger, E.P., Garland, J., Heard, S.O., ... Healthcare Infection Control Practices Advisory Committee. (2011). Guidelines for the prevention of intravascular catheter-related infections. *Clinical Infectious Diseases, 52,* E162–E193. doi:10.1093/cid/cir257

Perruchoud, C., Bovy, M., Rutschmann, B., Durrer, A., & Buchser, E. (2013). Silicone septum leakage at the origin of a drug overdose in a patient implanted with an intrathecal pump. *Neuromodulation, 16,* 467–470. doi:10.1111/j.1525-1403.2012.00523.x

Rosen, S.M., Bromberg, T.A., Padda, G., Barsa, J., Dunbar, E., Dwarakanath, M.D., ... Deer, T. (2013). Intrathecal administration of Infumorph® vs. compounded morphine for treatment of intractable pain using the Prometra® programmable pump. *Pain Medicine, 14,* 865–873. doi:10.1111/pme.12077

Saulino, M., & Gofeld, M. (2014). "Sonology" of programmable intrathecal pumps. *Neuromodulation, 17,* 696–698. doi:10.1111/ner.12159

Saulino, M., Kim, P.S., & Shaw, E. (2014). Practical considerations and patient selection for intrathecal drug delivery in the management of chronic pain. *Journal of Pain Research, 7,* 627–638. doi:10.2147/JPR.S65441

Smyth, C.E., Jarvis, V., & Poulin, P. (2014). Brief review: Neuraxial analgesia in refractory malignant pain. *Canadian Journal of Anesthesia, 61,* 141–153. doi:10.1007/s12630-013-0075-8

Strandness, T., Wiktor, M., Varadarajan, J., & Weisman, S. (2015). Migration of pediatric epidural catheters. *Pediatric Anesthesia, 25,* 610–613. doi:10.1111/pan.12579

Tandon, M., & Pandey, C.K. (2015). No rent is small for migration of epidural catheter into sub-arachnoid space. *Indian Journal of Anaesthesia, 59,* 133–135. doi:10.4103/0019-5049.151384

Toledano, R.D., & Tsen, L.C. (2014). Epidural catheter design: History, innovations, and clinical implications. *Anesthesiology, 121,* 9–17. doi:10.1097/ALN.0000000000000239

Wesemann, K., Coffey, R.J., Wallace, M.S., Tan, Y., Broste, S., & Buvanendran, A. (2014). Clinical accuracy and safety using the SynchroMed II intrathecal drug infusion pump. *Regional Anesthesia and Pain Medicine, 39,* 341–346. doi:10.1097/AAP.0000000000000107

Wilkes, D. (2014). Programmable intrathecal pumps for the management of chronic pain: Recommendations for improved efficiency. *Journal of Pain Research, 7,* 571–577. doi:10.2147/JPR.S46929

Zencirci, B. (2010). Postdural puncture headache and pregabalin. *Journal of Pain Research, 3,* 311–314. doi:10.2147/jpr.s9445

Chapter 14

Intraperitoneal Catheters

Miriam Rogers, EdD, MN, RN, AOCN®

I. History (Helm, 2012)
- A. Initially developed to access the peritoneal cavity for drainage of ascites fluid and for peritoneal dialysis
- B. Insertion techniques, access methods, and materials have evolved over time, but requirements for accessing the device and maintenance care under sterile conditions have not changed.
- C. As early as 1923, equipment used for other purposes, such as metal trocars and glass cannulas for surgical drains, was adapted to access the peritoneal cavity. The rigidity of these materials led to problems of leakage, infection, and catheter occlusion.
- D. In the 1940s and 1950s, discovery of less rigid materials, such as nylon and polyvinyl, improved the drainage of peritoneal fluid, yet infection and leakage remained a problem.
- E. In the 1960s, a silicone rubber model became the prototype of the current peritoneal catheters. This model featured a coiled intraperitoneal (IP) end with multiple perforations extending 23 cm from the tip and a long subcutaneous (SC) tunnel.
- F. In 1965, an improved peritoneal catheter was created for peritoneal dialysis, allowing for frequent access of abdominal cavity. A Dacron cuff was placed subcutaneously and a second external cuff was used, allowing for direct secure connection to external devices.
- G. Implanted SC ports were first used for peritoneal access in the early 1980s.
- H. Research continues on catheter modifications in an effort to decrease infection, leakage, and obstructive complications.

II. Device characteristics (Helm, 2012) (see Figure 14-1)
- A. Permanently or temporarily placed in the abdominal cavity
- B. Used intermittently or continuously
- C. Designed to provide sterile access into the abdominal cavity

III. Device features (Anastasia, 2012; Ellsworth, 2016; Gynecologic Oncology Group, n.d.; Helm, 2012)

- A. Overview
  1. Implanted SC or tunneled devices
  2. Contain a single lumen or have multiple holes (fenestrated) that permit increased distribution of solutions
  3. Available with or without cuff
- B. An implanted SC port is secured in the abdomen with the portal body placed over a bony prominence (Anastasia, 2012; Ellsworth, 2016; Gynecologic Oncology Group, n.d.; Helm, 2012).
  1. Materials: A titanium or plastic portal body has a self-sealing silicone septum and may have preattached or an attachable radiopaque polyurethane or silicone single-lumen or fenestrated catheter.
  2. The septum diameter is 12.7 mm and is accessed with a noncoring needle.
  3. The attached catheter is 8–16 Fr, with lengths ranging from 31 to 48 cm.
  4. The cuff is located between the IP and the SC sections of the catheter (if used).
- C. External tunneled catheters placed through abdominal wall with external access (Anastasia, 2012; Ellsworth, 2016; Gynecologic Oncology Group, n.d.; Helm, 2012; Piraino et al., 2011; Ques et al., 2013)
  1. Placed for paracentesis or delivery of medications into the peritoneum over variable amounts of time, such as a course of IP che-

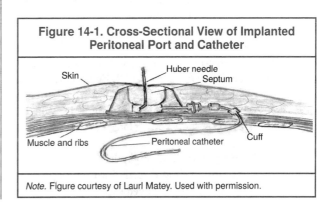

Figure 14-1. Cross-Sectional View of Implanted Peritoneal Port and Catheter

Skin — Huber needle — Septum

Muscle and ribs — Peritoneal catheter — Cuff

Note. Figure courtesy of Laurl Matey. Used with permission.

motherapy or palliative frequent paracentesis at end of life

2. Materials: Silicone or polyurethane with radiopaque stripe
3. Consist of three parts that are available in multiple styles, sizes, and configurations to adapt to body habitus: infant (31 cm), child (37 cm), and adult (42–47 cm) lengths
    a) The external segment generally is 20 cm.
    b) The SC segment is the shortest, ranging from 2–10 cm.
    c) The intra-abdominal segment is the longest, ranging from 31–48 cm.
4. The internal portion of the catheter may be coiled or straight with outer diameters ranging from 8–15 Fr. Coiled catheters decrease the incidence of catheter migration.
5. May have single or double Dacron cuffs on the catheter to secure its position, and may prevent infection within the IP cavity
    a) One cuff: Located between the external exit site and SC segments, placed 2–3 cm from the catheter exit site, deep subcutaneously to prevent cuff infection and extrusion
    b) Two cuffs: One located between the external exit site and SC segments and one between the SC and intra-abdominal segments, anchored to the rectus sheath, making a watertight seal to prevent leakage and infection
6. Available with clamps

IV. Device advantages and disadvantages (see Table 14-1)
V. Patient selection criteria (Al-Quteimat & Al-Badaineh, 2013; Anastasia, 2012; Echarri Gonzalez, Green, & Muggia, 2011; Ellsworth, 2016; Grosso et al., 2014; Jaaback, Johnson, & Lawrie, 2016; Robella et al., 2014; Ryan, Lyons, Hansen, & O'Gorman, 2013; Small, 2013; Sun et al., 2013)
    A. IP antineoplastic therapy; delivers a high concentration of drug directly into the peritoneal space, allowing prolonged exposure
    B. Palliation of metastasis such as abdominal carcinomatosis and intermittent drainage of ascites (Malayev, Levene, & Gonzalez, 2012; Ryan et al., 2013)
    C. IP chemotherapy is rarely used in the pediatric population. If a pediatric patient requires an IP catheter, it is most likely being used for peritoneal dialysis.
    D. A patient able to tolerate large volumes of IP fluid. The volume of fluid for IP treatment must be adjusted to the size of the patient.
    E. A patient or caregiver able to care for an external catheter

VI. Insertion techniques (Abdel-Aal, Gaddikeri, & Saddekni, 2011; Ellsworth, 2016; Kim et al., 2015; Ryan et al., 2013)
    A. Preassessment
        1. Prior to placement, ensure that contraindications do not exist, informed consent is obtained, preplacement is completed, laboratory studies are verified, and a medication/chemotherapy order is reviewed (see Appendix 4).
        2. Techniques, timing, and placement are varied. No standard approach has been established.
        3. Prior omentectomy is recommended to facilitate distribution of fluid drainage or instillation.
    B. External tunneled catheter considerations
        1. Inserted by a surgeon or interventional radiologist using maximum sterile barrier precautions under fluoroscopy with local or general sedation; can be placed at any time over the course of disease, from initial surgery through end-of-life care
        2. The catheter tip is directed toward the cul-de-sac of the pelvis, the peritoneum is closed, and a SC tunnel is made. The catheter exits through the anterior abdominal wall.
        3. The entire IP segment of the catheter, with its multiple exit holes or single lumen, must be placed in the peritoneum to avoid drug extravasation.
        4. The external portion of the catheter is placed away from the initial puncture site and sutured in place.
        5. The external portion of the catheter is placed off the side of the midline to provide easy access for the patient.
        6. Change postoperative dressing 24 hours after placement, unless excess soiling occurs.
    C. Implanted SC port (Dawson et al., 2011; Ellsworth, 2016; Helm, 2012; Kim et al., 2015; Risson et al., 2012)
        1. Inserted by a surgeon or interventional radiologist using maximum sterile barri-

Table 14-1. Advantages and Disadvantages of Intraperitoneal Devices		
Type	**Advantages**	**Disadvantages**
External tunneled peritoneal catheters	Serve as a semipermanent access device that allows cyclic treatments over a long period of time Decrease risk of visceral or bowel perforation when compared to temporarily placed intraperitoneal catheters for peritoneal access Permit faster fluid infusion rate: 2 L in 10–15 minutes Permit rapid drainage of fluid Allow for collection of fluid samples Allow for high-pressure forced irrigation or manipulation to loosen fibrin clots Access is less painful to the patient. Can be removed at the bedside or as outpatient if a cuff is used Available repair kits for the external portion Inexpensive catheter Patient and caregivers can learn how to care for the catheter and how to drain fluid for palliation of ascites.	Increase risk of infection because of external portion; exposed tubing provides direct access to peritoneal cavity. Increase risk of leakage around the exit site Insertion must be performed in the operating room. Increase risk of dislodgment Require maintenance: Dressing changes, exit site, and catheter care Increase cost because of necessary maintenance supplies May require more office visits or use of home health agency, adding to cost Inconvenience: Limit ability to swim, bathe, and wear certain clothing Can have a negative influence on the patient's body image
Implanted peritoneal ports	Serve as a semipermanent access device that allows cyclic treatments over a long period of time Potentially decrease risk of infection because of lack of external portion No risk of accidental removal Do not require dressing or flushing between treatments No restrictions on activity, bathing, or swimming Increase patient acceptance because of lack of external component	Must be surgically placed and removed in the operating room Require a needlestick to access device, which may cause discomfort to the patient Do not allow for high-pressure forced irrigation or manipulation to dislodge fibrin Slower infusion rate: 2 L in 30–45 minutes because of needle size limitations Decrease rate of fluid return: 2 L in 1–2 hours Inability to drain off or aspirate fluid because of needle size limitations More expensive with insertion

ers under fluoroscopy and conscious sedation or general anesthesia

2. Placed similarly as described in the external catheter procedure

3. After closure of the peritoneum, a SC tunnel is made to the selected port site over a bony prominence (preferably over the costal margin) to stabilize access.

D. Insertion complications (Ellsworth, 2016; Helm, 2012; Kim et al., 2015; Piraino et al., 2011) (see Table 14-2)

1. Pain: May require analgesics

2. Bleeding: Large amounts of blood in abdominal fluid. Bleeding may be significant enough to require blood transfusions or surgery to remove or replace the catheter, or it may be sign of perforation or blood vessel or tumor erosion. Consult a surgeon or interventional radiologist immediately.

3. Bowel perforation: Severe abdominal pain, fever, and tense abdomen. Consult a surgeon or interventional radiologist immediately.

4. Peritonitis: Fever, nausea, vomiting, severe abdominal pain, and cloudy peritoneal fluid. Consult the provider; cultures may be sent. Otherwise, antibiotics and analgesics, as ordered.

E. Postprocedure care: Assess for abdominal postsurgical complications (Ellsworth, 2016; Helm, 2012; Kim et al., 2015).

VII. Unique maintenance and care: Determine the type of IP access device implanted and review the manufacturer's instructions prior to use (Anastasia, 2012; Ellsworth, 2016; Gynecologic Oncology Group, n.d.; Helm, 2012; Piraino et al., 2011; Ques et al., 2013; Warady et al., 2012) (see Appendices 2, 4, 7, 12, and 13 and Figure 14-2).

A. Prior to accessing or caring for catheters or ports, verify scope of practice with the individual state board of nursing and institutional guidelines.

B. RNs managing peritoneal devices must be knowledgeable of the principles of drug administration and care of patients with these devices.

C. Maintain maximum sterile technique to prevent catheter tunnel infection and peritonitis. Use of sterile mask and gloves is highly recommended because of the vulnerability of the patient population to infection.

D. Ensure that all tubing connections are Luer lock. Label all lines close to the patient as feasible. Secure the catheter to prevent kinks and ten-

Table 14-2. Complications of Peritoneal Therapies and Interventions			
Complication	**Etiology**	**Signs/Symptoms**	**Interventions**
Patient discomfort	Increased fluid volume in abdomen	Abdominal distention	Loosen clothing. Administer analgesics, as ordered. Provide reassurance that problems are temporary. Evaluate the patient's size and adjust fluid volume and rate.
	Fluid loculation	Shortness of breath Abdominal pain	Administer oxygen and elevate the head of the bed. Change the patient's position. Administer analgesics, as ordered.
	Rapid fluid infusion	Abdominal or rectal pressure Complaints of pain	Warm fluid before instillation. Slow the rate of infusion.
		Shivering, complaints of cold feeling	Use warming blanket. Offer warm PO fluids.
Inflow failure	Needle misplacement Implanted port inversion	Inability to infuse solution or difficulty flushing Inability to access	Assess port and needle placement. Deaccess and reaccess port.
	Catheter kinks Blood or fibrin clots in catheter Obstruction of catheter by abdominal adhesions or omental blockage Catheter migration Fluid loculation Tumor progression	Inability to infuse solution or difficulty flushing	Reposition patient. Flush vigorously with sterile 0.9% normal saline (NS). Prepare for an imaging study to check catheter position. If catheter is in place but unable to irrigate, instill tissue plasminogen activator (tPA). If still no success, the catheter may need to be removed.
Outflow failure	Fibrin sheath formation creating a one-valve effect Omental adhesion or tumor causing outflow blockage of catheter Catheter migration	Inability to sample peritoneal fluid for diagnosis or specimen collection	Reposition the patient; attempt to flush with 20 ml NS. If still unsuccessful, attempt to withdraw a fluid sample after 30 minutes. Notify the provider if no improvement occurs.
		Inability to drain solution, although able to infuse solutions	Assure the patient that the fluid will eventually absorb.
		Ascites fluid may require paracentesis for removal.	Prepare the patient for an imaging study to diagnose the problem. If the catheter still infuses, future treatments may continue, as ordered, without the drainage of contents. tPA may be ordered.
Drug extravasation	Separation of port from catheter Dislodgment of port needle from septum Migration of catheter out of the peritoneum	Inability to aspirate fluid Poor rate of infusion and difficulty flushing Local swelling around exit site or port diaphragm Patient complains of pain Erythema at the site	Stop the drug infusion. Notify the provider. Attempt to aspirate the drug, if possible. Prepare the patient for diagnostic studies to determine placement. The device may be removed.
Exit-site infection	Improper sterile technique when performing treatments, dressing changes, and catheter care Contamination of open area at exit site (usually from skin flora) An immunosuppressed patient Erosion of tunnel cuff through the skin	Marked erythema or discharge from exit site Increased scab formation Local tenderness around exit site or tunnel	Culture exudate. Administer PO or IV antibiotics, as ordered. Increase local measures: Clean exit site once or twice a day, and apply sterile dressing. If cuff erosion exists, the device will have to be removed.

(Continued on next page)

	Table 14-2. Complications of Peritoneal Therapies and Interventions *(Continued)*		
Complication	**Etiology**	**Signs/Symptoms**	**Interventions**
Tunnel infection	Same as for exit-site infection	Infection occurring between the two cuffs, manifesting as inflammation appearing along the tunnel line of the catheter	Same as for exit-site infection Decreased chance of resolution Catheter removal usually is required. Ultrasound will reveal fluid collection around the catheter. Administer oral or IV antibiotics, as ordered.
Peritonitis	Infection occurs because of improper sterile technique when accessing device, changing dressing, or performing therapies. Immunocompromised patients are at an increased risk for infection. Less likely cause: Catheter erosion into small or large bowel	Fever and chills Abdominal tenderness to light palpation Rebound tenderness Cloudy fluid Positive cultures Peritoneal fluid with white blood cells greater than 100 cells/mm^3	Send cultures. Administer IV or intraperitoneal (IP) antibiotics, as ordered. Administer analgesics. The catheter may need to be removed if infection does not resolve or recurs with the same organism.
Slow infusion rate of solution	Kinks in catheter or tubing Fibrin sheath formation Obstruction of catheter by adhesions, omentum, or tumor	Increased time to infuse solution is more than 2 hours/L.	If using a port, check needle placement and gauge. Increase height of bag. Irrigate catheter with 20 ml sterile NS. Change the patient's position.
Leakage at exit site	Incomplete healing of surgical wound Dislodgment of port needle from septum	Visible leakage of IP fluid around catheter or insertion site: Redness, local pain Dressings saturated	Stop the treatment immediately. Check needle placement. Notify the provider. Perform sterile exit-site catheter care and place a sterile dressing over the site. Imaging may be required to verify catheter placement.
Catheter migration and erosion into other pelvic organs	Fistulization of catheter into pelvic organs: Small or large intestine, vagina, or bladder	Leakage of IP fluid from vagina, rectum, or bladder Abdominal/pelvic pain; urinary urgency	Stop infusion. Notify the provider. Imaging may be required to verify catheter placement; device may be removed.
Bleeding at exit site (external catheter)	Excessive movement of external tubing Removal of a crust (scab) before the natural separation has occurred	Bleeding when performing exit-site care, when dressing is removed Blood-stained gauze	Apply local pressure with sterile gauze. Anchor tubing with securement device. Perform gentle exit-site care; do not pull or twist the catheter.

sion, which may lead to malposition. Consider a tension loop. Use specialized tubing without injection ports to prevent accidental injection of unintended medication.

E. Trace the tubing or catheter from the patient to the point of origin each time the catheter is accessed, at handoff, and at transitions to a new setting or service.

F. No definitive recommendations regarding methods of access, deaccess, and maintenance care of peritoneal devices can be made based on available evidence.

G. External catheters are accessed with a needleless system.

   1. Use maximum barrier precautions at all times.

   2. Apply mask. Open supplies, including syringe, needleless connector, catheter clamp, gauze, and gloves, onto a sterile field.

   3. Cleanse exit site, catheter, and needleless connector. Do not use alcohol long term, as it can cause discoloration and damage to the device. Do not use acetone-based cleaning solutions because they are incompatible with the polymer material used in the peritoneal device.

   4. Gently aspirate to confirm no blood return is present. If present, discontinue use and notify the provider. Flush the catheter with 20 ml 0.9% normal saline (NS).

Figure 14-2. Implanted Peritoneal Port Access

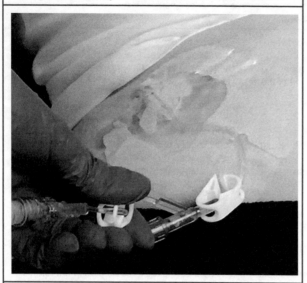

Note. Image courtesy of Laurl Matey. Used with permission.

5. Connect infusion tubing; start infusion and assess for leakage, ease of flow, SC infiltration, and pain.
6. Apply occlusive dressing and secure with a stress loop, attaching to the abdomen to prevent excess pulling.
7. Change dressing 24 hours postoperatively or with excess soiling. Dressings are changed three times a week; needleless connectors are changed after each use, if damaged, or if contaminated.

H. An implanted port requires a noncoring needle to access, regardless of implantation site.
1. Use maximum barrier precautions at all times.
2. Apply sterile mask and open supplies, including syringe, noncoring needle, needleless connector, gauze, and gloves, onto a sterile field.
3. After accessing port, gently aspirate to confirm that no blood return is present. If present, discontinue procedure and notify provider. Flush with 20 ml NS. Assess for leakage, ease of flow, SC infiltration, and pain. Withdraw peritoneal specimen, as ordered. Often, peritoneal ports may not yield a specimen. Use of heparinized solution flush after NS remains controversial.
4. Apply sterile occlusive dressing over access site after needle is removed, if needed.
5. An implanted port does not require dressing change and access site cleaning when not in use.

I. Administration considerations

1. After access, peritoneal fluid may be drained or allowed to be absorbed per provider order. In patients with gynecologic cancers receiving IP treatment, fluid typically is not drained in order to provide absorption into the systemic circulation.
2. Drugs considered irritants and vesicants to the venous system have a similar effect on the peritoneum, causing pain, burning, and sclerosing and may be difficult for the patient to tolerate. These agents may be selected for their sclerosing effect rather than their chemotherapy effect.
3. Drugs that have a high local toxicity that causes pain and the tendency to create adhesions are not used for planned multicourse therapies.

VIII. Special considerations (Al-Quteimat & Al-Badaineh, 2013; Anastasia, 2012; Chan, Morris, Rao, & Chua, 2012; Ellsworth, 2016; Gynecologic Oncology Group, n.d.; Helm, 2012; Neuss et al., 2013; Sun et al., 2013)
A. If ascites is present, drain fluid prior to infusion of chemotherapy to promote comfort and tolerance. Attach a peritoneal drainage bag for collection of fluid.
B. Warming IP fluid to body temperature has not been determined to be more tolerable than room temperature. No definitive recommendation regarding methods to warm fluid can be made with available evidence.
C. Infuse fluids, as ordered, through specialized tubing without injection ports.
1. Ensure position by infusing a small amount of NS, observing for leakage, difficult flow, or extravasation. Proceed with therapy if no issues are noted.
2. When fluid has infused, close the clamp for the duration of dwell time. During that time, assist the patient to turn from side to side every 15–30 minutes to improve distribution throughout the abdomen.
3. If the fluid will not be drained, flush the catheter with 20 ml NS and disconnect.
4. If fluid is to be drained, open the drainage clamp and allow fluid to drain by gravity. If fluid will not drain, reposition the patient, instruct the patient in performing the Valsalva maneuver, apply manual pressure to the abdomen, or irrigate the catheter with NS. Drainage is more rapid with an external catheter. An implanted port may or may not allow drainage of fluid.
D. Hyperthermic IP chemotherapy: Administered in specialized gynecologic oncology centers in

the operating room at the time of surgery. The complexity and risks associated with this procedure require special training and precautions (Dubé et al., 2015; Robella et al., 2014; Small, 2013; Wademan et al., 2012).

    1. Highly concentrated, heated chemotherapy is delivered directly to the abdomen during surgery without the need for a permanent device.

    2. Allows for higher chemotherapy dose

    3. Heating solution may improve absorption of chemotherapy and destroy microscopic cells. Once the solution circulates throughout abdomen, it is drained and the incision is closed.

E. Palliative management of ascites (Malayev et al., 2012)

    1. Patients and caregivers are taught how to perform drainage of peritoneal fluid using an external catheter in the home. Infection risks increase over time.

    2. Educate the patient and caregiver about external catheter maintenance (Piraino et al., 2011; Ques et al., 2013; Ryan et al., 2013).

      a) Exit-site, catheter, and cap care

      b) Dressing change three times a week

      c) Weekly cap and clamp change

      d) Signs and symptoms of infection

      e) Signs and symptoms to call provider, such as acute pain, infection, changes in condition, decrease or increase in ascetic fluid amounts

IX. Removal technique (Helm, 2012; Milczek, Klasa-Mazurkiewicz, & Wydra, 2015)

A. Whether an advanced practice nurse can remove temporary catheters depends on the individual state board of nursing and individual institution. Training and competency records must be maintained.

B. External catheters are removed by a surgeon or interventional radiologist under local anesthesia. Inspect the catheter for intactness following removal.

C. Implanted SC ports are removed by a surgeon or interventional radiologist under local anesthesia.

X. Complications (Chan et al., 2012; Ellsworth, 2016; Emoto et al., 2012; Gynecologic Oncology Group, n.d.; Helm, 2012; Kim et al., 2015; Milczek et al., 2015; Piraino et al., 2011; Ques et al., 2013; Ryan et al., 2013; Sun et al., 2013; Warady et al., 2012) (see Table 14-2)

A. The risk of infection increases over time with repeated access.

B. An inflammatory reaction can occur when instilling chemotherapy agents into the abdomen and also may contribute to catheter complications.

XI. Education and documentation: Review patient education, including aspects of drugs, infusion, access, potential for systemic effects, and the need to wear loose clothing with an expandable waistline (see Chapter 17).

XII. Practicum on IP catheters (see Appendix 13)

The author would like to acknowledge Lois Anaya Winkelman, RN, MS, AOCN®, for her contribution to this chapter that remains unchanged from the previous edition of this book.

References

Abdel-Aal, A.K., Gaddikeri, S., & Saddekni, S. (2011). Technique of peritoneal catheter placement under fluoroscopic guidance. *Radiology Research and Practice, 2011,* 141707. doi:10.1155/2011/141707

Al-Quteimat, O.M., & Al-Badaineh, M.A. (2013). Intraperitoneal chemotherapy: Rationale, applications, and limitations. *Journal of Oncology Pharmacy Practice, 20,* 369–380. doi:10.1177/1078155213506244

Anastasia, P. (2012). Intraperitoneal chemotherapy for ovarian cancer. *Oncology Nursing Forum, 39,* 346–349. doi:10.1188/12.ONF.346-349

Chan, D.L., Morris, D.L., Rao, A., & Chua, T.C. (2012). Intraperitoneal chemotherapy in ovarian cancer: A review of tolerance and efficacy. *Cancer Management and Research, 4,* 413–422. doi:10.2147/CMAR.S31070

Dawson, S.J., Hicks, R.J., Johnston, V., Allen, D., Jobling, T., Quinn, M., & Rischin, D. (2011). Intraperitoneal distribution imaging in ovarian cancer patients. *Internal Medicine Journal, 41,* 167–171. doi:10.1111/j.1445-5994.2009.02112.x

Dubé, P., Sideris, L., Law, C., Mack, L., Haase, E., Giacomantonio, C., …McCart, J.A. (2015). Guidelines on the use of cytoreductive surgery and hyperthermic intraperitoneal chemotherapy in patients with peritoneal surface malignancy arising from colorectal or appendiceal neoplasms. *Current Oncology, 22,* e100–e112. doi:10.3747/co.22.2058

Echarri Gonzalez, M.J., Green, R., & Muggia, F.M. (2011). Intraperitoneal drug delivery for ovarian cancer: Why, how, who, what, and when? *Oncology (Williston Park), 25,* 156–165, 170.

Ellsworth, P.I. (2016). *Peritoneal dialysis catheter insertion.* Retrieved from http://emedicine.medscape.com/article/1829737-overview

Emoto, S., Ishigami, H., Hidemura, A., Yamaguchi, H., Yamashita, H., Kitayama, J., & Watanabe, T. (2012). Complications and management of an implanted intraperitoneal access port system for intraperitoneal chemotherapy for gastric cancer with peritoneal metastasis. *Japan Journal of Clinical Oncology, 42,* 1013–1019. doi:10.1093/jjco/hys129

Grosso, G., Rossetti, D., Coccolini, F., Bogani, G., Ansaloni, L., & Frigerio, L. (2014). Intraperitoneal chemotherapy in advanced epithelial ovarian cancer: A survey. *Archives of Gynecology Obstetrics, 290,* 425–434. doi:10.1007/s00404-3252-2

Gynecologic Oncology Group. (n.d.). *Intraperitoneal chemotherapy administration using an implanted port.* Retrieved from http://www.gog.org/IPChemoEd/NursingGuidelines.PDF

Helm, C.W. (2012). Ports and complications for intraperitoneal chemotherapy delivery. *BJOG: An International Journal of Obstetrics and Gynaecology, 119,* 150–159. doi:10.1111/j.1471-0528.2011.03179.x

Jaaback, K., Johnson, N., & Lawrie, T.A. (2016). Intraperitoneal chemotherapy for the initial management of primary epithelial ovarian cancer. *Cochrane Database of Systematic Reviews, 2016*(1). doi:10.1002/14651858.CD005340.pub3

Kim, J.S., Kim, H.C., Kim, S.W., Yang, D.M., Ryu, J.K., Rhee, S.J., & Kwon, S.H. (2015). Complications related to medical devices of the abdomen and pelvis: Pictorial essay. *Japanese Journal of Radiology, 33*, 177–186. doi:10.1007/s11604-015-0400-y

Malayev, Y., Levene, R., & Gonzalez, F. (2012). Palliative chemotherapy for malignant ascites secondary to ovarian cancer. *American Journal of Hospital Palliative Care, 29*, 515–521. doi:10.1177/1049909111434044

Milczek, T., Klasa-Mazurkiewicz, D., & Wydra, D. (2015). Complications associated with 9–10 Fr venous access port use in adjuvant intraperitoneal chemotherapy after a cytoreductive surgery in ovarian cancer patients. *Advances in Medical Science, 60*, 216–219. doi:10.1016/j.advms.2015.03.001

Neuss, M.N., Polovich, M., McNiff, K., Esper, P., Gilmore, T.R., LeFebvre, K.B., … Jacobson, J.O. (2013). 2013 updated American Society of Clinical Oncology/Oncology Nursing Society Chemotherapy Administration Safety Standards including Standards for the Safe Administration and Management of Oral Chemotherapy. *Oncology Nursing Forum, 40*, 225–233. doi:10.1188/13.ONF.40-03AP2

Piraino, B., Bernardini, J., Brown, E., Figueiredo, A., Johnson, D.W., Lye, W.-C., … Szeto, C.-C. (2011). ISPD position statement on reducing the risks of peritoneal dialysis–related infections. *Peritoneal Dialysis International, 31*, 614–630. doi:10.3747/pdi.2011.00057

Ques, A.A., Campo, M.V., Arribas, C.M., Marcos, B.B., Ramos, C.Q., del Barrio, O.R., … Marenco, M.T. (2013). Effectiveness of different types of care for the peritoneal dialysis catheter exit site: A systematic review. *JBI Database of Systematic Reviews and Implementation Reports, 11*, 133–179. doi:10.11124/jbisrir-2013-1088

Risson, J.-R., Macovei, I., Loock, M., Paquette, B., Martin, M., & Delabrousse, E. (2012). Cirrhotic and malignant ascites: Differential CT diagnosis. *Diagnostic and Intervention Imaging, 93*, 365–370. doi:10.1016/j.diii.2012.02.008

Robella, M., Vaira, M., Marsanic, P., Mellano, A., Borsano, A., Cinquegrana, A., … DeSimone, M. (2014). Treatment of peritoneal carcinomatosis from ovarian cancer by surgical cytoreduction and hyperthermic intraperitoneal chemotherapy (HIPEC). *Minerva Chirurgica, 69*(1), 27–35.

Ryan, Y., Lyons, K., Hansen, J., & O'Gorman, A. (2013). Tunneled peritoneal catheters for the palliative therapy of malignant ascites. *Family Medicine and Community Health, 1*(1), 17–22. doi:10.15212/FMCH.2013.0103

Small, T. (2013). Introduction of hyperthemic intraoperative intraperitoneal chemotherapy (HIPEC) to the surgery program. *ORNAC Journal, 32*(2), 12–17, 28–33.

Sun, V., Otis-Green, S., Morgan, R., Wakabayashi, M., Hakim, A., Callado, M.E., … Grant, M. (2013). Toxicities, complications, and clinical encounters during intraperitoneal chemotherapy in 17 women with ovarian cancer. *European Journal of Oncology Nursing, 17*, 375–380. doi:10.1016/j.ejon.2012.10.005

Wademan, M., Ha, J., Singh, H., Markan, Y., Sharma, P., Kasamon, K., … Boutros, C. (2012). Current indications, techniques and results of cytoreductive surgery with hyperthermic intraperitoneal chemotherapy for intra-abdominal malignancies. *Surgery: Current Research, 2*, 125. doi:10.4172/2161-1076.1000125

Warady, B.A., Bakkaloglu, S., Newland, J., Cantwell, M., Verrina, E., Neu, A., … Schaefer, F. (2012). Consensus guidelines for the prevention and treatment of catheter-related infections and peritonitis in pediatric patients receiving peritoneal dialysis: 2012 update. *Peritoneal Dialysis International, 32*(Suppl. 2), S32–S86. doi:10.3747/pdi.2011.00091

Chapter 15

Pleural Catheters

Heather Thompson Mackey, RN, MSN, ANP-BC, AOCN®

I. History (Walcott-Sapp & Sukumar, 2015)
   A. The oldest documented use of a tube for thoracic drainage dates back to the time of Hippocrates in the fifth century B.C., when metal tubes were used to drain empyema from the chest cavity to promote health by restoring balance to the "humors" of the body.
   B. In subsequent years, chest tubes in varying forms were used to help remove infection and fluid, most extensively among soldiers in various wars from the time of the Crusades to modern day. In 1961, the first plastic chest tube was introduced, and thoracostomy was established as a standard of care for surgical and trauma patients during the Vietnam War.
   C. Modern day pleural catheters, including chest tubes and indwelling pleural catheters, are used in a variety of clinical applications, including both drainage and instillation in children and adults.
II. Device characteristics (Bhatnagar & Maskell, 2014; Cooke & David, 2013; Mahmood & Wahidi, 2013) (see Figure 15-1)
   A. Plastic, hollow cylindrical catheter with drainage side holes inserted through the chest wall into the pleural cavity between the visceral (lining the outer surface of each lung) and parietal (lining the thoracic cavity) pleura
   B. Used to drain air and fluid (including blood and empyema) from the pleural cavity
III. Device features (Cooke & David, 2013; Kuhajda et al., 2014; Mahmood & Wahidi, 2013; Myers & Michaud, 2013)
   A. Defined by size, shape, and manner of insertion and securement
      1. Gauges range from 6–40 Fr. Gauges ranging from 6–26 Fr are most commonly used in children. Gauges ranging from 20–40 Fr are most commonly used in adults. Smaller tubes typically are used for drainage of air and larger tubes for drainage of fluid.
         a) Large-bore chest tubes: > 14 Fr
         b) Small-bore chest tubes: ≤ 14 Fr

Figure 15-1. Pleural Catheters With Drainage Holes

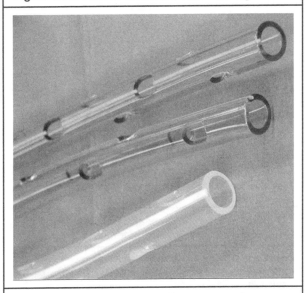

Note. Image by Bentplate84. This file is licensed under the Creative Commons Attribution 2.5 Generic license (https://creativecommons.org/licenses/by/2.5/deed.en). Retrieved from https://commons.wikimedia.org/wiki/File%3AChest_Tube_Drainage_Holes.jpg.

      2. Shape includes both straight tubes and coiled ("pigtail") catheters. Pigtail catheters are curved at the distal end to better secure in place.
   B. Can be classified based on insertion method
   C. Catheter materials (Cooke & David, 2013)
      1. Large-bore catheters are made of polyvinyl chloride and typically are stiff. Small-bore catheters, including pigtail and indwelling pleural catheters, are made of silicone and are more flexible.
      2. Silicone is preferred because of its better visualization on x-ray, less pleural inflammation, and more drainage holes than other catheters.
   D. Tunneled (long-term) versus nontunneled (short-term) catheters
      1. Large-bore chest tubes and pigtail catheters are not tunneled under the skin; they are inserted and secured with sutures.

2. Indwelling (tunneled) pleural catheters are small-bore catheters with a one-way valve system at the proximal hub. These are placed similarly to other types of chest tubes but tunneled to secure in place. A polyester cuff located on the catheter aids in securement.

3. Radiopaque markings are present along the catheter.

4. Heparin-coated catheters are available to help reduce thrombus formation and increase ease of insertion.

5. Heimlich valves (i.e., simple one-way valves) may be attached to large-bore chest tubes to provide intermittent temporary suction. Long-term indwelling pleural catheters contain a one-way valve at the proximal tip.

IV. Device advantages and disadvantages (Azan, Lim, & Guthrie, 2014; Gillen & Lau, 2013; Hogg et al., 2011; Lenker, Mayer, & Bernard, 2015; Mahmood & Wahidi, 2013; Myers & Michaud, 2013) (see Figure 15-2)

V. Patient selection criteria (Azan et al., 2014; Gilbert et al., 2015; Gillen & Lau, 2013; Hogg et al., 2011; Kheir, Shawwa, Alokla, Omballi, & Alraiyes, 2015;

Kuhajda et al., 2014; Lenker et al., 2015; Mahmood & Wahidi, 2013; Myers & Michaud, 2013; Rodriguez-Panadero & Romero-Romero, 2011)

A. Patient age, performance status, and surgical candidacy in general do not restrict the placement of pleural catheters.

B. Contraindications: Situations where lung is completely adherent to chest wall

1. Infection overlying the insertion site
2. History of multiple pleural adhesions
3. Presence of emphysematous blebs or scarring, coagulopathies, or platelet defects; correct coagulopathies and thrombocytopenia
4. Chest mass or tumor

C. Indications

1. Pneumothorax: Presence of air in the pleural cavity; may vary in size and can be spontaneous or related to illness, injury, or treatment
2. Hemothorax: Presence of blood
3. Malignant pleural effusion (MPE): Collection of malignant pleural fluid between the visceral and parietal pleura. Approximately 75% of MPEs result from lung and breast cancer (Gilbert et al., 2015; Gillen & Lau, 2013; Kheir et al., 2015; Lenker et al., 2015; Yu, 2011).

    a) Treatment usually includes tube thoracostomy, drainage, and sclerosis (i.e., chemical pleurodesis) of pleural space to prevent or slow recurrence following thoracentesis.

    b) Pleurodesis involves instillation of drug or sclerosing agent into pleural space that is irritating to the membranes, causing pleuritis. The inflammatory process causes the visceral and parietal pleura to adhere to one another, obliterating the pleural space and preventing reaccumulation of fluid.

    c) Historically, large-bore chest tubes were required for pleurodesis; small-bore catheters have now been shown to be as effective, with a minimum of 10–14 Fr recommended (Davies et al., 2012; Light, 2011; Roberts et al., 2010; Yu, 2011).

    d) For patients with recurrent MPE refractory to pleurodesis, tunneled small-bore pleural catheters can be used with fluid drainage bags to allow for outpatient management.

    e) Nontunneled chest tubes are used in patients with short life expectancies (Cooke & David, 2013; Stokes, 2007).

Figure 15-2. Advantages and Disadvantages of Pleural Catheters

Advantages	Disadvantages
• Allow for drainage of air and fluid from the pleural space	• Must be inserted by physician, advanced practice nurse, or physician assistant
• Provide a mechanism for instillation of medications and chemical treatments directly to the pleural space	• May involve discomfort with insertion
• Can be inserted at the bedside (short-term catheters)	• May cause pneumothorax, bleeding, infection, kinking, obstruction, or air leak
• May be used in many patient care settings	• Small-bore catheters have a lower flow rate, which affects their ability to quickly resolve large air or fluid accumulations. Thicker fluids are more likely to clog small-bore catheters as compared to large-bore chest tubes.
• Do not require operating room time	
• Small-bore catheters are useful in the outpatient population and allow for increased mobility. Placement of small-bore catheters using the Seldinger catheter-over-wire technique is less painful and does not require tissue dissection.	• External placement of chest tube and requirement for suction and water seal can limit mobility in some patients.
• Small-bore catheter placement is preferred in more stable patients and offers decreased risk of hemorrhage for those who are anticoagulated or with bleeding defects (Azan et al., 2014).	

D. Pleural catheter selection: Determined by indication and patient factors, such as size and health condition. Catheters are selected based on intended purpose, expected length of therapy, viscosity of fluid, fluid components, and the experience of the provider (Cooke & David, 2013).

   1. Large-bore chest tubes.
      a) Medical–surgical or trauma requiring short-term management of pneumothorax, hemothorax, drainage of pleural effusion and postsurgical drainage
      b) Instillation of medications or sclerosing agents
   2. Small-bore chest tubes
      a) Long-term management of MPEs, removal of empyema, or recurrent pleural effusions
      b) Pneumothorax or hemothorax management (Protic et al., 2010; Rahman et al., 2010; Rivera et al., 2009)

VI. Insertion techniques (Bhatnagar & Maskell, 2014; Cooke & David, 2013; Gillen & Lau, 2013; Hogg et al., 2011; Kuhajda et al., 2014; Mahmood & Wahidi, 2013; Myers & Michaud, 2013; Wiegand, 2011) (see Figure 15-3)

A. Prior to insertion, verify scope of practice with the individual state board of nursing and institutional guidelines.

B. Credentialing and ongoing competency validation is required.

C. Pleural catheters are inserted by a surgeon, interventional radiologist, or advanced practice registered nurse (APRN) using maximum sterile barrier precautions under local or general sedation.

D. Prior to placement, ensure that contraindications do not exist, informed consent is obtained, a preplacement assessment is completed, laboratory studies are verified, and the medication/chemotherapy order is reviewed (see Appendix 4).

E. Use fluoroscopy or ultrasound to assist positioning of the chest tubes (Gillen & Lau, 2013; Shojaee & Argento, 2014).

F. Insert into the "triangle of safety" (i.e., area bordered anteriorly by the lateral border of the pectoralis major, posteriorly by the lateral border of the latissimus dorsi, and inferiorly by a horizontal line at the level of the fifth intercostal space) (Havelock, Teoh, Laws, Gleeson, & BTS Pleural Disease Guideline Group, 2010).

   1. Gather required supplies.
   2. Position the patient.
   3. Wash hands.
   4. Maintain maximum sterile barrier precautions.
   5. Cleanse skin, allowing it to air-dry (see Appendix 2).
   6. Administer a local anesthetic, as needed (Bhatnagar & Maskell, 2014; Kuhajda et al., 2014) (see Appendix 7).
   7. Insertion site and technique of temporary catheters will vary.
      a) Typically inserted at the second intercostal space for pneumothorax as air rises to the top of the pleural space. When hemothorax or pleural effusion is present, insertion is made at the sixth to eighth intercostal space, midaxillary line, as fluid falls to the bottom of the pleural space.
      b) Insertion using blunt dissection: Use a scalpel to make a small incision at the insertion site. Insert a closed clamp to perform a blunt dissection. Palpation of the pleural space is made with the finger. Insert the chest tube and advance into the pleural space.
      c) Insertion using a trocar (i.e., single-use device): Pierce the pleural space following incision into the skin. This method holds a higher risk of complications, including chest penetration and damage to intrathoracic structures because of the increased force required for insertion.
      d) Once in place, connect the chest tube immediately to suction, the thoracic

Figure 15-3. Pleural Catheter Placement

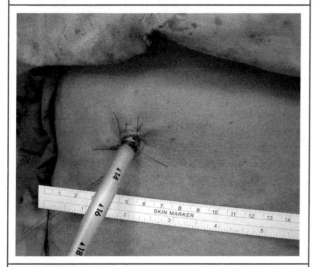

Note. From Chen et al., 2012. This file is licensed under the Creative Commons Attribution 2.5 Generic license (https://creativecommons.org/licenses/by/2.5/deed.en). Retrieved from https://commons.wikimedia.org/wiki/File:VATS_03.jpg.

_____
_____
_____
_____
_____
_____
_____

drainage system, or a clamp close to the patient's skin to prevent air from entering the pleural space. Three-chamber water seal systems commonly are used with chest tubes in the inpatient setting.

e) Suture the chest tube into place and secure it to the patient's skin distal to the insertion site with tape or a securement device. Apply sterile dressing.

8. Indwelling (tunneled) intrapleural catheter insertion: Use Seldinger technique; insert at the fourth to eighth intercostal space, midaxillary line.

a) Insert a blunt intrapleural needle (i.e., introducer) through the skin incision into the intercostal space 3–4 inches from the posterior midline. The needle, with the bevel tilted upwards, is directed medially at a 30°–40° angle to the skin over the superior edge of the patient's rib.

b) Ask the patient to hold breath as the needle punctures through the intercostal muscles while gently aspirating on the attached syringe.

c) Advance the introducer needle slowly until penetration into the parietal pleura. Aspiration from the syringe should produce air or fluid (depending on indication for use).

d) Introduce the guidewire through the introducer needle into the pleural space. Once the guidewire is in place, withdraw the introducer. Pass the chest tube catheter over the guidewire into the desired position within the pleural space; carefully withdraw the guidewire.

e) Introduce the tunneled catheters into the pleural space using a modified Seldinger technique through two small skin incisions. Incisions usually are 7–10 cm apart, allowing easy access to the drain and sufficient length of tunnel to reduce chance of dislodgment (Bhatnagar & Maskell, 2014).

f) Coil the external portion of the catheter to prevent pulling or kinking and suture into place.

g) Apply sterile dressing.

9. Confirm placement.

a) If ultrasound guidance is not used for insertion, perform a chest x-ray to confirm chest tube placement.

b) For intrapleural catheters, aspirate the catheter following suturing to the patient's skin. If resistance is met, this indicates proper placement into the pleural space. If air or blood is obtained, this indicates placement in the lung or blood vessel, respectively. Obtain a chest x-ray to evaluate for pneumothorax resulting from catheter insertion.

10. Label dressing with time, date, and initials of placement.

11. Monitor the patient's vital signs every 15 minutes for the first hour and then as needed, based on institutional policy.

12. Document the catheter type, size, date, time, provider name, and the patient's response in the patient medical record.

G. Insertion complications: A small pneumothorax is commonly seen on a chest x-ray and usually does not require intervention (Cooke & David, 2013).

1. Malposition is the most common complication (Kuhajda et al., 2014).

2. Complications are extremely rare with indwelling pleural catheter placement (Bhatnagar & Maskell, 2014).

3. Complications include bleeding, infection, subcutaneous (SC) emphysema, injury to the lung or diaphragm, and re-expansion pulmonary edema.

VII. Unique maintenance and care (Gillen & Lau, 2013; Hogg et al., 2011; Kuhajda et al., 2014; Myers & Michaud, 2013) (see Appendices 12 and 14)

A. Prior to accessing, verify scope of practice with the individual state board of nursing and institutional guidelines.

B. RNs managing pleural devices must be knowledgeable of the principles of drug administration and care of patients with these devices.

C. Ensure that all tubing connections are Luer lock. Label all lines close to the patient as feasible. Secure the catheter to prevent kinks and tension, which may lead to malposition. Consider tension loop. Use specialized tubing without injection ports, as indicated, to prevent accidental injection of unintended medication.

D. Trace the tubing or catheter from the patient to the point of origin each time the catheter is accessed, at handoff, and at transitions to a new setting or service.

E. Inspect the catheter insertion site and palpate for tenderness, crepitus, or SC emphysema at least daily through the intact dressing.

F. The catheter is not routinely changed unless complications such as obstruction or infection develop.

G. Dressing changes: Change if wet, soiled, or non-occlusive. Use maximum sterile barrier precautions to change dressing.
1. Split 4 × 4 gauze dressings are used around the catheter exit site.
2. Apply occlusive dressing over the split gauze dressing.
3. Do not use petroleum gauze because of its increased risk of suture failure (Muffly et al., 2012).
4. Avoid getting the exit site wet. Shower only with the exit site covered with sterile, watertight occlusive dressing (Gillen & Lau, 2013).
5. Change gauze-only dressings every 48 hours; change sterile occlusive dressings at least weekly.

H. To avoid the creation of high-negative intraluminal pressure that can lead to damage of the lung tissue, do not strip chest tubes. In the event of clots or debris in the tubing, the tube can be gently "milked" by pinching the tubing around the clot to help move the clot into the drainage system, as appropriate.

I. Flush small-bore tunneled pleural catheter to dislodge clots and debris from the lumen of the tube. Use 30 ml of 0.9% normal saline (NS) every 6–8 hours to help prevent tube blockage (Yarmus & Feller-Kopman, 2012).

J. Fibrinolytics have been used in management of obstructions and are performed by experienced providers (Lui, Thomas, & Lee, 2016; Thomas et al., 2015; Vial et al., 2016).
1. Dilute 2–6 mg of tissue plasminogen activator into 25–100 ml NS and instill into tube; allow a dwell time of at least 1–2 hours in the pleural space while the tube remains clamped (Hogg et al., 2011).
2. Unclamp and allow to drain.

K. Drainage of tunneled pleural catheters can be performed by patients and caregivers in the outpatient setting after receiving education and training. Follow the drainage procedure outlined by the device manufacturer. A drainage kit may be used by the manufacturer (Bhatnagar & Maskell, 2014; Gillen & Lau, 2013).
1. Infection risk increases with repeated access. Pleural fluid typically is drained every one to two days.
2. Normally, discomfort occurs when fluid is being drained; however, if the pain is severe or does not stop with slowing or discontinuing the drainage procedure, the provider should be notified as soon as possible, as this may be indicative of infection or other complications.
3. Avoid removing large amounts of fluid at one time.
4. Tunneled pleural catheters
   a) Use maximum sterile barrier precautions.
   b) Remove the catheter valve hubcap and discard. Cleanse the catheter hub. Attach the end of the catheter to the access end of the sterile drainage tubing or the vacuum bottle or bag.
   c) Once locked into place, remove the support clip on the bottle and puncture the foil seal, establishing the vacuum.
   d) Unclamp the catheter, if present; fluid will drain into the vacuum bottle.
   e) Once the fluid has stopped draining, clamp the catheter (if present) and remove the access tip from the catheter value. Cleanse the valve; a new sterile catheter valve cap is placed and locked into position.
   f) Record the time, date, and amount of fluid.

L. Intrapleural chemotherapy (den Hollander et al., 2014; Gilbert et al., 2015; Kheir et al., 2015; Thomas et al., 2014)
1. Can be administered using a temporary thoracentesis needle or through chest tubes and intrapleural catheters
2. Typically performed by a trained physician or nurse practitioner
   a) Situate the patient in Fowler or high Fowler position.
   b) Drain pleural fluid prior to instillation of infusion agent.
   c) Use maximum sterile barrier precautions and observe safe handling technique.
   d) Administer medication into the catheter and clamp.

e) After prescribed dwell time, drain fluid and dispose using safe handling technique.

VIII. Removal technique (Bhatnagar & Maskell, 2014; Cooke & David, 2013; Kuhajda et al., 2014; Wiegand, 2011)

A. Can be removed by a surgeon, interventional radiologist, or possibly an APRN. APRN removal depends on the individual state board of nursing and institutional guidelines. Training and competency records must be maintained.

B. The device is removed when signs and symptoms of infection are present, an obstruction cannot be relieved, damage has occurred, or when the device is no longer required for therapy.

1. Temporary catheters typically are removed within one week of placement to reduce infection risk.

2. Indwelling catheters can remain indefinitely (Bhatnagar & Maskell, 2014).

C. Prior to removal, chest tubes typically are clamped or removed from suction intermittently (while leaving the tube to water seal) to assess for signs of respiratory compromise indicating that the tube should not be removed. A serial chest x-ray may be used to determine if removal is appropriate.

D. Temporary catheter removal

1. Gather supplies.
2. Premedicate with analgesics.
3. Clamp the catheter and discontinue suction.
4. Wash hands.
5. Position the patient.
6. Use maximum sterile barrier precautions.
7. Hold the chest tube in place with sterile forceps and cut the suture anchoring the chest tube to the patient's skin.
8. Ask the patient to perform the Valsalva maneuver after a few deep breaths.
9. Hold an occlusive dressing over the insertion site and remove the catheter; stop immediately if resistance is met. Immediately cover the site with occlusive dressing. Tie off the stay suture (e.g., sutures placed by some providers at the time of insertion to help secure the catheter) and close the suture using square knots, if present. Otherwise, close with butterfly wound closure strips.
10. Apply a sterile occlusive dressing.
11. Discard used supplies and remove gloves.
12. Wash hands.

E. Indwelling pleural catheter removal: Follow the procedure for temporary catheter removal above.

1. Locate the SC polyester cuff of catheter along the tunnel site. Mark the skin, as needed, to indicate location.

2. A small incision is made over the cuff and is dissected away from the underlying tissue.

3. Close the incision site over the cuff area with butterfly closures.

4. Cover the insertion site with gauze and secure the dressing with tape.

F. Postprocedure

1. Obtain the patient's vital signs and assess respiratory status.

2. Obtain a chest x-ray, as ordered.

3. Monitor the patient's respiratory status postprocedure and document observations and actions.

IX. Complications (Bhatnagar & Maskell, 2014; Cooke & David, 2013; Fysh, Wrightson, Lee, & Rahman, 2012; Gillen & Lau, 2013; Hogg et al., 2011; Kuhajda et al., 2014; Lui et al., 2016; Mahmood & Wahidi, 2013; Myers & Michaud, 2013; Rodriguez-Panadero & Romero-Romero, 2011; Thomas et al., 2014; Yarmus & Feller-Kopman, 2012) (see Figure 15-4)

A. Both chest tubes and indwelling pleural catheters can develop pneumothorax, infection, bleeding, kinking, obstruction, air leak, cellulitis of tract site, pain, and tumor seeding.

B. Small-bore catheters are more likely to develop tube blockage by debris and clots.

C. Breakage: Rubber-tipped clamps should be kept at the patient's bedside or within reach at all times. If the catheter breaks, clamps should be applied as close to the insertion site as possible. The provider should be immediately notified.

D. Dislodgment

1. Cover the site immediately with sterile gauze and tape into place.

2. Notify the provider immediately; monitor the patient for signs and symptoms of tension pneumothorax.

X. Education and documentation (see Chapter 17)

XI. Practicum on pleural catheters (see Appendix 14)

Figure 15-4. Potential Complications of Pleural Catheters

Early	Late
• Pneumothorax	• Catheter dislodgment
• Postprocedure pain	• Clot, debris, or loculation
• Bleeding	• Infection, superficial cellulitis, empyema
• Lung injury	• Metastases along catheter tract
• Pleural fluid leakage	• Fracture of the catheter
	• Fibrosis and scarring around catheter cuff

Note. Based on information from Bhatnagar & Maskell, 2014; Cooke & David, 2013; Gillen & Lau, 2013; Lui et al., 2016; Thomas et al., 2015; Vial et al., 2016.

References

Azan, B., Lim, G., & Guthrie, M. (2014). Pigtail insertion. Retrieved from http://epmonthly.com/article/pigtail-insertion

Bhatnagar, R., & Maskell, N.A. (2014). Indwelling pleural catheters. *Respiration, 88*, 74–85. doi:10.1159/000360769

Cooke, D.T., & David, E.A. (2013). Large-bore and small-bore chest tubes: Types, function, and placement. *Thoracic Surgery Clinics, 23*, 17–24. doi:10.1016/j.thorsurg.2012.10.006

Davies, H.E., Mishra, E.K., Kahan, B.C., Wrightson, J.M., Stanton, A.E., Guhan, A., … Rahman, N.M. (2012). Effect of an indwelling pleural catheter vs chest tube and talc pleurodesis for relieving dyspnea in patients with malignant pleural effusion: The TIME2 randomized controlled trial. *JAMA, 307*, 2383–2389. doi:10.1001/jama.2012.5535

den Hollander, B.S., Connolly, B.L., Sung, L., Rapoport, A., Zwaan, C.M., Grant, R.M., … Temple, M.J. (2014). Successful use of indwelling tunneled catheters for the management of effusions in children with advanced cancer. *Pediatric Blood and Cancer, 61*, 1007–1012. doi:10.1002/pbc.24902

Fysh, E.T., Wrightson, J., Lee, Y.C., & Rahman, N.M. (2012). Fractured indwelling pleural catheters. *Chest, 141*, 1090–1094. doi:10.1378/chest.11-0724

Gilbert, C.R., Lee, H.J., Skalski, J.H., Maldonado, F., Wahidi, M., Choi, P.J., … Yarmus, L. (2015). The use of indwelling tunneled pleural catheters for recurrent pleural effusions in patients with hematologic malignancies: A multicenter study. *Chest, 148*, 752–758. doi:10.1378/chest.14-3119

Gillen, J., & Lau, C. (2013). Permanent indwelling catheters in the management of pleural effusions. *Thoracic Surgery Clinics, 23*, 63–71. doi:10.1016/j.thorsurg.2012.10.005

Havelock, T., Teoh, R., Laws, D., Gleeson, F., & BTS Pleural Disease Guideline Group. (2010). Pleural procedures and thoracic ultrasound: British Thoracic Society pleural disease guideline 2010. *Thorax, 65*(Suppl. 2), ii61–ii76. doi:10.1136/thx.2010.137026

Hogg, J.R., Caccavale, M., Gillen, B., McKenzie, G., Vlaminck, J., Fleming, C.J., & Friese, J.L. (2011). Tube thoracostomy: A review for the interventional radiologist. *Seminars in Interventional Radiology, 28*, 39–47. doi:10.1055/s-0031-1273939

Kheir, F., Shawwa, K., Alokla, K., Omballi, M., & Alraiyes, A.H. (2015). Tunneled pleural catheter for the treatment of malignant pleural effusion: A systematic review and meta-analysis. *American Journal of Therapeutics, 23*, e1300–e1306. doi:10.1097/MJT.0000000000000197

Kuhajda, I., Zarogoulidis, K., Kougioumtzi, I., Huang, H., Li, Q., Dryllis, G., … Zarogoulidis, P. (2014). Tube thoracostomy; Chest tube implantation and follow up. *Journal of Thoracic Disease, 6*(Suppl. 4), S470–S479. doi:10.3978/j.issn.2072-1439.2014.09.23

Lenker, A., Mayer, D.K., & Bernard, S.A. (2015). Interventions to treat malignant pleural effusions. *Clinical Journal of Oncology Nursing, 19*, 501–504. doi:10.1188/15.CJON.501-504

Light, R.W. (2011). Pleural controversy: Optimal chest tube size for drainage. *Respirology, 16*, 244–248. doi:10.1111/j.1440-1843.2010.01913.x

Lui, M.M.S., Thomas, R., & Lee, Y.C.G. (2016). Complications of indwelling pleural catheter use and their management. *BMJ Open Respiratory Research, 3*, e000123. doi:10.1136/bmjresp-2015-000123

Mahmood, K., & Wahidi, M.M. (2013). Straightening out chest tubes: What size, what type, and when. *Clinics in Chest Medicine, 34*, 63–71. doi:10.1016/j.ccm.2012.11.007

Muffly, T.M., Couri, B., Edwards, A., Kow, N., Bonham, A.J., & Paraíso, M.F. (2012). Effect of petroleum gauze packing on the mechanical properties of suture materials. *Journal of Surgical Education, 69*, 37–40. doi:10.1016/j.jsurg.2011.06.012

Myers, R., & Michaud, G. (2013). Tunneled pleural catheters: An update for 2013. *Clinics in Chest Medicine, 34*, 73–80. doi:10.1016/j.ccm.2012.12.003

Protic, A., Barkovic, I., Bralic, M., Cicvaric, T., Stifter, S., & Sustic, A. (2010). Targeted wire-guided chest tube placement: A cadaver study. *European Journal of Emergency Medicine, 17*, 146–149 doi:10.1097/MEJ.0b013e3283307b35

Rahman, N.M., Maskell, N.A., Davies, C.W., Hedley, E.L., Nunn, A.J., Gleeson, F.V., & Davies, R.J. (2010). The relationship between chest tube size and clinical outcome in pleural infection. *Chest, 137*, 536–543. doi:10.1378/chest.09-1044

Rivera, L., O'Reilly, E., Sise, M.J., Norton, V.C., Sise, C.B., Sack, D.I., … Anteveil, J. (2009). Small catheter tube thoracostomy: Effective in managing chest trauma in stable patients. *Journal of Trauma, 66*, 393–399. doi:10.1091/TA.0b013e318173f81e

Roberts, M.E., Neville, E., Berrisford, R.G., Antunes, G., Ali, N.J., & BTS Pleural Disease Guideline Group. (2010). BTS Pleural Disease Guidelines. *Thorax, 65*(Suppl. 2), ii32–ii40. doi:10.1136/thx.2010.13694

Rodriguez-Panadero, F., & Romero-Romero, B. (2011). Management of malignant pleural effusions. *Current Opinion in Pulmonary Medicine, 17*, 269–273. doi:10.1097/MCP.0b013e3283474015

Shojaee, S., & Argento, A.C. (2014). Ultrasound-guided pleural access. *Seminars in Respiratory Critical Care Medicine, 35*, 693–705. doi:10.10055/s-0034-1395794

Stokes, L.S. (2007). Percutaneous management of malignant fluid collections. *Seminars in Interventional Radiology, 24*, 398–408. doi:10.1055/s-2007-992328

Thomas, R., Budgeon, C.A., Kuok, Y.J., Read, C., Fysh, E.T.H., Bydder, S., & Lee, Y.C.G. (2014). Catheter tract metastasis associated with indwelling pleural catheters. *Chest, 146*, 557–562. doi:10.1378/chest.13-3057

Thomas, R., Piccolo, F., Miller, D., MacEachern, P.R., Chee, A.C., Huseini, T., … Lee, Y.C. (2015). Intrapleural fibrinolysis for the treatment of indwelling pleural catheter-related symptomatic loculations: A multicenter observational study. *Chest, 148*, 746–751. doi:10.1378/chest.14-2401

Vial, M.R., Ost, D.E., Eapen, G.A., Jimenez, C.A., Morice, R.C., O'Connell, O., & Grosu, H.B. (2016). Intrapleural fibrinolytic therapy in patients with nondraining indwelling pleural catheters. *Journal of Bronchology and Interventional Pulmonology, 23*, 98–105. doi:10.1097/LBR.0000000000000265

Walcott-Sapp, S., & Sukumar, M. (2015). A history of thoracic drainage: From ancient Greeks to wound sucking drummers to digital monitoring. Retrieved from http://www.ctsnet.org/article/history-thoracic-drainage-ancient-greeks-wound-sucking-drummers-digital-monitoring

Wiegand, D.J.L.-M. (Ed.). (2011). *AACN procedure manual for critical care* (6th ed.). St. Louis, MO: Elsevier Saunders.

Yarmus, L., & Feller-Kopman, D. (2012). Pneumothorax in the critically ill patient. *Chest, 141*, 1098–1105. doi:10.1378/chest.11-1691

Yu, H. (2011). Management of pleural effusion, empyema, and lung abscess. *Seminars in Interventional Radiology, 28*, 75–86. doi:10.1055/s-0031-1273942

Chapter 16

Ambulatory Infusion Pumps

Andrea B. Moran, RN, APRN

I. History (Fry, 2012; McKeag, 2015)
  A. The first ambulatory pump was marketed in the late 1950s to infuse the chemotherapy agent 5-fluorouracil. Lightweight pumps were created to allow treatment outside of the hospital.
  B. Initially, a mechanical windup watch motor with a rotary peristaltic mechanism was used as a power source.
  C. Over the next two decades, pump manufacturers developed smaller, more cost-effective pumps. In the early 1980s, the computerized ambulatory drug delivery system pump was developed. The use of home infusion therapy grew, and manufacturers introduced ambulatory infusion pumps.
  D. In the early 1990s, multi-therapy pumps were programmed to administer various infusions.
  E. By the 2000s, "smart" pumps were developed with the ability to store dosing guidelines and provide warnings to clinicians for potentially unsafe infusions.
II. Device characteristics (Broadhurst, 2012; Emergency Care Research Institute [ECRI], 2014; Freemantle, Clark, & Crosby, 2011; Lee, 2014; Mohseni & Ebneshahidi, 2014)
  A. Parenteral agent delivery is peristaltic (see Figure 16-1), syringe driven (see Figure 16-2), or elastomeric (see Figure 16-3).
  B. The small size of the pump allows the patient to carry or wear in a pouch.
  C. Home use gives the patient freedom of movement while receiving prescribed therapy.
  D. Reliable delivery of accurate volumes and consistent flow for small fluid volumes; reliability is preserved if refilled repeatedly.
III. Device features (ECRI, 2014; Mohseni & Ebneshahidi, 2014)
  A. Sizes are compact and small.
    1. Peristaltic pumps: 1–3 pounds
    2. Syringe pumps: 1–7 pounds
    3. Elastomeric pumps: 0.5–2 pounds
  B. The device provides continuous or intermittent infusion for medications and nutrition in flow rates varying from 0.02–300 ml/hour.

C. Pumps are designed for small volumes, such as an antibiotic, or for large volumes, such as total parenteral nutrition (TPN).
D. Reservoirs are available as bags, cassettes, elastomeric balloons, or syringes.
E. Peristaltic pumps are used to administer a variety of fluids, medications, or TPN in intermittent or continuous modes. High volumes and higher flow rates can be accommodated by peristaltic pumps.
F. Syringe pumps typically are used to administer highly concentrated drugs or antibiotics.
G. Elastomeric pumps consist of an elastomeric membrane containing the drug inside a protective shell (conformable elastomer or rigid plastic).

Figure 16-1. Peristaltic Ambulatory Pump

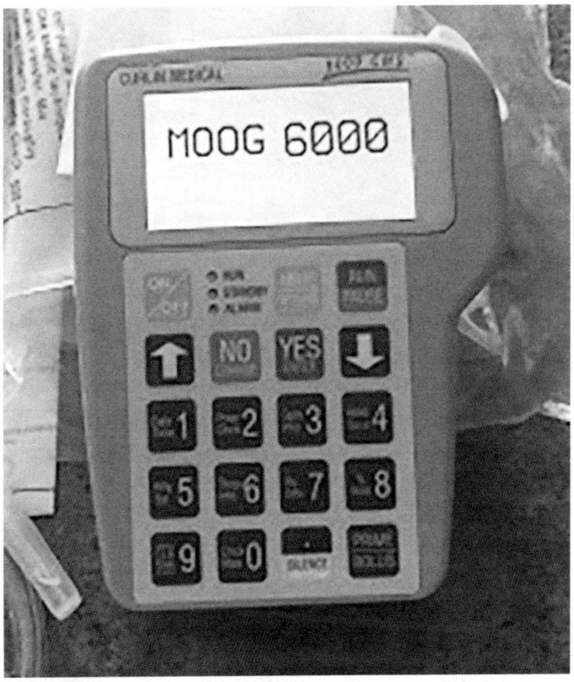

Note. Image courtesy of Joan Bradley. Used with permission.

Figure 16-2. Syringe Infusion Pump

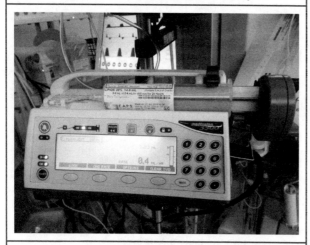

Note. Image courtesy of Andrea Moran. Used with permission.

Figure 16-3. Elastomeric Pump

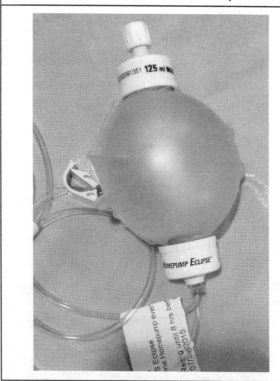

Note. Image courtesy of Andrea Moran. Used with permission.

1. Membranes are made of natural and synthetic material, such as isoprene rubber, latex, and silicone.
2. Membranes can be single layered or multilayered.
H. Operational procedures: See the specific pump manufacturer for detailed instructions (Broad-

hurst, 2012; Weisman, Missair, Pham, Gutierrez, & Gerbhard, 2014; West, 2014).
1. Power source
   a) Peristaltic pumps
      (1) Alkaline batteries
      (2) Rechargeable battery packs
      (3) Nine-volt batteries
   b) Syringe pumps provide a constant force to plunger, creating constant pressure within the syringe.
      (1) Nonelectronic with constant flow and no-bolus or free-flow features
      (2) Lithium-ion battery
   c) Elastomeric balloons use an elastomeric membrane to generate infusion pressure.
2. Method of infusion and rate regulation: Flow rates should remain within 5% of the rate provided by the manufacturer (ECRI, 2015).
   a) Linear peristaltic/rotary peristaltic
      (1) The mechanism propels fluid forward using appendages that move in a wave-like motion.
      (2) The rotary rotates the tubing between a cam (or disk) and cylinder to move fluid forward with a specific rocking or reciprocating motion.
      (3) The rate is programmed into the pump as continuous or intermittent. Some have an optional programmed bolus feature.
      (4) Delivery capability is 1–3,000 ml/day, with program flexibility of milliliters, milligrams, or micrograms.
      (5) A dual channel is available for simultaneous infusion.
   b) Syringe infusions
      (1) A motor-driven gear mechanism propels fluid by forcing a plunger or piston on the syringe barrel.
      (2) The rate is regulated by the size of the syringe and speed of the motor.
   c) Elastomeric
      (1) An elastomeric membrane generates infusion pressure when filled with fluid. As gravity or positive pressure causes the membrane to deflate, fluid is forced out.
      (2) Rate regulation is controlled by an inline orifice or flow restric-

tor within the administration set and is affected by the pressure gradient across the flow restrictor and by fluid viscosity.

(3) The type of membrane determines the pressure generated on the fluid when stretched. Multilayered membranes can generate higher pressure compared to single-layered membranes.

(4) Infusion rate is 0.5–500 ml/hour (Mohseni & Ebneshahidi, 2014).

3. Alarm system
   a) Peristaltic pumps: Available with audible or visual alarms for occlusion, air in line, low reservoir volume, low battery, and pump malfunction
   b) Syringe pumps: Intermittent audible tone when infusion ends or with occlusion
   c) Elastomeric: No alarm system

4. Advantages and disadvantages of ambulatory infusion pumps (see Table 16-1)

IV. Patient selection criteria (Kumpf & Tillman, 2012)
   A. In general, patient age and performance status do not restrict use.

1. Pediatrics: Smaller, less-obtrusive pump devices may better enable participation in school or outdoor activities.
2. Neonatal and pediatrics primarily use syringe pumps.
3. Older adults: Consider weight of pump and reservoir for the patient.
4. Consider ability of the patient or caregiver to provide pump care and troubleshooting for complications.

   B. All disease states are appropriate for treatment or symptom management medications administered by an ambulatory pump.
   C. Administration of therapy (McKeag, 2015; Newston & Ingram, 2014; Pajarón et al., 2015; Schaepelynck et al., 2011; West, 2014): Medications can be delivered by an ambulatory pump to any body system (e.g., venous, arterial, epidural, subcutaneous, peritoneal).
   1. TPN: Continuous or cyclic therapy
   2. Antibiotics
   3. Pain management
   4. Chemotherapy
   5. Insulin
   6. Hydration

V. Unique maintenance and care: Refer to manufacturer instructions for operational procedure prior to use.

Table 16-1. Advantages and Disadvantages of Ambulatory Infusion Pumps

Type of Pump	Advantages	Disadvantages
Peristaltic	Provide intermittent and continuous infusions Used for all types of therapy Alarm features Wide range of infusion rates and volumes Easy-to-read displays for adjustments and troubleshooting Pump memory available Smart pump technology	Require programming Potentially cumbersome and heavy to carry pouches when full Free-flow risk Labor intensive
Syringe	Lightweight and portable Cost-effective Easy to use Require little or no maintenance Ability to visualize drug flow Alarm features Disposable syringe Smart pump technology	Can fracture or break if dropped Limited volumes Not for large-volume infusions Drug stability factor Require adequate manual dexterity to maintain syringe and tubing Free-flow risk
Elastomeric	Lightweight, portable, and concealable Easy to use No programming No maintenance Reservoir and tubing attached Disposable Simple directions No batteries	Difficult to fill, especially those with multilayer membranes Admixture considerations Drug stability factor Require calculation of concentrations and volumes Limited infusion rates Not for large-volume infusions Not all insurances reimburse No alarms

A. Continuous infusion minimizes necessity to disconnect the system, which obviates the requirement to flush the access device.

B. Intermittent infusion requires the access device to be flushed with 10–20 ml 0.9% normal saline after drug is completed and the appropriate lock solution is administered.
   1. For some devices, such as the syringe and elastomeric device, the patient or caregiver may need to disconnect the pump after flushing.
   2. Patient teaching is necessary to ensure proper disconnection from the pump.

C. Tubing and reservoir changes
   1. Peristaltic: The bag or cassette may be changed up to every seven days depending on drug, drug stability, and reservoir size. Reservoir covers are available.
   2. Syringe: The syringe (5–60 ml) will depend on the pump. Change syringe every 12–24 hours or at end of infusion.
   3. Elastomeric devices are disposable with each dose and available with or without filters. A filling device is available to fill the pump with the drug.
   4. The patient and caregiver can be taught to change the cassette or syringe or connect the elastomeric devices.
   5. Reservoirs, syringes, or elastomeric devices may necessitate one home or clinic visit per day to change the drug reservoir. Or, these devices may be changed every three to seven days depending on the drug and treatment plan. Some patients may need to go to the clinic to have the pump reservoir changed, depending on insurance coverage or the ability to care for the pump.
   6. Tubing for TPN should be changed every 24 hours.

D. Drug calculations
   1. Ascertain drug concentration required for stability for dose in a reservoir.

2. The drug dose must be stable for the duration of the infusion at room temperature.
3. The rate of infusion is programmed into the pump according to the drug concentration.
4. Dose error reduction systems (DERSs) are available and referred to as smart syringe pumps and peristaltic pumps (ECRI, 2015; Harding, 2011; Kastrup, Balzer, Volk, & Spies, 2012; McKeag, 2015; Orto, Hendrix, Griffith, & Shaikewitz, 2015; Schraagen & Verhoeven, 2013).
   a) DERSs provide guided manual programming using pump-based software.
   b) Drug libraries are downloaded to the pump.
   c) The software checks programmed doses against preset limits stored in drug libraries.

E. Because elastomeric pumps do not have alarms, they can be weighed several times a day to detect potential infusion abnormalities.
   1. Monitor for reduction in balloon size, indicating a reduction in volume.
   2. A recent study showed significant variations when patients weighed their elastomeric pumps at home, suggesting measuring errors.
   3. No definitive recommendation can be made regarding weighing elastomeric pumps. More research is needed to prove that weighing elastomeric pumps to monitor proper infusion is an adequate safety measure (Cormack, Iliov, & Kluger, 2015).

F. Educate patients and caregivers to maintain pump data logs to record pump settings, setting changes, alarm activations, and when batteries are changed or charged (ECRI, 2015; Prakash et al., 2014).

VI. Complications
   A. Occlusion
      1. An empty reservoir can cause an occlusion and increase the risk of a clot formation. Instruct the patient on how to disconnect the pump or to return to the clinic to have the pump disconnected.
      2. Kinked tubing: Secure a tension loop to prevent kinking and occlusion.
      3. IV catheter infiltration: Teach the patient signs of infiltration and how to stop the pump from continuing to infuse. The clinic should be called immediately.
      4. Pump malfunction: Provide the patient and caregiver contact information for the clinic and the pump manufacturer in the event of an emergency.

a) Most troubleshooting can be conducted over the phone. If the pump malfunction cannot be corrected, the patient should be instructed to stop the pump and return to the clinic for a backup pump.

b) Some pump companies will allow a second pump to be kept at the patient's home to be used as a backup.

c) Exposure to radiation may lead to electronic pump malfunction. Ensure pumps are shielded from radiation or disconnected (if feasible). After exposure to radiation (including x-rays), infusion pumps should be checked to ensure proper functioning. If possible, use elastomeric pump for patients undergoing radiation to avoid this complication (Bak et al., 2013).

B. Incorrect programming of pump (ECRI, 2015; Kastrup et al., 2012; McKeag, 2015; Orto et al., 2015; Prakash et al., 2014; Schraagen & Verhoeven, 2013)

1. Causes: Bypassing programming procedure alert messages (i.e., safeguards of the pump, input of incorrect pump settings)

2. Verify pump settings with another nurse to ensure accuracy prior to connecting to patient.

3. Barcode technology on the drug bag, cassette, or syringe allows information to be compared with the patient's prescribed information.

4. Label each syringe, cassette, or bag with drug, rate of infusion, and patient's name.

5. Smart pump technology is recommended to minimize the risk of incorrect dosing (ECRI, 2015).

a) Technology warns users of incorrect medicine orders, calculation errors, and misprogramming.

b) Soft limits require confirmation prior to initiating the infusion if preset limits differ from the program.

c) Hard limits will not allow infusion if preset limits differ from the program.

d) Some pumps are available to store alerts and log information, which can be analyzed to improve drug libraries and subsequent clinical practice.

6. Check pumps frequently to ensure correct infusion.

C. Incorrect flow rate of elastomeric pump (Cormack et al., 2015; Grissinger, 2013; Mohseni & Ebneshahidi, 2014; Wang, Moeller, & Ding, 2012; Weisman et al., 2014)

1. Back pressure in the pump can occur as a result of vertical displacement of the device to the infusion set. Keep the device steady in the carrying case.

2. Use a filling device to measure medication accurately and avoid underfilling or overfilling.

3. Variations in atmospheric pressure can cause flow rate to increase.

4. Variations in temperature may affect rate. In general, an increase or decrease in flow rate can occur by 2%–3% for every one degree of temperature increase or decrease for water-based solutions.

5. Increased viscosity of the drug will decrease the flow rate.

VII. Education and documentation (see Chapter 17)

References

Bak, K., Gutierrez, E., Lockhart, E., Sharpe, M., Green, E., Costa, S., … Warde, P. (2013). Use of continuous infusion pumps during radiation treatment. *Journal of Oncology Practice, 9,* 107–111. doi:10.1200/JOP.2012.000717

Broadhurst, D. (2012). Transition to an elastomeric infusion pump in home care: An evidence-based approach. *Journal of Infusion Nursing, 35,* 143–151. doi:10.1097/NAN.0b013e31824d1b7a

Cormack, J.R., Iliov, A., & Kluger, R. (2015). Unreliability of weighing elastomeric pumps for determining volume of fluid infused. *American Journal of Health-System Pharmacy, 72,* 602–604. doi:10.2146/ajhp140556

Emergency Care Research Institute. (2014). ECRI's Institute infusion pump test criteria. Retrieved from https://www.ecri.org/components/HDJournal/Pages/Infusion-Pump-Test-Criteria.aspx?tab=2

Emergency Care Research Institute. (2015). *Infusion pumps, large-volume.* Executive summary. Retrieved from https://www.ecri.org/Pages/default.aspx

Freemantle, A., Clark, D., & Crosby, V. (2011). Safer ambulatory syringe drivers: Experiences of one acute hospital trust. *International Journal of Palliative Nursing, 17,* 86–91. doi:10.12968/ijpn.2011.17.2.86

Fry, A. (2012). Insulin delivery device technology 2012: Where are we after 90 years? *Journal of Diabetes Science and Technology, 6,* 947–953. doi:10.1177/193229681200600428

Grissinger, M. (2013). Improved safety needed in handling elastomeric reservoir balls used for pain relief. *Pharmacy and Therapeutics, 38,* 243–245.

Harding, A.D. (2011). Use of intravenous smart pumps for patient safety. *Journal of Emergency Nursing, 37,* 71–72. doi:10.1016/j.jen.2010.07.006

Kastrup, M., Balzer, F., Volk, T., & Spies, C. (2012). Analysis of event logs from syringe pumps: A retrospective pilot study to assess possible effects of syringe pumps on safety in a university hospital critical care unit in Germany. *Drug Safety, 35,* 563–574.

Kumpf, V.J., & Tillman, E.M. (2012). Home parenteral nutrition: Safe transition from hospital to home. *Nutrition in Clinical Practice, 27,* 749–757. doi:10.1177/0884533612464888

Lee, P.T. (2014). Syringe driver safety issues: An update. *International Journal of Palliative Nursing, 20,* 115–119. doi:10.12968/ijpn.2014.20.3.115

McKeag, N. (2015). Infusion pumps: Constantly evolving. *British Journal of Nursing, 24*(Suppl. 10), S6. doi:10.12968/bjon.2015.24.Sup10.S6

Mohseni, M., & Ebneshahidi, A. (2014). The flow rate accuracy of elastomeric infusion pumps after repeated filling. *Anesthesia and Pain Medicine, 4*, e14989. doi:10.5812/aapm.14989

Newston, C., & Ingram, B. (2014). Ambulatory chemotherapy for teenagers and young adults. *British Journal of Nursing, 23*, S36, S38–42.

Orto, V., Hendrix, C.C., Griffith, B., & Shaikewitz, S.T. (2015). Implementation of a smart pump champions program to decrease potential patient harm. *Journal of Nursing Care Quality, 30*, 138–143. doi:10.1097/NCQ.0000000000000090

Pajarón, M., Fernández-Miera, M.F., Allende, I., Arnaiz, A.M., Gutiérrez-Cuadra, M., Cobo-Belaustegui, M., … Sanroma, P. (2015). Self-administered outpatient parenteral antimicrobial therapy (S-OPAT) for infective endocarditis: A safe and effective model. *European Journal of Internal Medicine, 26*, 131–136. doi:10.1016/j.ejim.2015.01.001

Prakash, V., Koczmara, C., Savage, P., Trip, K., Stewart, J., McCurdie, T., … Trbovich, P. (2014). Mitigating errors caused by interruptions during medication verification and administration: Interventions in a simulated ambulatory chemotherapy setting. *BMJ Quality and Safety, 23*, 884–892. doi:10.1136/bmjqs-2013-002484

Schaepelynck, P., Darmon, P., Molines, L., Jannot-Lamotte, M.F., Treglia, C., & Raccah, D. (2011). Advances in pump technology: Insulin patch pumps, combined pumps and glucose sensors, and implanted pumps. *Diabetes and Metabolism, 37*(Suppl. 4), S85–S93. doi:10.1016/S1262-3636(11)70972-7

Schraagen, J.M., & Verhoeven, F. (2013). Methods for studying medical device technology and practitioner cognition: The case of user-interface issues with infusion pumps. *Journal of Biomedical Informatics, 6*, 181–195. doi:10.1016/j.jbi.2012.10.005

Wang, J., Moeller, A., & Ding, Y.S. (2012). Effects of atmospheric pressure conditions on flow rate of an elastomeric infusion pump. *American Journal of Health-System Pharmacy, 69*, 587–591. doi:10.2146/ajhp110296

Weisman, R.S., Missair, A., Pham, P., Gutierrez, J.F., & Gebhard, R.E. (2014). Accuracy and consistency of modern elastomeric pumps. *Regional Anesthesia and Pain Medicine, 39*, 423–428. doi:10.1097/AAP.0000000000000130

West, C. (2014). The use of syringe drivers in the community: Considerations for palliative care providers. *International Journal of Palliative Nursing, 20*, 56–59. doi:10.12968/ijpn.2014.20.2.56

Chapter 17

Education, Documentation, and Legal Issues for Access Devices

Heather Thompson Mackey, RN, MSN, ANP-BC, AOCN®

I. Education
- A. Education should be individualized to the patient's and caregiver's age, developmental and cognitive level, cultural influences, and language and learning preferences. Assess and address factors such as emotional state, sensory deficits, functional limitations, educational level, and other barriers to learning (Polovich, Olsen, & LeFebvre, 2014).
- B. Provide the patient and caregiver with comprehensive education about the specific access device being used, with subsequent documentation of education made in the medical record (see Figures 17-1 and 17-2). Such education includes the following:
  1. Indications
  2. Type of device and insertion procedure
  3. Potential complications
  4. Signs and symptoms to report to the healthcare team
  5. Demonstration of self-care skills, as appropriate
  6. Resources for supplies and emergency care
  7. Care and maintenance instructions
  8. Method of instruction used (e.g., verbal explanation, demonstration, return demonstration, written instructions, educational video, websites, online instructions) (see Figure 17-3)
  9. Assessment of the patient's and caregiver's level of understanding with return demonstration of care provided, as needed
II. Staff training and education: Improves access device competency; document in personnel records (O'Grady et al., 2011) (see Figure 17-2).
- A. Educational activities should address the following:
  1. Appropriateness of access device management within the nurse's scope of practice
  2. Insertion and access procedures
  3. Care and maintenance procedures
  4. Assessment of catheter function, potential complications, and interventions
  5. Elements of patient and family education about access devices
  6. Standards of care, including institutional policies pertaining to access devices
  7. Risk management strategies to decrease exposure to legal threats associated with access device use
- B. Comprehensive competency documentation that demonstrates gap analysis of learning needs for nurses may assist training validation.
- C. Documentation of regular continuing education opportunities can maintain and update knowledge, including advances made in access device technology.
III. Patient documentation (DeLa Cruz, Caillouet, & Guerrero, 2012; Doyle-Lindrud, 2015; Polovich et al., 2014)
- A. Legibly document accurate and descriptive information in a timely manner regarding the patient, access device, and nursing care provided.
- B. Follow standards outlined in institutional policies and evidence-based practice guidelines.
- C. Documentation (Gallieni et al., 2011) (see Appendices 4, 5, and 12)
  1. Assessment
     - a) Rationale for device
     - b) Type, purpose, and duration of therapy; previous access device complications; and comorbidities that could affect the functioning of the access device
  2. Interventions
     - a) Insertion
       (1) Informed consent
       (2) Date and time of insertion
       (3) Type of device inserted: Include name, manufacturer, lot or serial number, gauge, length, and size.

(4) Location of insertion site: Specify vein, artery, or body cavity, if appropriate.
(5) Type of anesthetic, as appropriate
(6) Type of cleansing agent
(7) Presence of blood return or other body fluid, as appropriate
(8) Complications
(9) Method of securement and type of dressing
(10) Confirmation of placement

b) Use of access device
(1) Date, time, and purpose of use
(2) Methods used to evaluate proper functioning prior to use
(3) Complications, if any
(4) Notification of provider if complication assessed
(5) Strategies used to manage complications
3. Care and maintenance of access device (DeLa Cruz et al., 2012)

Figure 17-1. Essentials for Patient and Caregiver Education

	Completed (date/time and initials)
1. Indications for access device	
Venous access devices:	
• Administration of IV medications and therapies	
• Administration of IV fluids	
• Blood sampling for routine laboratory studies	
Specialty access devices (specific to type of catheter placed):	
• Infusion of medications and therapies	
• Drainage or withdrawal of bodily fluids	
2. Type of device inserted	
• Specific type of catheter placed (name, manufacturer, lot or serial number)	
• Details of catheter (gauge, length, size)	
3. Review of potential complications of access device	
• Breakage	
• Infection	
• Malposition	
• Obstruction preventing flushing or withdrawal of blood or body fluids	
4. Signs and symptoms of access device complications to monitor for and report	
• Breakage in catheter	
• Inability to flush or withdraw	
• Temperature greater than 100.5°F (38°C)	
• Chills when flushing catheter, as appropriate	
• Redness or tenderness at insertion site (based on anatomical location of catheter)	
5. Demonstration of self-care skills related to access device, as appropriate	
6. Identification of community resources for supplies and emergency care related to access device, if appropriate	
7. Care and maintenance of device	
• Keeping dressing clean and dry and changing immediately if wet	
• Dressing change procedure, if appropriate	
• Flushing procedure, if appropriate	
• Other maintenance procedures, as appropriate	
8. Additional resources for the patient and caregiver	

Figure 17-2. Essentials for Competency Documentation	
	Completed (date/time and initials)
Assessment of Access Device	
1. Need for access device and type of device needed	
2. Regular assessment findings of the patient and device • Type • Purpose • Duration of therapy • Previous access device problems • Other health problems	
Insertion of Access Device	
1. Informed consent prior to insertion	
2. Date, time, and setting of insertion	
3. Type of device inserted, including • Name • Manufacturer • Lot or serial number • Gauge or length and size	
4. Location of insertion device	
5. Preparation of insertion site including local anesthetic, as appropriate	
6. Presence of blood return or other body fluid; ability to flush	
7. Complications of insertion procedure	
8. Method used to secure device and type of dressing used	
9. Confirmation of catheter placement and location (e.g., ultrasound; x-ray, if appropriate; location of catheter tip)	
Use of Access Device	
1. Date, time, and purpose for device use	
2. Methods used to evaluate proper functioning of device prior to use	
3. Complications noted with use, if any	
4. Notification of provider, if troubleshooting needed	
5. Strategies used to manage complications	
6. Compliance with regulatory agency standards and guidelines	
Care and Maintenance of Access Device	
1. Dressing change	
2. Flushing procedure	
3. Needleless connector change	
4. Use of clamps on the device or extension tubing, as appropriate	
5. Assessment of insertion site and exit site; intactness of device	
Removal of Access Device	
1. Indication for removal	
2. Date and time of removal	
3. Type of device removed and description of device following removal	
4. Procedure used for removal and observations of complications during device removal	
5. Patient teaching about postremoval care and potential complications	

Figure 17-3. Example of a Patient Education Sheet: Venous Access Devices (VADs)

When to contact your healthcare professional:
You have a VAD in place. It may be totally implanted under your skin, or you may have one or two tubings (lumens) on your chest or in your arm. The device will be used for your IV medications, delivery of fluids, or to draw blood for monitoring of laboratory tests. Your nurse will let you know how he or she will use the device and will show you how to care for your device.
There are several things you will need to let your nurse or doctor know about if they should occur.

Fever of 100.5°F (38°C) or higher or chills when flushing catheter	The VAD is placed in a large vein in your chest. Bacteria can enter the bloodstream through the catheter and cause a bloodstream infection (sepsis). **THIS IS AN EMERGENCY** and you should call your healthcare professional immediately. Phone # clinic: Phone # after hours:
Redness or tenderness at insertion site or up the arm	This can be a sign of infection or irritation of the vein. Notify your doctor's office as soon as possible, especially if you have a fever.
Inability to flush a lumen	If you are administering your IV therapy at home and are unable to flush the line, do not force it. If your catheter has clamps, make sure they are open. Try flushing again. If you are still unable to flush the line, you will need to contact your home healthcare nurse or your doctor's office immediately.
Breakage of line	If you have tubing coming from your arm or your chest and the tubing breaks, immediately clamp the tubing closest to your body and contact your doctor's office or go to the nearest emergency department.

---

    a) Dressing change: Type and procedure used
    b) Flushing: Type, volume, and frequency
    c) Needleless connector: Type and frequency
    d) Date of assessment, intactness of device, and any subjective information
  4. Removal of access device
    a) Indication for removal
    b) Date and time
    c) Type of device removed and description after removal, including catheter tip
    d) Removal procedure used and complications, if any
    e) Wound or catheter tip culture, as ordered
    f) Patient education about postremoval care, potential complications, and what to report to the provider
IV. Legal issues
  A. Scope
    1. Historically, nurses were not named in medical malpractice suits, as they were not felt to be true professionals, but rather individuals who simply followed the orders provided by others (e.g., physicians). This has changed in the latter part of the 20th century with the establishment of nursing as a discipline and with the increased recognition of nursing's ability to be autonomous and independent (Karno, 2011).
    2. Today, nurses are responsible for providing increasingly complex care across a variety of delivery systems, such as preventive, acute, and end-of-life care; rehabilitation; and survivorship (Brant & Wickham, 2013).
    3. In an effort to provide the highest quality cancer care, nurses have a "steadfast commitment to patient care, improved safety and quality, and better outcomes" (Institute of Medicine [IOM], 2010, p. xi).
    4. Nurses have a responsibility to critically evaluate patient factors and exercise good judgment in patient care (Alexander & Webster, 2010; Dychter, Gold, Carson, & Haller, 2012).
    5. Malpractice claims against nurses have risen over the past decade, accounting for 2 in every 100 payments (Reising, 2012). Oncology nursing is a specialty that carries a higher risk for nursing malpractice because of the nature of the work (Masoorli, 2005).
    a) Performance of invasive procedures
    b) Administration of infusion therapy, including vesicant chemotherapy
    c) Low-volume, high-risk interventions
  B. Legal standard of care
    1. The concept of legal standard of care specific to nursing is considered the level of care that a reasonably prudent nurse would provide in the same or similar circumstances where behavior is evaluated against a similarly experienced and educated nurse who possesses ordinary skills, knowledge, and abilities (Karno, 2011).

2. A reasonably prudent nurse whose conduct sets the standard is a person of average and ordinary caution and skill (Karno, 2011).
3. Several characteristics related to access devices and nursing should be considered when evaluating care (Alexander & Webster, 2010).
    a) The standard of care is a reasonable expectation of nursing care.
    b) The standard of care is measurable (e.g., a nurse trained to access an implanted port should know what site care is needed prior to access to prevent catheter-related bloodstream infections).
    c) The standard of care is valid based on location of care (e.g., a nurse practicing in a state that permits insertion of peripherally inserted central catheters [PICCs] should be able to perform insertion and care following appropriate training).
    d) The standard of care must be applicable based on the current state of knowledge.
4. Standards
    a) Voluntary (e.g., professional standards)
    b) Required nationally
    c) Required by individual state laws
    d) Required by individual institutional practices
    e) Regulated by a combination of these standards or governing bodies
C. Negligence
    1. *Negligence* is the failure to implement the standard of care a reasonably prudent person would provide in the same or similar circumstances (Karno, 2011). When it affects a nurse, it is referred to as professional negligence or malpractice.
    a) Acts of negligence can result from committing an act (commission) or failure to act (omission). Examples include failing to monitor a vesicant infusion via a peripheral IV site that results in extravasation (omission) or flushing of an implantable port with 10 ml of 1,000 IU/ml of heparin instead of the flush prescribed (commission).
    b) *Negligence per se*, or negligence as a matter of law, occurs when an individual violates a duty required by a law. In the case of nursing, if a nurse inserts a PICC without training, this practice would be beyond the scope of his or her state practice act and considered negligence per se.

2. To prove professional negligence of a nurse, certain elements must be established by the plaintiff, or the person bringing the suit against the nurse:
    a) The nurse had a **duty** to the plaintiff.
    b) The nurse violated, or **breached**, a standard of care.
    c) The breach **caused** the plaintiff's injury.
    d) **Damages** resulted from breach of the standard of care.
3. Nine common areas of nursing negligence, or malpractice, exist in the nursing care of an infusion patient or patient with an access device (Alexander & Webster, 2010; Dychter et al., 2012; Gilbar, 2014; Karno, 2011; Ranchon et al., 2011; Reising, 2012).
    a) Failure to administer medication appropriately (e.g., giving the wrong medication; giving medication at the wrong time; giving an incorrect dose of medication, including chemotherapy; giving a contraindicated medication via a venous access device [VAD], such as administering vincristine through an epidural or intrathecal access device)
    b) Failure to use equipment in a competent manner (e.g., improper VAD selection or access technique used, improper use of infusion pumps or administration sets)
    c) Failure to assess and monitor (e.g., failing to monitor an infusion site during vesicant administration, failing to assess a device insertion site for evidence of infection)
    d) Failure to act (e.g., failure to administer prescribed medication to treat a life-threatening condition)
    e) Failure to communicate (e.g., failure to share abnormal assessment findings or a patient's deteriorating condition with the provider)
    f) Failure to document (e.g., neglecting to document blood return status prior to

vesicant administration despite physically checking for blood return)

g) Failure to prevent infection (e.g., lack of adherence to organizational policies and procedures with dressing changes to an access device, not using sterile technique for PICC insertion)

h) Failure to appropriately identify and label access device line(s) (e.g., patient with a venous port and a peritoneal port) (see Figure 17-4)

i) Negligent conduct of another (e.g., assisting or allowing the negligence of another healthcare provider)

D. Risk management strategies (Alexander & Webster, 2010; DeLa Cruz et al., 2012; Karno, 2011)

1. Adherence to standard of care

a) One of the primary actions nurses can take to limit their exposure to legal suits is to practice within established standards of care.

b) Nurses must maintain knowledge of the legal and voluntary standards that govern their practice, regularly reviewing these requirements that include, but are not limited to, their individual job description, state nurse practice act, Occupational Safety and Health Administration regulations, Joint Commission standards, and organizational policies and procedures.

c) Nurses must provide comprehensive nursing care at all times and must not

---

Figure 17-4. Intraperitoneal and Venous Ports in Close Proximity Without Labeling

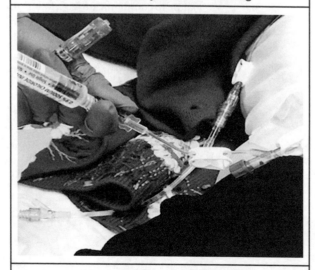

Note. Image courtesy of Laurl Matey. Used with permission.

---

practice outside their scope of practice or job setting. Nurses also must be aware of limitations to nursing practice as related to insertion, access, manipulation, or removal of specific access devices as defined by state board of nursing promulgated laws.

d) Nurses must maintain competency with current access devices and their management and undergo an in-depth assessment at regular intervals to ensure that their practice is consistent with current standards of care. Nurses must identify and participate in regular continuing nursing education opportunities for their personal and professional development.

e) Nurses must regularly identify learning gaps and seek education to meet learning needs (IOM, 2010).

2. Patient rights (Gallieni et al., 2011)

a) A critical nursing responsibility is to ensure that patient rights (e.g., informed consent, refusal of treatment, discharge planning, freedom from restraints, confidentiality) are maintained at all times.

b) One of the most effective proactive risk mitigation strategies is *informed consent*, a process of detailed discussion and decision making between a provider and a patient. Patients must be educated regarding the nature of the procedure; on reasonable alternatives; and the risks, benefits, and uncertainties of access devices. Documentation must reflect that the patient has received the information and agreed to the insertion of a device. For consent to be valid, a patient must have decision-making capacity; if the patient is incapacitated or incompetent to make decisions, consent must be provided by the surrogate decision maker.

c) Patients may refuse an access device, and providers are legally required to honor their decision, including any advance directives.

d) Discharge planning must begin as soon as possible to adequately prepare patients.

e) Information about patients must be kept private and confidential at all times.

3. Documentation (Doyle-Lindrud, 2015)

a) Accurate and comprehensive documentation that is objective, timely, and legible is imperative.

b) Documentation increasingly is challenging in the current environment of electronic medical records (EMRs) and "checkbox" documentation.

c) The reliability of a medical record is discredited because of inconsistencies, unexplained time gaps, omissions, or changes made to the record.

d) Documentation commonly is the only effective evidence that actions provided by a nurse meet the legal standard of care when caring for a patient (Alexander & Webster, 2010).

4. Unusual occurrence reports
    a) Learning documents without punitive intent
    b) Help provide factual, specific information concerning an event that may increase risk of harm to the patient

5. Professional liability insurance
    a) Most healthcare facilities and agencies carry insurance against negligent acts by their employees performed within the course of the job. In some cases, the interest of the nurse may conflict with another employee named in a litigation; nurses must determine when or if maintaining an individual liability insurance policy would be of personal benefit.
    b) Purchasing an individual liability insurance policy requires consideration of risks and benefits, including evaluation of personal liability risk, contractual obligations between the nurse and the insurer, and the availability of personal assets to compensate for a patient's injury in the event the institution or agency does not provide coverage or when the injury occurs outside the employee's job (e.g., volunteer work).

6. Continuing competence and professional improvement
    a) *Continued competence* is defined as "the ongoing ability to render safe, direct nursing care, or the ongoing ability to make sound judgments upon which nursing care is based" (Alexander & Webster, 2010, p. 58).
    b) Strategies such as continuing nursing education, self-assessment, professional certification and recertification, chart

audits, and clinical simulations mitigate legal risks.

E. Special considerations
    1. EMR: A variety of unanswered legal and ethical concerns exist with the growing use and implementation of EMRs (Doyle-Lindrud, 2015; Sittig & Singh, 2011).
        a) With the development of health information exchanges, healthcare providers have greater access to information beyond their institutions. Subsequently, the volume of records and information available can be cumbersome and difficult to review.
        b) EMRs may increase a provider's legal responsibility and accountability. Computer audits can provide extensive information on which provider had access to a patient's record and what actions were taken.
        c) Liabilities arise when data, such as laboratory values, are imported into a medical record automatically without a provider reviewing (and acting upon) the information.
        d) Documentation made by cutting and pasting from previous notes could contribute to error in the EMR.
        e) EMRs raise ethical issues concerning the ownership of protected health information. De-identified data sets of patients have been sold by various EMR vendors, raising questions of what happens to data if reidentified. Breaching of systems and firewalls allows the opportunity for data to be stolen with ramifications beyond the Health Insurance Portability and Accountability Act as it relates to identify theft and fraud.

The author would like to acknowledge Debra J. McCorkindale, RN, BSN, for her contribution to this chapter that remains unchanged from the previous edition of this book.

References

Alexander, M., & Webster, H. (2010). Legal issues of infusion nursing. In A.M., Corrigan, L. Gorski, J. Hankins, & R. Perucca (Eds.), *Infusion nursing: An evidence-based approach* (3rd ed., pp. 49–59). St. Louis, MO: Elsevier Saunders.

Brant, J.M., & Wickham, R. (Eds.). (2013). *Statement on the scope and standards of oncology nursing practice: Generalist and advanced practice.* Pittsburgh, PA: Oncology Nursing Society.

DeLa Cruz, R.F., Caillouet, B., & Guerrero, S.S. (2012). Strategic patient education program to prevent catheter-related bloodstream infection [Online exclusive]. *Clinical Journal of Oncology Nursing, 16,* E12–E17. doi:10.1188/12.CJON.E12-E17

Doyle-Lindrud, S. (2015). The evolution of the electronic health record. *Clinical Journal of Oncology Nursing, 19,* 153–154. doi:10.1188/15. CJON.153-154

Dychter, S.S., Gold, D.A., Carson, D., & Haller, M. (2012). Intravenous therapy: A review of complications and economic considerations of peripheral access. *Journal of Infusion Nursing, 35,* 84–91. doi:10.1097/ NAN.0b013e31824237ce

Gallieni, M., Martina, V., Rizzo, M.A., Gravellone, L., Mobilia, F., Giordano, A., ... Genovese, U. (2011). Central venous catheters: Legal issues. *Journal of Vascular Access, 12,* 273–279. doi:10.5301/JVA.2011.7745

Gilbar, P.J. (2014). Intrathecal chemotherapy: Potential for medication error. *Cancer Nursing, 37,* 299–309. doi:10.1097/ NCC.0000000000000108

Institute of Medicine. (2010). *The future of nursing: Leading change, advancing health.* Washington, DC: National Academies Press.

Karno, S. (2011). Nursing malpractice/negligence and liability. In P. Grant & D. Ballard (Eds.), *Law for nurse leaders: A comprehensive reference* (pp. 249–280). New York, NY: Springer.

Masoorli, S. (2005). Legal issues related to vascular access devices and infusion therapy. *Journal of Infusion Nursing, 28*(Suppl. 3), S18–S21. doi:10.1097/00129804-200505001-00004

O'Grady, N.P., Alexander, M., Burns, L.A., Dellinger, E.P., Garland, J., Heard, S.O., ... Healthcare Infection Control Practices Advisory Committee. (2011). Guidelines for the prevention of intravascular catheter-related infections. *Clinical Infectious Diseases, 52,* E162–E193. doi:10.1093/cid/cir257

Polovich, M., Olsen, M., & LeFebvre, K.B. (Eds.). (2014). *Chemotherapy and biotherapy guidelines and recommendations for practice* (4th ed.). Pittsburgh, PA: Oncology Nursing Society.

Ranchon, F., Salles, G., Späth, H., Schwiertz, V., Vantard, N., Parat, S., ... Rioufol, C. (2011). Chemotherapeutic errors in hospitalised cancer patients: Attributable damage and extra costs. *BMC Cancer, 11,* 478. doi:10.1186/1471-2407-11-478

Reising, D.L. (2012). Make your nursing care malpractice-proof. *American Nurse Today, 7.*

Sittig, D.F., & Singh, H. (2011). Legal, ethical, and financial dilemmas in electronic health record adoption and use [Online exclusive]. *Pediatrics, 127,* e1042–e1047. doi:10.1542/peds.2010-2184

Appendices

Appendices

Author	Design/Sample	Intervention/Variables Examined	Findings
\multicolumn{4}{c}{**Appendix 1. Summary of Evidence for Access Device–Related Recommendations: 2011–Present***}			

Appendix 1. Summary of Evidence for Access Device–Related Recommendations: 2011–Present*

Author	Design/Sample	Intervention/Variables Examined	Findings
\multicolumn{4}{c}{**Ultrasound/Fluoroscopy Insertion Techniques**}			
Brass et al., 2015	Design: Meta-analysis Sample: 35 studies with 5,108 participants; short- and long-term VADs	Evaluation of safety and efficacy of two-dimensional US or Doppler US versus traditional landmark technique in adults and children	Subclavian vein puncture: A two-dimensional US reduced the risk of arterial puncture and hematoma formation. No evidence was found to suggest a difference in total or other complications, overall or first-time success rates, number of attempts until success, or the time taken to insert the catheter. No evidence was found to suggest a difference in outcomes with use of a US device. Femoral vein puncture: Minimal evidence was available. No evidence was found to suggest a difference in complication rates, time taken for insertion, arterial puncture, or hematoma formation with use of two-dimensional US; however, success on the first attempt was more likely with two-dimensional US, and a small increase in overall success rate was noted. The use of US guidance for insertion of subclavian or femoral catheters was not supported. The authors cautioned that the reviewed studies were not of optimum quality; current evidence is insufficient to support the use of US-guided catheter insertion.
Bowen et al., 2014	Design: Retrospective analysis Sample: 351 CVADs** placed in the internal jugular vein	Evaluation of US guidance for complication rate and costs	US guidance proved to have reduced complications and costs and elimination of postprocedural chest x-rays.
Ahn et al., 2012	Design: Retrospective analysis Sample: 1,254 central venous ports implanted via the internal jugular vein using US and fluoroscopy guidance	Evaluation of US and fluoroscopy guidance for technical success and complication rates	Technical success rate was 99.9% with a 5% complication rate. Complications included infection, thrombotic malfunction, nonthrombotic malfunction, venous thrombosis, and wound problems.
Lamperti et al., 2012	International evidence-based recommendations on US-guided vascular access: Systematic literature review	Literature on US vascular access for central, peripheral, and arterial short- and long-term catheters from January 1985 to October 2010	Recommendations suggest that two-dimensional vascular screening prior to CVAD cannulation and real-time US needle guidance with a long axis/in-plane technique optimize the probability of correct needle placement. US guidance also can be used for peripheral and arterial cannulation, to assess for the catheter's tip position, and for immediate and life-threatening complications. Educational courses and training are required to achieve competence and minimal skills when cannulation is performed with US guidance.
Teichgräber et al., 2011	Design: Retrospective analysis Sample: 3,160 implanted port catheter systems	Evaluation of successful insertion and complication rates after US-guided port implantation	US-guided port implantation via the internal jugular vein route had low postprocedural complications; 922,599 catheter days were evaluated and 374 (11.8%) adverse events were reported, with the most common being BSI catheter-induced venous thrombosis and catheter migration.

(Continued on next page)

Appendix 1. Summary of Evidence for Access Device–Related Recommendations: 2011–Present* *(Continued)*

Author	Design/Sample	Intervention/Variables Examined	Findings
	**Intracavitary Electrocardiography Insertion Techniques**		
Rossetti et al., 2015	Design: Case-controlled cohort Sample: 309 patients with different catheters (e.g., PICC, short-term CVAD, long-term CVAD)	Evaluation of safety and accuracy of IC-ECG in pediatric patients for the placement of CVADs	No complications were reported; IC-ECG is safe and accurate in pediatric patients. Accuracy is 95.8% and is higher (98.8%) when using a dedicated ECG monitor.
Walker et al., 2015	Design: Systematic literature review Sample: 5 studies involving 729 participants	Comparison of IC-ECG–guided catheter placement with surface anatomy–guided insertion plus chest x-ray confirmation to assess accurate catheter tip placement	IC-ECG–guided insertion was significantly more accurate than surface anatomy–guided insertion. The authors concluded that IC-ECG–guided catheter insertion could potentially eliminate the requirement of a postprocedural chest x-ray to assess catheter tip placement.
Wang et al., 2015	Design: Prospective, nonrandomized Sample: 1,160 patients with cancer with PICCs or CVADs** placed in the internal jugular vein	Evaluation of sensitivity and specificity amplitude changes in P-waves of IC-ECGs to assess the tip placement of CVADs	Amplitude change of P-wave proves good sensitivity and excellent specificity; better sensitivity was observed in the placement of centrally inserted versus peripherally inserted VADs.
	**Placement Confirmation Imaging**		
Walker et al., 2015	*See Intracavitary Electrocardiography Insertion Techniques*		
Bowen et al., 2014	*See Ultrasound/Fluoroscopy Insertion Techniques*		
Thomopoulos et al., 2014	Design: Retrospective analysis Sample: 891 participants with implanted port placement	Evaluation of the necessity of a systematic postoperative chest x-ray following implanted port insertion under fluoroscopic guidance	A very low incidence of immediate complications was identified in chest x-rays. The authors concluded a chest x-ray should be performed postprocedurally only in cases of clinical suspicion of malposition.
	**Transparent Versus Gauze and Tape Dressings**		
Chico-Padrón et al., 2011	Design: Randomized, case controlled Sample: 2 subsamples of 75 patients: (1) 50 patients with short- and medium-peripheral catheters, including 21 patients with gauze and 29 with transparent dressings, and (2) 25 patients with central catheters**, including 13 patients with gauze and 12 with transparent dressings Device: Gauze and tape; transparent polyurethane dressing	Comparison of safety and costs of transparent versus gauze dressings in IV short- and medium-peripheral catheters and intravascular central catheters	No significant differences were found in complication rates between the types of dressings. Increased costs were associated with gauze versus transparent dressings due to the increased frequency of dressing changes needed with gauze.

(Continued on next page)

Appendix 1. Summary of Evidence for Access Device–Related Recommendations: 2011–Present* *(Continued)*

Author	Design/Sample	Intervention/Variables Examined	Findings
O'Grady et al., 2011	Guidelines for the prevention of intravascular catheter-related infections, 2011: Systematic literature review	Systematic literature review and expert work group committees of representatives from healthcare member services and professional organizations to update evidence and recommendations to include changes from the previous edition in 2002 to 2011	Guidelines suggest no difference in use of transparent or gauze and tape dressing; the choice of dressing could be matter of preference.
Pedrolo et al., 2011	Design: Randomized, case controlled Sample: 21 nontunneled CVADs Device: Gauze and tape; transparent polyurethane dressings	Comparison of stability, rate of catheter-related infections, local reaction, and exudate absorption	No significant differences were found in catheter-related infections, dressing stability, or exudate absorption. Local reactions were more prevalent in the gauze and tape dressings.
Chlorhexidine-Impregnated Dressings or Sponges			
Karpanen et al., 2016	Design: Randomized Sample: Skin samples, sutures, CVC intradermal and tip samples; CHG-impregnated dressing group (n = 136); nonantimicrobial dressing group (n = 137)	Comparison of transparent film dressing incorporating a 2% CHG gel with a nonantimicrobial dressing	A significantly reduced number of microorganisms was recovered from the CVC insertion site, suture site, sutures, and catheter surface in the CHG-impregnated dressing group compared with the nonantimicrobial dressing group.
Kerwat et al., 2015	Design: Prospective, nonrandomized Sample: 308 patients and 337 catheters; nontunneled catheters receiving regional anesthesia (peripheral nerve block) Device: CHG-impregnated sponge or dressing	Comparison of the rate of bacterial colonization at the insertion site and the catheter tip of catheters dressed with a CHG-impregnated sponge or dressing with conventional dressing	CHG-impregnated dressings significantly reduced bacterial colonization of the catheter tip and of the insertion site of epidural and peripheral regional catheters.
Ullman et al., 2015	Design: Systematic review Sample: 22 studies involving 7,436 participants	Different interventions and comparisons involving sterile gauze, standard polyurethane, CHG-impregnated dressings, silver-impregnated dressings, hydrocolloid dressing, second-generation gaseous permeability standard polyurethane, and sutureless securement devices	Medication-impregnated dressing products, defined as only CHG-impregnated dressings as either a patch or a whole dressing, reduced the incidence of CVAD-related BSI relative to all other dressing types.
Pedrolo et al., 2014	Design: Randomized, case-controlled cohort Sample: 85 patients with short-term CVADs Device: CHG-impregnated dressing, gauze and tape dressing	Comparison of BSI rates, local reactions, and dressing fixation between the two types of dressings	No statistical differences were found in BSIs, local reaction, or fixation between the types of dressings.

(Continued on next page)

Appendix 1. Summary of Evidence for Access Device–Related Recommendations: 2011–Present* *(Continued)*				
Author	**Design/Sample**	**Intervention/Variables Examined**	**Findings**
Safdar et al., 2014	Design: Meta-analysis Sample: 9 randomized trials Device: CHG-impregnated sponge or dressing used with various short- and long-term VADs and short-term temporary arterial catheters	Evaluation of CHG-impregnated sponge dressing for prevention of catheter colonization and catheter-related BSI Topical skin antisepsis preinsertion included studies comparing CHG 0.5% in 70% EtOH; 10% povidone-iodine versus 70% alcohol; alcohol-povidone-iodine 10%; alcohol spray; CHG alone, 4% aqueous povidone-iodine scrub followed by 5% povidone-iodine in 70% EtOH; or did not report	A significant reduction in catheter colonization and catheter-related infections resulted with the use of the dressing.
Timsit et al., 2012	Design: Prospective, randomized Sample: 1,879 patients with intravascular catheters inserted for an expected duration of > 48 hours Device: CHG-impregnated dressing, highly adhesive dressing, and standard dressing	Comparison of CHG-impregnated dressing, highly adhesive dressing, and standard dressing for catheter colonization and catheter-related infections in patients in ICUs	CHG-impregnated dressings showed a significantly lower catheter-related infection rate (67%) and catheter-related BSI rate (60%) compared to non–CHG-impregnated dressings. Highly adhesive dressings decreased dressing detachment rates but increased skin colonization and catheter colonization without influencing catheter-related infections or catheter-related BSI rates.
Cleansing Agents: Before Accessing Port			
Kao et al., 2014	Design: Prospective, case-controlled cohort Sample: 396 patients, consecutive Device: Implanted ports	Comparison of CHG and povidone-iodine for prevention of BSI associated with accessing implantable venous ports, including type of bacteria and time to infection rates	No significant difference was found in preventing port-associated BSIs. CHG: A significant improvement was found in time to first BSI caused by gram-positive bacteria; no significant preventive effects were found on time to first BSI caused by gram-negative bacteria or fungi.
Cleansing Agents: Before Accessing Needleless Connectors or Hubs			
Moreau & Flynn, 2015	Design: Systematic literature review Sample: 140 studies and 34 abstracts Device: NC hubs	Evaluation of NC disinfection practices, influence of hub contamination on infection, and measure of education and compliance	Following insertion, the greatest risk of catheter contamination is the NC, with 33%–45% of the sample contaminated and compliance with disinfection protocols as low as 10%. Reduction of 48%–86% in infections was noted with use of passive alcohol disinfection caps. No optimal technique or disinfection can be recommended. Recommendations given: 1. Use CHG-alcohol, povidone-iodine, an iodophor, or 70% alcohol as antisepsis on NCs, stopcocks, and access ports. 2. Scrub connectors with 70% alcohol for 5–60 seconds to decrease infection risk.
Hong et al., 2013	Design: Experimental model Sample: In vitro Device: MaxPlus® MP1000 positive pressure NCs	Comparison of different scrub times (swipe, 5, 15, or 30 seconds) of CHG-alcohol compared to alcohol to determine residual disinfectant activity	Alcohol swipe did not adequately disinfect NCs. CHG-alcohol and alcohol performed similarly at > 5-second scrubs. CHG-alcohol resulted in residual disinfectant activity for up to 24 hours.

(Continued on next page)

Appendix 1. Summary of Evidence for Access Device–Related Recommendations: 2011–Present* *(Continued)*

Author	Design/Sample	Intervention/Variables Examined	Findings
Sweet et al., 2012	Design: Observations before and after trial Sample: Central line days in oncology unit prior to and after intervention; types include tunneled and implanted port VADs, nontunneled short-term VADs, and PICCs. Activity: Cleaning of hubs was changed from using alcohol wipes to using alcohol-impregnated port protectors.	Comparison of number of days to CLABSI rates in the preintervention versus the postintervention time periods	The intervention period (3,005 catheter days) experienced one CLABSI; the historical period (6,851 catheter days) experienced 16 CLABSIs. Use of the alcohol-impregnated port protectors and needleless neutral pressure connectors significantly reduced the rates of CLABSIs in the oncology population.
Simmons et al., 2011	Design: Experimental Sample: In vitro Device: CVC hubs*	Comparison of cleaning duration and reduction in bacterial load when using alcohol disinfection at 3, 10, and 15 seconds	No significant difference in bacterial load was found between each of the three levels of disinfection duration; however, any disinfection significantly decreased the bacterial load as compared to controls.
Cleansing Agents: Before Catheter Site Care and Dressing Changes			
Bilir et al., 2013	Design: Prospective, randomized, case controlled Sample: 109 patients Device: CVC** and arterial catheters**, CHG, octenidine, and povidone-iodine	Comparison of CHG, octenidine, and povidone-iodine for prevention of catheter-related infections (colonization and rate of sepsis)	The CHG cohort demonstrated no catheter-related sepsis or colonization. The octenidine and povidone-iodine cohorts demonstrated a 10.5% catheter-related sepsis rate; colonization was 26.3% in the povidone-iodine cohort and 21.5% in the octenidine cohort.
Atahan et al., 2012	Design: Prospective, randomized, case controlled Sample: 50 patients, convenience Device: CVADs** inserted in the operating suite	Evaluation of the effect of multiple disease and demographic variables, including use of CHG solution or povidone-iodine on the development of catheter colonization and related BSIs in CVCs	A significant reduction was found in catheter-related BSIs and colonization with the use of CHG compared to povidone-iodine antiseptic solution. No other statistically significant differences were found. Variables included patient age and gender, presence of malignancy and coexisting diseases, catheter duration, use of total parenteral nutrition, and blood products.
Girard et al., 2012	Design: Prospective, randomized Sample: 806 catheters, longitudinal convenience Device: CVADs** in patients in an ICU	Comparison of alcoholic povidone-iodine with CHG antiseptic solution for prevention of central venous device infections (colonization and incidence)	When switched from povidone-iodine to CHG, a significant reduction in colonization was noted, but no significant difference was found in CVC-related infection or bacteremia. Povidone-iodine was associated with higher risk of colonization and infection.
Cleansing Agents: Epidural Catheters			
Kulkarni & Awode, 2013	Design: Prospective, randomized Sample: n = 60 (50 epidural) Device: Epidural; CVAD**	Comparison of cost, efficacy, and side effects of 10% povidone-iodine and 2% CHG for skin disinfection prior to insertion	Findings suggest no differences in all variables.
Krobbuaban et al., 2011	Design: Prospective, randomized Sample: 98 patients Device: Epidural catheters used for regional anesthesia	Comparison of CHG-alcohol and povidone-iodine for skin disinfection (cultures of insertion site and immediately following antisepsis) prior to neuraxial blockade procedure	The incidence of positive skin culture was significantly lower in CHG cohort compared to povidone-iodine cohort in cultures taken immediately after skin infection (35% versus 10%, respectively).

(Continued on next page)

Appendix 1. Summary of Evidence for Access Device–Related Recommendations: 2011–Present* *(Continued)*

Author	Design/Sample	Intervention/Variables Examined	Findings
		Flushing Protocols: CVADs	
Gorji et al., 2015	Design: Prospective, randomized, double-blind Sample: 84 patients with triple-lumen CVADs** inserted via subclavian or through jugular routes in the ICU Agent: 3 ml heparinized saline and 10 ml NS flushes	Blinded comparison of 3 ml heparinized saline flush or 10 ml NS flush following medication administration; catheters evaluated every 8 hours for blood return and flushing for 21 days	No significant differences in catheter patency between the two solutions were found. The use of heparin had no effect on prolonging catheter survival.
Ferroni et al., 2014	Design: Experimental, in vitro Sample: 576 polyurethane short-term CVADs Activity: Flushing technique	Comparison of efficacy of pulsatile versus continuous flushing versus no flushing (positive control) to prevent bacterial colonization in polyurethane short venous access catheters contaminated with *Staphylococcus aureus*	Significantly higher *Staphylococcus aureus* endoluminal contamination was found with continuous flushing versus pulsatile flushing.
López-Briz et al., 2014	Design: Systematic literature review Sample: 6 studies (1,433 participants) with various CVADs (PICC; port; double-, triple-, and quadruple-lumen CVADs) Agent: Heparin and 0.9% sodium chloride	Comparison of heparin at varying concentrations versus 0.9% sodium chloride intermittent flushing for prevention of occlusion in CVCs in adults	No conclusive evidence of differences in occlusion rates was found between using heparin saline versus using sodium chloride intermittent flushing. No differences in catheter survival, rate of thrombosis, rate of infection, mortality, bleeding rates, or heparin-induced thrombocytopenia were found.
Lyon & Phalen, 2014	Design: Prospective, randomized, one-way, single-blinded post-test with control Sample: 90 homecare patients (no cancer diagnoses) with PICCs Agent: 3 flushing protocols and the use of alteplase	Flushing protocols: 10 ml NS, medication administration, 10 ml NS flush; 10 ml NS, medication administration, 10 ml NS, 3 ml heparinized saline (100 IU/ml); 10 ml NS, medication administration, 10 ml NS, 5 ml heparinized saline (10 ml) Variables evaluated: Sluggishness, occlusion, missed medication doses, catheter replacement, additional nursing visits, and the use of alteplase	The saline flush group had the highest incidence of occlusions requiring alteplase. The higher concentration heparin flush group and the saline flush group had comparable episodes of sluggishness. The lower concentration heparin flush group had the least number of episodes of occlusions and use of alteplase.
Goossens et al., 2013	Design: Randomized, open label Sample: 802 patients with cancer with newly inserted implanted venous ports Agent: 3 ml (100 IU/ml) heparin and NS	Comparison of 3 ml (100 IU/ml) heparin lock versus a saline lock for incidence of catheter-related bacteremia, occurrence of functional problems, and blood withdrawal occlusion Both groups received flush with 10 ml NS before and after blood sampling.	No significant difference was found in blood withdrawal occlusion, catheter-related bacteremia, and occurrence of functional problems between the two solutions. The authors concluded that NS is an effective solution if combined with consistent, pulsatile flushing technique followed by a positive pressure locking technique.
Schallom et al., 2012	Design: Randomized, open label Sample: 341 patients with multilumen CVADs** in the ICU and the burn/trauma ICU Agent: NS and saline-heparin combination	Evaluation of CVC lumen patency comparing 10 ml NS flush q 8 hours versus 10 ml NS flush followed by 3 ml of heparin (10 IU/ml) lock flush solutions q 8 hours	No significant difference in catheter occlusion was found between the two solutions.

(Continued on next page)

Appendix 1. Summary of Evidence for Access Device–Related Recommendations: 2011–Present* *(Continued)*			
Author	**Design/Sample**	**Intervention/Variables Examined**	**Findings**
Flushing Protocols: Arterial Catheters			
Robertson-Malt et al., 2014	Design: Retrospective analysis of 7 studies Sample: 606 participants in randomized, controlled, and quasi-randomized trials (7 studies) with temporary arterial catheters in ICUs Agent: Heparin	Comparison of heparin at various concentrations versus saline alone for patency and functionality of catheter Concentrations: 1–2 IU/ml under continuous pressure, 3 ml/hour under continuous pressure, and 4 IU/ml under continuous pressure of heparin; 100 IU/ml was studied.	Available evidence is of poor quality with the risk of bias. Due to a high degree of variability in study designs, meta-analysis was not possible. Findings do not support the addition of heparin (100 IU/ml) to a maintenance solution of NS (pressurized to deliver 3 ml/hour).
Catheter Occlusion: tPA Locks or Infusions to Restore Function of Occluded VADs			
Ponce et al., 2015	Design: Prospective, case-controlled cohort Sample: 339 tunneled CVADs placed for hemodialysis in 247 patients across two centers Agent: Alteplase	Evaluation of the incidence of thrombotic obstruction of tunneled CVADs and the efficacy of treatment with alteplase; secondary aims were to identify factors associated with thrombotic occlusion.	Approximately 87% of patients experienced successful reversal of occlusion using alteplase protocols. The number of catheter days, presence of diabetes, and exit-site infections were associated with thrombotic occlusions.
van der Merwe, 2015	Design: Observational case series Sample: 3 nonconsecutive patients diagnosed with acute thrombosed arteriovenous fistula Agent: tPA	Demonstration of the successful use of tPA to decrease clot burden in arteriovenous fistula in the dialysis patient	Objective evidence was found of a decrease in clot burden on US or fistulogram in all patients; however, this was a small sample size and more research is needed.
Ernst, 2014	Design: Retrospective analysis Sample: 34,579 records of patients treated for a CVAD occlusion	Comparison of length of stay, costs, and readmissions associated with the use of alteplase to treat catheter occlusions	Alteplase-treated patients had lower daily and total postocclusion costs as compared to patients who received catheter replacement.
Manns et al., 2014	Design: Prospective, randomized Sample: Hemodialysis catheters Agent: rtPA 1 mg per lumen, rtPA/heparin-locking solutions, and heparinized solution only	Comparisons of weekly rtPA in each lumen and twice-weekly rtPA/heparin-locking solutions to determine risks of malfunction and bacteremia compared to heparin administered three times a week alone; costs of each regimen were evaluated.	A twice-weekly rtPA/heparin lock protocol used in each lumen of the catheters demonstrated a mean overall cost and efficacy similar to that of a three-times-per-week heparin lock protocol.
Ragsdale et al., 2014	Design: Retrospective analysis Sample: Data from 150 occlusion events in critically ill pediatric patients who had CVADs**	Evaluation of the safety and efficacy of alteplase infusions and dwells to clear partially occluded catheters	Alteplase infusions are as efficacious as dwells in this population to clear partially occluded catheters. If infusion is used, more occlusions are resolved in older and larger patients and in those with catheters less than 7 days. If dwell is used, more occlusions are resolved in smaller catheters. Safety for both infusion and dwell is acceptable.
Vercaigne et al., 2012	Design: Prospective, randomized, parallel arm multicenter Sample: 82 patients with CVADs placed for hemodialysis Agent: Alteplase	Comparison of the safety and efficacy of an alteplase dwell over 30–90 minutes versus a new push protocol to restore function to occluded catheters and to increase blood flow in catheters with less than 200 ml/min flow to > 300 ml/min flow	The alteplase push protocol was as safe and effective and more practical than the dwell protocol. Approximately 65% of catheters receiving the dwell protocol achieved the 300 ml/min endpoint, compared to 82% of the catheters in the push protocol achieving the 300 ml/min endpoint. Study limitations included small sample size.

(Continued on next page)

Appendix 1. Summary of Evidence for Access Device–Related Recommendations: 2011–Present* *(Continued)*			
Author	**Design/Sample**	**Intervention/Variables Examined**	**Findings**
Tebbi et al., 2011	Design: Phase III, single arm Sample: 246 patients with dysfunctional CVADs** Agent: Tenecteplase	Evaluation of the safety and efficacy of tenecteplase in restoring function to CVADs	Approximately 72% of patients achieved restoration of function within 120 minutes of the first dose; 81% received restoration after two doses. Frequencies were similar among adults and pediatric patients. The authors concluded that one or two doses of tenecteplase showed efficacy and safety in catheter function restoration.
Catheter Occlusion Prophylaxis			
Akl et al., 2014	Design: Systematic review Sample: 12 studies with 2,823 participants with CVADs** (adults and children) Agent: Various combinations of comparisons of low-dose vitamin K antagonists (warfarin), low-molecular-weight heparin, unfractionated heparin, or fondaparinux versus no intervention or versus placebo	Evaluation of the relative efficacy and safety of anticoagulation for thromboprophylaxis in people with cancer with a CVAD	Compared with no anticoagulation, a significant reduction was found in symptomatic DVT with heparin and asymptomatic DVT with vitamin K antagonists. The authors warned that benefits must outweigh harms when considering anticoagulation in this population.
Lavau-Denes et al., 2013	Design: Phase III, open label, randomized Sample: 407 patients with CVADs** Agent: Low-molecular-weight heparin, warfarin, or no prophylaxis	Comparison of the two kinds of prophylaxis and no prophylaxis on incidence of thrombotic events	Prophylaxis showed a benefit regarding catheter-related and noncatheter-related DVT without an increase in side effects. No difference was found in prophylactic efficacy between warfarin and low-molecular-weight heparin.
Kahn et al., 2012	Consensus Guidelines: American College of Chest Physicians, 9th ed. Design: Systematic literature review	Consensus recommendations based on previous editions, systematic literature review, and expert opinion	Work provides recommendations of evidence-based anticoagulant therapy, prevention of venous thromboembolism, diagnosis of DVT, and antithrombotic therapy in specific populations (e.g., surgical, nonsurgical, atrial fibrillation, neonates and children, ischemic stroke, cardiovascular disease, pregnancy).
Catheter Occlusion Prevention: Heparin-Bonded Catheters			
Shah & Shah, 2014	Design: Retrospective analysis Sample: 2 studies involving 287 pediatric participants (randomized and quasi-randomized trials) Device: Heparin-bonded catheters and nonheparin-bonded or antibiotic-impregnated catheters with CVADs**	Evaluation of the efficacy of heparin-bonded catheters for prolongation of patency	No difference was found in catheter-related thrombosis with the use of heparin-bonded catheters compared to nonheparin-bonded catheters.
Peripheral IV Maintenance and Dwell Time			
Webster et al., 2015	Design: Systematic review Sample: 7 trials with a total of 4,895 patients	Clinically indicated versus routine replacement of peripheral catheters	No significant difference was found in catheter-related BSI or phlebitis rates between those catheters routinely replaced or when clinically indicated. The authors recommended a policy change for catheter replacement only when clinically indicated.

(Continued on next page)

Appendix 1. Summary of Evidence for Access Device–Related Recommendations: 2011–Present* *(Continued)*

Author	Design/Sample	Intervention/Variables Examined	Findings
Paşalioğlu & Kaya, 2014	Design: Cross-sectional study Sample: 439 peripheral catheters (103 patients) in one infectious disease inpatient unit (Turkey) hospitalized > 1 day	Evaluation of the effect of indwell time on phlebitis development in peripheral venous catheters	Phlebitis was detected in 41.2% of peripheral IV catheters; 35.8% of catheters did not work properly; treatment ended and the catheter was removed in 3.6% of patients; and 19.4% of catheters were removed after more than 120 hours. Only grades 2 and 3 phlebitis were observed. The risk of phlebitis if the catheter was in place less than 48 hours was 5.8 times more likely than that of patients with catheters in place 49–96 hours, and 2.8 times more likely than that of patients with catheters in place for 97–120 hours.
Rickard et al., 2012	Design: Randomized Sample: 3,283 patients (5,907 catheters), including 1,593 clinically indicated and 1,690 routine replacement	Comparison of routine replacement (every 72 hours) versus clinically indicated replacement of peripheral catheters	No significant difference was found between the two groups. Mean dwell time for catheters was 99 hours when replaced as clinically indicated and 70 hours when routinely replaced. Phlebitis occurred in 114 of 1,593 (7%) patients in the clinically indicated group and in 114 of 1,690 (7%) patients in the routine replacement group. The authors recommended replacement of peripheral catheters as clinically indicated.

Infection: Sterile Versus Aseptic Catheter or Dressing Care

Flynn et al., 2015	Design: Comparative case design Sample: 150 bone marrow transplant patients with tunneled venous catheters Activity: ANTT and sterile technique	Evaluation of catheter-related BSI rates when ANTT versus sterile technique is used when changing NCs	The authors cautioned a small sample size and concluded that results imply that ANTT is not associated with increased catheter-related BSI, and that quality and consistent ANTT is a safe method for management of tunneled venous catheters.

Infection: Catheter and Insertion Site Selection

Ge et al., 2012	Design: Meta-analysis Sample: 1,513 participants with cancer receiving long- and short-term central hemodialysis catheters Activity: Route of insertion	Evaluation of insertion routes and risks for complications in long- and short-term CVCs and short-term hemodialysis catheters	Subclavian and internal jugular central venous access routes have similar risks and complications in long-term catheterization. A subclavian route is preferable to a femoral route in short-term catheterization (lower risk of colonization and thrombotic complications). Femoral and internal jugular routes have similar risks of catheter-related complications in short-term hemodialysis catheterization, except jugular routes have higher risks of mechanical complications.
O'Grady et al., 2011	2011 Guidelines for the Prevention of Intravascular Catheter-Related Infections Design: Systematic literature review	Systematic literature review and expert work group committees comprising representatives from healthcare member services and professional organizations to update evidence and recommendations to include changes from the previous edition in 2002 to 2011	Numerous recommendations were made regarding education, training, and staffing to ensure appropriate infection control measures; removal; insertion site; hand hygiene; catheter insertion protocols, dressing, and maintenance; and avoidance of routine use of anticoagulant therapy to decrease CLABSI.

(Continued on next page)

Appendix 1. Summary of Evidence for Access Device–Related Recommendations: 2011–Present* *(Continued)*

Author	Design/Sample	Intervention/Variables Examined	Findings
Infection: Antibiotic Use (Prophylaxis or Lock)			
Kubiak et al., 2014	Design: Retrospective analysis Sample: Patient records of those treated for CLABSI with adjunctive ethanol-lock therapy for CVAD salvage in combination with systemic antimicrobial treatment; 68 patient records; included long-term tunneled silicone, implanted port (polyurethane), PICC (polyurethane), and patients with both implanted port and PICC Activity: Review	Evaluation of adjunctive 70% ethanol-lock therapy for safety and possible efficacy for CLABSI	No adverse events were found with the use of ethanol-lock therapy. The authors reported that it warranted further investigation.
Schoot et al., 2013	Design: Systematic literature review Sample: 132 pediatric patients with tunneled CVADs among multiple studies Device/Agent: Urokinase lock solution, systemic antibiotics, ethanol lock solutions	Comparison of efficacy of addition of urokinase-lock or ethanol-lock protocols to systemic antibiotics in the treatment of VAD-related infections compared to a control group Secondary endpoint: Adverse events associated with lock protocols	No significant effect was found with urokinase or ethanol lock in addition to systemic antibiotics. Study limitations included low power and short follow-up.
van de Wetering et al., 2013	Design: Systematic literature review Sample: 11 trials with a total of 828 patients with cancer (adults and children)	Evaluate the efficacy of administering antibiotics prior to the insertion of long-term CVCs, flushing or locking long-term CVCs with a combined antibiotic and heparin solution, or both to prevent gram-positive, catheter-related infections	Most studies were found to be at a low or unclear risk of bias. No benefit was found in administering antibiotics before the insertion of long-term CVCs to prevent gram-positive, catheter-related infections. Flushing or locking long-term VADs with a combined antibiotic and heparin solution appeared to reduce gram-positive, catheter-related sepsis in people at risk of neutropenia from chemotherapy or bone marrow disease.
Infection: Impregnated Catheter			
Lai et al., 2013	Design: Systematic literature review Sample: 56 studies (11 types of antimicrobial impregnations; 16,512 catheters) Device: Any type of impregnated catheter against either nonimpregnated catheters or catheters with another impregnation	Evaluation of the efficacy of antimicrobial-impregnated catheters for the prevention of infection, thrombosis/thrombophlebitis, bleeding, and erythema or tenderness at the insertion site	The use of antimicrobial-impregnated catheters improved outcomes, showing decreased rates of catheter-related BSI and catheter colonization. The magnitude of benefit is varied according to catheter type and setting; significant benefit is seen in ICU settings. Limited evidence exists to support their use to reduce clinically diagnosed sepsis or mortality. Findings suggested caution in routinely recommending across all settings.

(Continued on next page)

Appendix 1. Summary of Evidence for Access Device–Related Recommendations: 2011–Present* *(Continued)*			
Author	**Design/Sample**	**Intervention/Variables Examined**	**Findings**
Infection: Needleless Connectors			
Flynn et al., 2015	*See Infection: Sterile Versus Aseptic Catheter or Dressing Care*		
Martinez et al., 2015	Design: Prospective, nonrandomized Sample: Neutropenic hematology patients with long-term, tunneled Hickman® catheter	Effect of NC bundle on catheter-related BSIs	Use of the bundle (a neutral pressure mechanical valve connector, more frequent changes of the connector [twice weekly and after each blood sample for a new fever episode], and a more efficient 2% CHG solution to clean the connectors) significantly reduced BSIs and catheter-related BSI rates.
Moureau & Flynn, 2015	*See Cleansing Agents: Before Accessing Needleless Connectors or Hubs*		
Sandora et al., 2014	Design: Comparative analysis Sample: Pediatric stem cell transplant recipients	Comparison of NC change frequency and CLABSI rate Collection periods: Baseline sampling during which the connector was changed every 96 hours regardless of the infusate it was exposed to; or the connector was changed every 24 hours with blood or lipid infusions; or a third sampling that mirrored the first study group	NCs changed every 24 hours when blood or lipids are infused are associated with increased CLABSI rates.
Tabak et al., 2014	Design: Meta-analysis Sample: 7 studies; 4 in ICUs, 1 in a home health setting, and 2 in long-term acute care settings	Evaluation of the risk for CLABSI associated with the use of a new NC with an improved engineering design	Newer design, positive-displacement connectors (connection with visible fluid path to assess efficacy of flush technique; a solid, flat, smooth access surface that is easily disinfected; an open fluid pathway that facilitates high flow and avoids hemolysis; a tight septum seal; and a single-part activation of the fluid path) are associated with lower CLABSI risk.
Sherertz et al., 2011	Design: Comparative analysis Sample: Blood samples from three different NC designs	Comparison of three different NC designs for catheter-related BSI	Blood samples from the Clearlink™ connectors met the Centers for Disease Control and Prevention criteria for BSIs; however, these patients were asymptomatic.
Removal of VAD With Infection			
Lorente et al., 2014	Design: Prospective, multicenter, observational Sample: 384 patients with CVADs** in ICUs that suspected catheter-related infections	Evaluation of clinical practice concerning CVADs when catheter-related infection is suspected	No statistical difference was found in mortality in patients with confirmed catheter-related BSIs according to the catheter removal at the moment of suspicion versus removal of catheter at any point later. The authors concluded that immediate removal of the CVAD with the suspected infection may not be necessary in all patients.

(Continued on next page)

Author	Design/Sample	Intervention/Variables Examined	Findings
Appendix 1. Summary of Evidence for Access Device–Related Recommendations: 2011–Present* *(Continued)*			
Blood Sampling From VADs for Blood Cultures			
Herrera-Guerra et al., 2015	Design: Comparative, prospective, nonrandomized Sample: Blood culture results from double- or triple-lumen or acute hemodialysis CVADs 24 patients eligible during the study period	Comparison of pooled blood cultures from each catheter lumen versus individually cultured venous catheter lumens	Sampling multiple lumens from a central line and incubating them in the same culture bottle is as effective as individual culture bottles in the diagnosis of either colonization or of catheter-related BSI.
Winokur et al., 2014	Design: Nonrandomized Sample: 62 pediatric patients with cancer	Analysis of 5 ml normally discarded blood assessed for pathogens	A correlation between positive blood cultures from the usual blood samples with the normally discarded specimen was found in all cases. In four cases, the normally discarded specimen demonstrated earlier time to positivity compared to the usual care specimen.
Blood Sampling From VADs for Coagulation Studies			
Dalton et al., 2015	Design: Systematic literature review Sample: 12 studies/326 participants with various CVADs (e.g., tunneled; implanted port; double- and triple-lumen; valved tunneled; PICC; hemodialysis tunneled; or other CVAD not specified)	Best practices determined for collecting coagulation studies from CVADs	Significant variability was found in sampling techniques and discard volume practices. The only reliable method for obtaining coagulation test results from CVADs is to flush then waste or discard blood sample prior to obtaining coagulation sample; however, this method has been studied only in PICCs.
Humphries et al., 2012	Design: Prospective, quasi-experimental Sample: 30 patients with heparinized PICCs Activity: Aseptic specimen drawing procedure from PICC; sample from venipuncture	Evaluation of an evidence-based procedure of drawing samples of coagulation testing from heparinized PICCs compared with blood results drawn from venipuncture	Blood samples from heparinized PICCs for coagulation tests were almost perfectly correlated with those drawn from venipunctures for prothrombin time, partial thromboplastin time, and fibrinogen in seconds and in milligrams; only the international normalized ratio samples suggested nonagreement.
Safety and Efficacy: Power Ports			
Goltz et al., 2014	Design: Retrospective analysis Sample: 729 patients with femoral vein implanted port with 1,979 catheter days analyzed	Evaluation of indication for, technical success of, and clinical outcome and safety of percutaneously implanted venous power ports in a femoral site	Indications were planned chemotherapy for breast and esophagus cancer and long-term central venous access for IV therapy. Technical success was 100%. One device was explanted as a result of infection. No early complications were noted. The authors concluded that if implantation of a totally implantable venous power port is not feasible in a standard chest, upper arm, or forearm site, femoral placement may be alternatively used safely and effectively.
Teichgräber et al., 2012	Design: Prospective, observational Sample: 78 ports/1,000 catheter days Device: Power-injectable central venous port system	Evaluation of the clinical benefit of power-injectable central venous ports	Complication rates of power-injectable central venous ports are comparable to standard port systems. Use of these ports for contrast injection should be increased.

(Continued on next page)

Appendix 1. Summary of Evidence for Access Device–Related Recommendations: 2011–Present* *(Continued)*			
Author	**Design/Sample**	**Intervention/Variables Examined**	**Findings**
General Principles			
Schiffer et al., 2013	Central Venous Catheter Care for the Patient With Cancer: American Society of Clinical Oncology Clinical Practice Guideline	Systematic literature review and expert work group to develop evidence-based recommendations specific to the care of patients with cancer who have CVCs.	Numerous recommendations were made regarding general management of short- and long-term CVCs.

* Full references from Appendix 1 are available in the Chapter 1 reference list.

** Additional specifics regarding type of access device are not specified.

ANTT—aseptic no-touch technique; BSI–bloodstream infection; CHG—chlorhexidine gluconate; CLABSI—central line–associated bloodstream infection; CVAD—central venous access device; CVC—central venous catheter; DVT—deep vein thrombosis; ECG—electrocardiogram; EtOH—ethanol; IC-ECG—intracavitary electrocardiography; ICU—intensive care unit; NC—needleless connector; NS—0.9% normal saline; PICC—peripherally inserted central catheter; rtPA—recombinant tissue plasminogen activator; tPA—tissue plasminogen activator; US—ultrasound; VAD—venous access device

				Appendix 2. Cleansing Agents				
Agent*	**Mode of Action**	**Gram-Positive Organisms**	**Gram-Negative Organisms**	**Tuberculosis**	**Fungi**	**Viruses**	**Residual Activity**	**Duration of Anti-Infective Effect**
Alcohol 70%	Denaturation of protein	Excellent	Excellent	Good	Good	Good	None	Brief
Iodophor 10% (povidone-iodine)	Oxidation/ substitution by free iodine	Excellent	Good	Good	Good	Good	Minimal	2 hours
Chlorhexidine (2% for all insertions; > 0.5% for all maintenance care)	Cell wall disruption	Excellent	Good	Poor	Fair	Good	Excellent	4–6 hours

Special Considerations*

Allergic reaction: Chlorhexidine (see Figures 1 and 2)	Prevention: Detailed history of previous allergic reactions. Consider allergy testing with specific immunoglobulin E to chlorhexidine or skin prick test if risks are present. Signs/Symptoms: • Mild irritant contact dermatitis • Allergic urticarial • Generalized erythema • Periorbital edema • Stomatitis • Vesicle formation • Bronchospasm • Life-threatening anaphylaxis Management: • Use povidone-iodine and alcohol for skin preparation. • If allergic to povidone-iodine, use alcohol or soap and water. • After procedure, ensure all preparation cleanser is removed from skin. • Management of anaphylaxis: Epinephrine, corticosteroids, IV fluid bolus
Chemical irritation: Chlorhexidine	Chlorhexidine gluconate manufacturer packaging warns of meningeal irritation if contact occurs when accessing intraventricular devices. Ensure skin is completely air-dried prior to access.
Contraindications: Alcohol	Alcohol is contraindicated for use with epidural and intrathecal devices prior to access.

*Ensure all products completely air-dry prior to access.

Figure 1. Chlorhexidine Allergic Skin Reaction to the Eyes	**Figure 2. Chlorhexidine Reaction to the Anterior Chest**
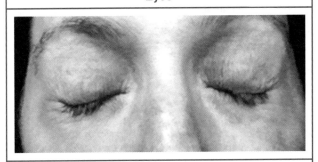	
Note. Image courtesy of Mady C. Stovall. Used with permission.	*Note.* Image courtesy of Mady C. Stovall. Used with permission.

References

Abdallah, C. (2015). Perioperative chlorhexidine allergy: Is it serious? *Journal of Anaesthesiology and Clinical Pharmacology, 31,* 152–154. doi:10.4103/0970-9185.155140

Guleri, A., Kumar, A., Morgan, R.J.M., Hartley, M., & Roberts, D.H. (2012). Anaphylaxis to chlorhexidine-coated central venous catheters: A case series and review of the literature. *Surgical Infections, 13,* 171–174. doi:10.1089/sur.2011.011

Hong, H., Morrow, D.F., Sandora, T.J., & Priebe, G.P. (2013). Disinfection of needleless connectors with chlorhexidine-alcohol provides long-lasting residual disinfectant activity. *American Journal of Infection Control, 41,* e77–e99. doi:10.1016/j.ajic.2012.10.018

Kao, H.-F., Chen, I.-C., Hsu, C., Chang, S.Y., Chien, S.-F., Chen, Y.-C., … Yeh, K.-H. (2014). Chlorhexidine for the prevention of bloodstream infection associated with totally implantable venous ports in patients with solid cancers. *Supportive Care in Cancer, 22,* 1189–1197. doi:10.1007/s00520-013-2071-5

Koch, A., & Wollina, U. (2014). Chlorhexidine allergy. *Allergo Journal International, 23,* 84–86. doi:10.1007/s40629-014-0012-6

Mimoz, O., Lucet, J.-C., Kerforne, T., Pascal, J., Souweine, B., Goudet, V., … Timsit, J.-C. (2015). Skin antisepsis with chlorhexidine-alcohol versus povidone iodine-alcohol, with and without skin scrubbing, for prevention of intravascular-catheter-related-infection (CLEAN): An open label, multicenter, randomised, controlled, two-by-two factorial trial. *Lancet, 21,* 2069–2077. doi:10.1016/S0140-6736(15)00244-5

Moka, E., Argyra, E., Siafaka, I., & Vadalouca, A. (2015). Chlorhexidine: Hypersensitivity and anaphylactic reactions in the perioperative setting. *Journal of Anaesthesiology and Clinical Pharmacology, 31,* 145–148. doi:10.4103/0970-9185.155138

Odedra, K.M., & Farooque, S. (2015). Chlorhexidine: An unrecognised cause of anaphylaxis. *Postgraduate Medicine Journal, 90,* 709–714. doi:10.1136/postgradmedj-2013-132291

Silvestri, D.L., & McEnery-Stonelake, M. (2013). Chlorhexidine: Uses and adverse reactions. *Dermatitis, 24,* 112–118. doi:10.1097/DER.0b013e3182905561

Sivathasan, N., & Goodfellow, P.B. (2011). Skin cleansers: The risks of chlorhexidine. *Journal of Clinical Pharmacology, 51,* 785–786. doi:10.1177/0091270010372628

Appendix 3. Terminology	
Term	**Definition**
Aseptic	Condition free from septic matter or free from organisms
Care bundles	Group of evidence-based interventions aimed at improving patient care processes and outcomes (e.g., maximum sterile barrier precautions on insertion, hand hygiene, chlorhexidine skin antisepsis, assessment of venous access device necessity).
Caregiver	Unpaid or paid individual who assists another individual with activities of daily living
Cathetergram	Also known as a dye study, performed when a central venous access device is improperly functioning (e.g., no blood return) to verify correct placement and patency; provides visualization of the integrity of the catheter
Clean	Condition free from debris or organisms
Contralateral	The side of the body that is opposite from the side in question
Epidural	Space between periosteum and dura matter, extending from base of skull to sacrum and containing adipose tissue, blood and lymph vessels, and spinal nerves
Hand hygiene	Handwashing with conventional soap and water or with alcohol-based hand rubs
Intrathecal	Space between dura mater and arachnoid membrane, containing cerebrospinal fluid (also called subdural)
Ipsilateral	Occurring on the side of the body in question
Long term	Greater than six weeks
Maximum sterile barrier precautions	Includes cap, mask, sterile gown, sterile gloves, and sterile full-body drape
Needleless connectors	An access point for infusion connections without the need for a needle; available in a variety of designs
Percutaneous	Procedure where access to an inner vein, artery, or organ is performed via a needle puncture through the skin, rather than an "open" surgical approach
Polyurethane	Firm, not stiff, material that softens and becomes pliable in the vein in response to body core temperature; provides exceptional tensile strength and flexibility, permitting thinner walled and greater internal diameter lumens for high flow rate catheters; thromboresistant
Protective caps	Connect to catheter hub or needleless connector to provide a physical barrier to contamination; available with passive disinfectant
Provider	Refers to the healthcare provider (e.g., physician, nurse practitioner, physician assistant)
Short term	Less than six weeks
Silicone	Flexible material that allows catheter to "float" within the vein, which may decrease damage to intima of the vessel; requires special insertion technique due to flexibility of material; thromboresistant
Sterile	Condition of being free from living microorganisms or germs
Temporary	Short-term dwelling; typically 1–3 days
Universal procedures	See Appendix 4

Appendix 4. Universal Concepts for Access Devices

Principle	Concepts	Additional Information
Professional	Procedures should be performed by personnel skilled in assessing signs of access device–related complications. Skilled personnel improve outcomes. Always evaluate the risks and benefits of the device selected, including estimated duration of use, intended purpose, and patient risk factors. Report manufacturer device defects.	Complications include erythema, swelling, tenderness, pain, induration, fever, chills, no blood return, and inability to withdraw or infuse fluid.
Hand hygiene and asepsis	Wash hands with conventional soap and water or alcohol-based hand rubs. Perform hand hygiene before and after palpation of catheter insertion or exit sites, and before and after any manipulation. Palpation of site should not occur after application of antiseptic unless asepsis is maintained. Wear clean or sterile gloves when changing dressings, as per device recommendations.	
Insertion	Ensure no contraindications exist for placement. Ensure informed consent is obtained prior to insertion of device. Ensure time-out procedures are used prior to placement of device. Preplacement assessment is completed. Laboratory studies are verified. Medication or antineoplastic agent is verified for accuracy. Strictly maintain hand hygiene. Assess for optimal insertion site; use of the femoral vein in adults is not recommended for IV lines. Use maximum sterile barriers for all devices except peripheral IVs (for which an aseptic no-touch technique may be used). Use a 2% chlorhexidine/alcohol preparation of the skin before insertion unless contraindicated or an allergy exists. Allow antiseptic to air-dry prior to insertion.	
Maintenance	Assess daily for the need for continued device use, and remove promptly when no longer needed. Use care bundles for all insertion, access, and maintenance activities. Monitor all exit sites on a regular basis visually or by palpation through an intact dressing. Organize care to minimize entries into the system. Maintain strict aseptic technique for all maintenance procedures. Scrub the hub of the needleless connector vigorously with appropriate antiseptic prior to use. Secure all tubing with a securement device. Do not use tape on tubing connections. Do not use topical antibiotics on insertion sites (except for hemodialysis catheters). Change dressing, IV tubing, or needleless connector when wet, soiled, contaminated, damaged, or nonadherent. Use > 0.5% chlorhexidine for daily skin cleansing (unless allergic).	Evidence-based sterile precautions exist for specific specialty access catheters (see Appendix 12). Tape can transmit bacterial contamination. Topical antibiotics increase risk of fungal infections and antimicrobial resistance.
Flushing	Flush with 0.9% normal saline (NS) before and after use, as indicated by device. Flush with 10–20 ml NS after blood withdrawal, as indicated by device. Never use excessive force. Use a 10 ml or larger syringe for central venous access devices (VADs). Some prefilled syringes contain less than 10 ml of fluid but have a 10 ml diameter syringe and are safe to use. Use a 3 ml diameter syringe for peripheral IVs and midline catheters. Flush vigorously, using pulsating (push-pause) technique, as indicated by device. NS is comparable to heparin lock for nonvalved VADs.	Blood return is not expected with specialty devices and is to be avoided with arterial devices. Pressure is inversely related to syringe size. High pressure increases the risk of catheter or septum rupture or separation. Maximum tolerated pressure may vary by device or if physiologic factors are present (e.g., fibrin sheath, clot).

(Continued on next page)

Appendix 4. Universal Concepts for Access Devices *(Continued)*		
Principle	**Concepts**	**Additional Information**
Blood sampling principles for venous devices	Obtain blood cultures from an implanted port with signs of an infection prior to initiation of antibiotic therapy. Use blood-sparing techniques when drawing blood samples. Organize work to minimize number of accesses of device; time blood sampling to coincide with other indications for accessing device, such as administration of another medication (e.g., antibiotic), if possible. During continuous infusion: Discontinue infusate(s) at least one minute before sampling. Clamp all lumens not being used for sampling on open-ended catheters. If results are grossly out of range, redraw sample from a peripheral vein. Coagulation studies: Inconclusive data to support peripheral sampling only; practices vary widely regarding sampling via peripherally or VADs. Some drugs can adhere to catheter wall; consider peripheral sampling.	Studies differ on whether sampling from heparin-locked catheters will confound results. Examples include aminoglycosides, cyclosporine, and gentamicin; may affect serum drug level results.
Blood sampling methods	Discard method (most common technique): • Withdraw and discard prior to collection of sample: Amounts vary from 3–10 ml (5–6 ml reported most frequently) for adults and 3–5 ml for children. • Flush with 10–20 ml of NS for adults and 3–10 ml for children. (Follow with heparin if necessary, as per catheter type.)	
	Vacutainer method: • Vacutainer is inserted into injection cap to obtain sample. • Withdrawal amount can be collected through vacutainer into empty blood collection tube.	Not routinely used
	Reinfusion method: • Discard sample is saved and reinfused after sample is collected. • Used often in neonate and infant populations	Not routinely used in adult population; caution is necessary to avoid reinfusion of clots.
	Mixing method: • Blood is withdrawn and immediately reinfused; repeated 3–4 times without removing syringe; then sample is taken. • Used in pediatric population	Not routinely used in adult population
Administration set	Ensure all components are compatible to minimize leaks and maintain integrity. Replacement (including secondary sets and add-on devices that are continuously used): • For equipment used to administer blood, blood products, fat emulsions (e.g., lipids), or total parenteral nutrition: Within 24 hours of initiation and every 24 hours thereafter • For equipment for propofol infusion: Every 6–12 hours and when the vial is changed • For equipment used to administer infusates: No more often than at 96-hour intervals Change needleless connectors after each use, if contaminated, or after breakage. Protective caps (connected to catheter hub or needleless connector, providing physical barrier to contamination): Change every 7 days, if contaminated or after breakage.	Some components may be incompatible with some infusates.

(Continued on next page)

Appendix 4. Universal Concepts for Access Devices *(Continued)*		
Principle	**Concepts**	**Additional Information**

Documentation	Ensure compliance with standards and policies.
	Rationale for device:
	• For insertion
	  – Informed consent
	  – Date and time of insertion
	  – Type of device and location of insertion
	  – Anesthetic, if used
	  – Presence of blood return or other body fluid
	  – Insertion complications, if any
	  – Dressing
	  – Confirmation of placement
	  – Patient education regarding catheter care, as indicated
	• For access
	  – Date, time, and purpose
	  – Evaluation of proper functioning
	  – Type of infusate
	  – Complications, if any; notify provider and implement strategies
	• For maintenance
	  – Evaluation of device; subjective information
	  – Type of dressing, frequency of tubing change
	  – Type, volume, frequency of flushing, as indicated
	  – Type, frequency of cap change, if any
	• For removal
	  – Date, time, and rationale
	  – Description of removal including catheter tip and assessment for catheter body intactness
	  – Wound or tip culture, if ordered
	  – Patient education regarding postprocedural care	

Patient preparation	Always ensure patient understanding of procedure to be performed. Always perform preprocedure assessment; consider any special needs regarding age, physical condition, or catheter type. Always answer any questions the patient or caregiver may have prior to initiation of procedure. Always perform time-out procedure to verify correct patient, correct site, and correct procedure.	

References

Joint Commission. (2013). CLABSI toolkit—Preventing central line–associated bloodstream infections: Useful tools, an international perspective. Retrieved from http://www.jointcommission.org/topics/clabsi_toolkit.aspx

Joint Commission. (2017). 2017 National Patient Safety Goals. Retrieved from http://www.jointcommission.org/standards_information/npsgs.aspx

Merrill, K.C., Sumner, S., Linford, L., Taylor, C., & Macintosh, C. (2014). Impact of universal disinfectant cap implementation on central line–associated bloodstream infections. *American Journal of Infection Control, 42,* 1274–1277. doi:10.1016/j.ajic.2014.09.008

O'Grady, N.P., Alexander, M., Burns, L.A., Dellinger, E.P., Garland, J., Heard, S.O., ... Healthcare Infection Control Practices Advisory Committee. (2011). Guidelines for the prevention of intravascular catheter-related infections. *Clinical Infectious Diseases, 52,* E162–E193. doi:10.1093/cid/cir257

Schiffer, C.A., Mangu, P.B., Wade, J.C., Camp-Sorrell, D., Cope, D.G., El-Rayes, B.F., ... Levine, M. (2013). Central venous catheter care for the patient with cancer: American Society of Clinical Oncology clinical practice guideline. *Journal of Clinical Oncology, 31,* 1357–1370. doi:10.1200/JCO.2012.45.5733

Appendix 5. Venous Devices

Characteristics	Peripheral Intravenous Line	Midline	Central Nontunneled	Peripherally Inserted Central Catheter	Tunneled	Implanted Port	Apheresis
Short or long term	Short term	Short term	Short term	Long term	Long term	Long term	Short or long term
Insertion and replacement or removal considerations	Use clean (not sterile) gloves and aseptic no-touch technique (ANTT). Do not touch access site after antiseptic is applied. Replace when there is a specific clinical indication.	Insertion may require specialized training. Maintain maximum sterile barrier precautions. Replace when there is a specific clinical indication.	Insertion requires specialized training. Avoid femoral site (adults). Maintain maximum sterile barrier precautions; highest risk of central line–associated bloodstream infection. Placement and tip location must be confirmed prior to use. Do not routinely replace. Do not remove on the basis of fever alone; use clinical judgment if infection is suspected. Use clean gloves for removal.	Insertion requires specialized training. Maintain maximum sterile barrier precautions. Placement and tip location must be confirmed prior to use. Do not remove on the basis of fever alone; use clinical judgment if infection is suspected. Use clean gloves for removal.	Perform in interventional radiology (IR) or operating room (OR) under conscious sedation or general anesthesia. Maintain maximum sterile barrier precautions. Placement and tip location must be confirmed prior to use. Do not remove on the basis of fever alone; use clinical judgment if infection is suspected.	Perform in IR or OR under conscious sedation or general anesthesia. Maintain maximum sterile barrier precautions. Placement and tip location must be confirmed prior to use. Do not remove on the basis of fever alone; use clinical judgment if infection is suspected.	Perform in IR or OR under conscious sedation or general anesthesia. Maintain maximum sterile barrier precautions. Placement and tip location must be confirmed prior to use.
Insertion skin preparation	Chlorhexidine gluconate (CHG) 2% is recommended; povidone-iodine or 70% alcohol can be used. Air-dry without fanning.	CHG 2% is recommended; povidone-iodine or 70% alcohol can be used. Air-dry without fanning.	CHG 2% is recommended; povidone-iodine or 70% alcohol can be used. Air-dry without fanning.	CHG 2% is recommended; povidone-iodine or 70% alcohol can be used. Air-dry without fanning.	CHG 2% is recommended; povidone-iodine or 70% alcohol can be used.	CHG 2% is recommended; povidone-iodine or 70% alcohol can be used.	CHG 2% is recommended; povidone-iodine or 70% alcohol can be used.

(Continued on next page)

Appendix 5. Venous Devices (Continued)

Characteristics	Peripheral Intravenous Line	Midline	Central Nontunneled	Peripherally Inserted Central Catheter	Tunneled	Implanted Port	Apheresis
Dressing and securement device change: Sterile transparent	Replace with IV change. Use ANTT. Wear either clean or sterile gloves.	Change 24 hours after insertion and at least every 7 days. Use ANTT. Wear either clean or sterile gloves.	Change 24 hours after insertion and at least every 7 days. Use ANTT. Wear either clean or sterile gloves.	Apply sterile dressing after insertion; change 24 hours after insertion to a transparent dressing and at least every 7 days until healed. Use ANTT. Wear either clean or sterile gloves.	Apply sterile dressing after insertion; change 24 hours after insertion to a transparent dressing and at least every 7 days until healed. No definitive evidence exists regarding necessity for any dressing on a well-healed exit site. Use ANTT. Wear either clean or sterile gloves.	Apply sterile dressing after insertion; change 24 hours after insertion and with needle change (if needle is in place). Use ANTT. Wear either clean or sterile gloves. For continuous access, change noncoring needle and dressing every 7 days or if nonocclusive.	Apply sterile dressing after insertion; change 24 hours after insertion to transparent and at least every 7 days until healed. Short-term catheters: Change at least every 7 days. Long-term catheters: No definitive evidence exists regarding necessity for any dressing on a well-healed exit site. Use ANTT. Wear either clean or sterile gloves.
Dressing and securement device change: Sterile gauze and tape	Every other day (QOD) or PRN if wet, soiled, or nonocclusive. Use ANTT.	QOD or PRN if wet, soiled, or nonocclusive. Use ANTT.	QOD or PRN if wet, soiled, or nonocclusive. Use ANTT.	QOD or PRN if wet, soiled, or nonocclusive. Use ANTT.	QOD or PRN if wet, soiled, or nonocclusive. Use ANTT.	QOD or PRN if wet, soiled, or nonocclusive. Use ANTT.	QOD or PRN if wet, soiled, or nonocclusive. Use ANTT. Exit site may bleed or ooze due to increased stiffness of the catheter.
Flush: 0.9% normal saline (NS)*	Flush 1–3 ml every 8, 12, or 24 hours when not in use, following blood sampling.	Flush 1–3 ml every 8, 12, or 24 hours when not in use, following blood sampling.	Flush 5–10 ml after each use, following blood sampling. May use NS 10 ml every 8 hours.	Flush 5–10 ml after each use; following blood sampling. Valved or closed tip: Flush 5–10 ml daily, QOD, or three times weekly.	Flush 5–10 ml after each use, following blood sampling. Valved or closed tip: Flush 5 ml daily, QOD, three times weekly.	Flush 5–10 ml after each use, following blood sampling. Flush 5 ml every 4–8 weeks if not in use for valved ports.	Flush 5–10 ml after each use.

(Continued on next page)

Appendix 5. Venous Devices (Continued)

Characteristics	Peripheral Intravenous Line	Midline	Central Nontunneled	Peripherally Inserted Central Catheter	Tunneled	Implanted Port	Apheresis
Flush: Heparin	N/A	N/A	Flush 10–100 IU/ml, 2–3 ml/day per lumen. Flush with NS, then heparin lock after use for intermittent infusions.	Flush 10–100 IU/ml, 3 ml/day; 3 ml/day QOD; or three times weekly; per lumen.	Flush 10–100 IU/ml, 3 ml/day; 3 ml QOD; 5 ml three times weekly; or 5 ml weekly; per lumen	Flush 10–100 IU/ml, 5 ml after each use per lumen; and every 4–8 weeks if not in use.	Flush 1,000 IU/ml, 1–2 ml/day after each use or every day.
Needleless connector (more frequently if damaged or signs of blood precipitate)	Replace with catheter change or after each use.	Replace with catheter change or after each use.	Replace after each use.	Replace after each use or weekly (if in use).	Replace after each use or weekly (if in use).	Replace after each use with continuous access. Replace following completion of multiple consecutive infusions.	Replace after each use.
Protective caps	N/A	N/A	Replace every 7 days or if damaged or contaminated.	Replace every 7 days or if damaged or contaminated.	Replace every 7 days or if damaged or contaminated.	N/A	Replace every 7 days or if damaged or contaminated.
Blood sampling	Discard 1 ml; varies due to dead space volume differences in products	Discard 1 ml; varies due to dead space volume differences in products Using midlines for blood specimen sampling remains controversial.	Clamp all lumens not being used for withdrawal; 3–5 ml discard; flush with 10–20 ml NS after sampling.	Clamp all lumens not being used for withdrawal; 3–5 ml discard; flush with 10–20 ml NS after sampling.	Discard 3–5 ml; flush with 10–20 ml NS after sampling.	Discard 3–5 ml; flush with 10–20 ml NS after sampling.	Clamp all lumens not being used for withdrawal; 3–5 ml discard; flush with 10–20 ml NS after sampling.

(Continued on next page)

Appendix 5. Venous Devices *(Continued)*

Characteristics	Peripheral Intravenous Line	Midline	Central Nontunneled	Peripherally Inserted Central Catheter	Tunneled	Implanted Port	Apheresis
Other (See specific chapter for details.)	Not indicated for continuous vesicant therapy or certain solutions	Not indicated for continuous vesicant therapy or certain solutions	Indicated for urgent fluid resuscitation and pressure monitoring	Can be used for all types of IV therapy Do not draw peripheral venipuncture blood samples, obtain blood pressures, or insert a peripheral IV catheter into the ipsilateral limb with a peripherally inserted central catheter.	Can be used for all types of IV therapy	Can be used for all types of IV therapy No recommendation can be made for frequency of replacing needles used for continuous access. Consideration of replacing needle should be evaluated every 7–10 days or if access is compromised. Do not draw peripheral venipuncture blood samples, obtain blood pressures, or insert a peripheral IV catheter into the ipsilateral limb with a peripheral implanted port.	Larger lumens than other venous access devices; if the heparinized saline is not aspirated and discarded prior to use, monitor coagulation levels, as this amount of heparin may lead to therapeutic serum levels.

* Flush with NS after each drug administration. NS volume is dependent on device used (e.g., 2–10 ml).

Appendix 6. Peripheral/Midline Venous Device Competency Documentation		
Skill	**Met**	**Not Met**
A. Preparing the Patient		
1. Explains the procedure to the patient and caregiver		
2. Performs preplacement assessment of the patient		
B. Inserting the Catheter		
1. Washes hands		
2. Organizes equipment		
3. Examines veins on both extremities		
4. Washes hands again; applies gloves. If inserting midline, uses maximum sterile barriers		
5. Applies local anesthetic, if ordered		
6. Applies tourniquet; cleanses site		
7. Stabilizes vein below venipuncture site with nondominant hand		
8. Observes for blood return; advances catheter into vein; pushes catheter off stylet, if used		
9. Releases tourniquet		
10. Occludes tip of catheter by pressing fingers of nondominant hand over vein to prevent retrograde bleeding		
11. Attaches to appropriate device for IV therapy		
12. Secures IV catheter with securement device		
13. Applies occlusive dressing over the insertion site		
14. Discards all equipment appropriately		
15. Washes hands		
16. Documents appropriately		
C. Blood Sampling		
1. Washes hands		
2. Organizes equipment		
3. Applies gloves		
4. Cleans connector with alcohol or chlorhexidine wipe using scrubbing motion and allows to dry		
5. Attaches prefilled syringe of 0.9% normal saline (NS) and checks for blood return using gentle aspiration		
6. Removes at least 1 ml of blood (or twice the catheter and add-on device volume) and discards		
7. Withdraws appropriate amount for laboratory test		
8. Flushes catheter with 1–3 ml NS		
9. Caps the catheter or connects to appropriate solution		
10. Discards all equipment appropriately		
11. Washes hands		
12. Documents appropriately		

(Continued on next page)

Appendix 6. Peripheral/Midline Venous Device Competency Documentation *(Continued)*		
Skill	**Met**	**Not Met**
D. Changing the Needleless Connector		
1. Washes hands		
2. Prepares appropriate equipment		
3. Applies gloves		
4. Changes needleless connector at appropriate frequency		
5. Discards all equipment appropriately		
6. Washes hands		
7. Documents appropriately		
E. Caring for the Insertion Site		
1. Washes hands		
2. Prepares appropriate equipment		
3. Applies gloves		
4. Removes old dressing carefully and discards dressing and gloves		
5. Washes hands		
6. Applies new gloves		
7. Cleanses exit site and allows to dry		
8. Applies appropriate dressing		
9. Discards all equipment appropriately		
10. Washes hands		
11. Labels dressing with date, time, and initials		
12. Documents appropriately		
F. Assessing and Intervening in Catheter Malfunction		
1. Assesses for infusion complications		
2. Is aware of signs and symptoms of phlebitis or infiltration		
3. Reassures the patient and prepares for intervention, if needed		
G. Documenting Findings and Patient Education		
1. Documents all assessment findings and procedures		
2. Evaluates the patient's and caregiver's education and response to teaching, including return demonstration of technical tasks and signs and symptoms of potential complications		

	Appendix 7. Topical Anesthetics		
Type	Application	Comments	Applicable Evidence
Alkane vapo-coolant spray	Spray a light mist onto skin from several inches away; allow to air-dry prior to access or insertion.	Frostbite can occur on excessively used or extremely sensitive skin. Spray evaporates rapidly; therefore, effect is transient.	Comparisons of swabs of chlorhexidine-disinfected/no spray and chlorhexidine-disinfected/applied spray IV insertion sites from 50 patients showed no increased risk of infection when spray is used as an anesthetic prior to peripheral IV cannulation following disinfection. When compared to nondisinfected skin, vapocoolant-treated skin had a significantly decreased colonization; however, it was not sufficient to be used as the sole disinfectant. Similar findings have been reported when compared to application of spray following 70% isopropyl alcohol skin preparation. Comparisons of spray to ice in pediatric patients undergoing IV catheter placement showed more satisfaction with the use of spray, which may have been more effective than ice as an analgesic.
Dry heat	Place dry heated towels wrapped around the extremity; commercial dry hot packs.	Avoid friable skin; no specific time interval is recommended.	Dry heat was found to be successful for pain relief during IV insertions when compared to moist heat. Dry heat resulted in more successful insertions on the first attempt and more comfortable cannulations as compared to moist heat applications.
Intradermal lidocaine (1% lidocaine without epinephrine)	Insert needle bevel up just proximal to intended insertion site.	Needlestick may cause discomfort; may be sensitive to lidocaine. Burning may occur during injection.	Use provided effective pain relief. Comparison of subcutaneous lidocaine to a lidocaine/tetracaine patch showed comparable pain control during arterial catheter insertions; lidocaine caused discomfort during injection. Use of an air-pressured delivery system rather than a needle to administer lidocaine prior to venipuncture resulted in less reported pain in children aged 1–6 years when compared with vapocoolant alone and with vapocoolant plus placebo air injection.
Transcutaneous electrical nerve stimulation (TENS)	Apply to radial side of wrist of dominant forearm 20 minutes before insertion.	Local erythema and itching may occur.	A comparison of an active TENS patient group and a placebo TENS group showed incidence of pain to be similar between the groups, but pain intensity was significantly lower in the active TENS group.
Transdermal cream	Apply thick layer 1–2 hours prior to access or IV insertion. Cover with transparent dressing. Remove completely and cleanse site prior to insertion or access.	Typical preparations are compounds of lidocaine and prilocaine. Local edema, pallor, or erythema may occur.	Cream has been researched in combination with oral paracetamol 40 mg/kg for children prior to one needle insertion; the addition of paracetamol provided no additive effect in reducing fear, distress, or pain when combined with topical anesthesia. A review of 12 clinical trials in pediatric and adult populations revealed nine pediatric and three adult cases of systemic toxicity (e.g., methemoglobinemia, central nervous system toxicity, cardiotoxicity). Factors increasing systemic toxicity risk include excessive dosing of cream, large application surface area, prolonged application time, compromised skin in treatment area, aged < 3 months or premature infant, and concomitant use of a methemoglobin-inducing agent.
Transdermal patch	Apply 20–30 minutes prior to IV insertion or access.	Erythema or edema may occur. Potential exists for systemic toxicity.	Patch may be comprised of tetracaine (4%) or tetracaine (7%) and lidocaine (7%) combination. Comparisons of each compound prove equivalent efficacy in pain management during venous cannulation.

* A provider order is required prior to application of any topical anesthetic.

References

Evans, J.G., Taylor, D.M., Hurren, F., Ward, P., Yeoh, M., & Howden, B.P. (2015). Effects of vapocoolant spray on skin sterility prior to intravenous cannulation. *Journal of Hospital Infection, 90,* 333–337. doi:10.1016/j.jhin.2015.03.010

Hedén, L., von Essen, L., & Ljungman, G. (2014). Effect of high-dose paracetamol on needle procedures in children with cancer: An RCT. *Acta Paediatrica, 103,* 314–319. doi:10.1111/apa.12509

Kiger, T., Knudsen, E.A., Curran, W., Hunter, J., Schaub, A., Williams, M.J., … Kwekkeboom, K. (2014). Survey of heat use during peripheral IV insertion by health care workers. *Journal of Infusion Nursing, 37,* 443–440. doi:10.1097/NAN.0000000000000074

Kim, S., Park, K., Son, B., & Jeon, Y. (2012). The effect of transcutaneous electrical nerve stimulation on pain during venous cannulation. *Current Therapeutic Research: Clinical and Experimental, 73,* 134–139. doi:10.1016/j.curtheres.2012.05.001

Lunoe, M.M., Drendel, A.L., Levas, M.N., Weisman, S.J., Dasgupta, M., Hoffmann, R.G., & Brousseau, D.C. (2015). A randomized clinical trial of jet-injected lidocaine to reduce venipuncture pain for young children. *Annals of Emergency Medicine, 66,* 466–474. doi:10.1016/j.annemergmed.2015.04.003

Mlynek, K., Lyahn, H., Richards, B., Schleicher, W., Bassiri Gharb, B., Procop, G., … Zins, J. (2015). Skin sterility after application of a vapocoolant spray part 2. *Aesthetic Plastic Surgery, 39,* 597–601. doi:10.1007/s00266-015-0509-5

Oman, K.S., Fink, R., Kleiner, C., Makic, M.B., Wenger, B., Hoffecker, L., … Cook, P. (2014). Intradermal lidocaine or bacteriostatic normal saline to decrease pain before intravenous catheter insertion: A meta-analysis. *Journal of Perianesthesia Nursing, 29,* 367–376. doi:10.1016/j.jopan.2013.12.008

Ravishankar, N., Elliot, S.C., Beardow, Z., & Mallick, A. (2012). A comparison of Rapydan® patch and Ametop® gel for venous cannulation. *Anaesthesia, 67,* 367–370. doi:10.1111/j.1365-2044.2011.07000.x

Ruetzler, K., Sima, B., Mayer, L., Golescu, A., Dunkler, D., Jaeger, W., … Hutschala, D. (2012). Lidocaine/tetracaine patch (Rapydan) for topical anesthesia before arterial access: A double-blind, randomized trial. *British Journal of Anesthesia, 109,* 790–796. doi:10.1093/bja/aes254

Tran, A.N., & Koo, J.Y. (2014). Risk of systemic toxicity with topical lidocaine/prilocaine: A review. *Journal of Drugs in Dermatology, 13,* 1118–1122.

Waterhouse, M.R., Liu, D.R., & Wang, V.J. (2013). Cryotherapeutic topical analgesics for pediatric intravenous catheter placement: Ice versus vapocoolant spray. *Pediatric Emergency Care, 29,* 8–12. doi:10.1097/PEC.0b013e31827b214b

Appendix 8. Nontunneled Device Competency Documentation		
Skill	**Met**	**Not Met**
A. Preparing the Patient		
1. Identifies the patient and verifies order for device placement		
2. Explains the procedure to the patient or caregiver		
3. Performs preplacement assessment of the patient		
4. Ensures that informed consent is obtained		
B. Assisting With Device Placement		
1. Administers premedications, as ordered, prior to procedure		
2. Obtains necessary equipment and prepares medications or pump, as ordered		
3. Maintains maximum sterile barrier precautions. Washes hands and applies sterile gloves, sterile gown, mask, and head covering.		
4. Assists the provider with placing line as requested, maintaining strict sterile technique; supports and reassures the patient		
5. Ensures confirmation and proper tip placement prior to use		
6. Evaluates the patient for postinsertion complications		
C. Accessing the Device		
1. Organizes maintenance care to minimize entry into the system		
2. Explains the procedure to the patient		
3. Assembles equipment and washes hands; applies clean gloves		
4. Ensures the catheter is clamped whenever the line is opened; uses only smooth-edged clamps or latex- or plastic-covered clamps		
5. Vigorously scrubs needleless connector with cleansing agent, and attaches syringe with 0.9% normal saline (NS) to flush		
6. Opens clamp, flushes catheter, and verifies positive blood return; then removes syringe and attaches IV tubing directly to catheter hub		
7. If therapy is intermittent IV push, attaches needleless connector using the SASH (saline, administer medication, saline, heparin) method		
D. Blood Sampling (Discard Method)		
1. Explains the procedure to the patient		
2. Washes hands and prepares appropriate equipment		
3. Applies gloves		
4. Removes 3–5 ml of blood and discards		
5. Removes necessary blood for testing		
6. Flushes the catheter with 10–20 ml NS		
7. Heparinizes catheter, if appropriate		

(Continued on next page)

Appendix 8. Nontunneled Device Competency Documentation *(Continued)*		
Skill	**Met**	**Not Met**
E. Changing the Needleless Connector		
1. Explains the procedure to the patient		
2. Washes hands, obtains necessary equipment, then applies gloves		
3. Ensures catheter is clamped		
4. Vigorously scrubs needleless connector with cleansing agent		
5. Scrubs hub, minimizing time catheter is opened		
6. Changes connector at appropriate frequency		
F. Caring for the Exit Site		
1. Explains the procedure to the patient		
2. Washes hands and obtains necessary equipment		
3. Applies gloves		
4. Removes old dressing carefully to minimize tugging on the line		
5. Inspects exit site for erythema, tenderness, edema, exudate, length of catheter protruding from the skin, and integrity of external portion of catheter; removes gloves		
6. Applies new gloves		
7. Cleanses exit site and applies appropriate dressing		
8. Secures tension loop or other securement to avoid catheter dislodgment		
9. Changes dressing at appropriate frequency		
G. Removing the Catheter per Licensing and Institutional Restrictions		
1. Verifies order for catheter removal and indication		
2. Explains the procedure to the patient		
3. Washes hands and assembles necessary equipment		
4. Applies gloves		
5. Removes old dressing and discards		
6. Applies new gloves		
7. Ensures all IV solutions are discontinued		
8. Instructs the patient to perform the Valsalva maneuver		
9. Grasps hub and gently and steadily pulls the catheter out until completely removed		
10. Applies pressure to the exit site until bleeding has stopped		
11. If catheter infection is suspected, ensures tip does not contact any surface, cuts tip off with sterile scissors, and places in a sterile container for culture, if ordered		
12. Applies occlusive dressing over exit site		
13. Measures catheter and compares to inserted length		
14. Inspects catheter for defects or jagged edges suggestive of breakage		

(Continued on next page)

Appendix 8. Nontunneled Device Competency Documentation *(Continued)*		
Skill	**Met**	**Not Met**
15. If length or appearance warrant, notifies healthcare provider and preserves line		
H. Assessing and Intervening in Catheter Malfunction		
1. Differentiates between infusion complications, fibrin sheath formation, catheter kinkage, and catheter malposition		
2. Is aware of signs and symptoms of infection		
3. Obtains order for necessary flush medications, as required (e.g., tissue plasminogen activator)		
4. Reassures the patient and prepares for diagnostic procedures, as indicated		
I. Documenting Findings and Patient Education		
1. Documents all assessment findings and procedures		
2. Evaluates the patient's and caregiver's education and response to teaching, including return demonstration of technical tasks and signs and symptoms of potential complications		

Appendix 9. Peripherally Inserted Central Catheter, Tunneled, and Apheresis (Long-Term) Venous Device Competency Documentation		
Skill	**Met**	**Not Met**
A. Preparing the Patient		
1. Explains the procedure to the patient and caregiver		
2. Performs preaccess assessment of the patient and catheter		
3. Ensures that informed consent is obtained		
4. Confirms catheter placement prior to use		
B. Accessing the Long-Term Venous Device		
1. Organizes catheter care to minimize entry into the system		
2. Maintains a strict aseptic technique		
3. Never leaves catheter open to air		
4. Uses only smooth-edged clamps or latex- or plastic-covered clamps, as appropriate		
5. Uses securement device to stabilize		
6. Washes hands		
7. Prepares appropriate equipment		
8. Applies gloves		
9. Cleanses the needleless connector vigorously; accesses catheter		
10. Flushes the catheter at appropriate frequency		
C. Infusing Fluids or Medications		
1. States appropriate medications/fluids and rates of infusion for device		
2. States two possible complications and appropriate interventions, as appropriate, for medication or fluid infused		
D. Blood Sampling (Discard Method)		
1. Follows procedure for accessing system		
2. Removes at least 3–5 ml of blood or solution and discards		
3. Clamps the catheter at appropriate times		
4. Withdraws the desired amount of blood		
5. Flushes the catheter with 10–20 ml of 0.9% normal saline after blood withdrawal		
E. Changing the Needleless Connector		
1. Washes hands		
2. Prepares appropriate equipment		
3. Applies gloves		
4. Cleanses catheter and applies connector using aseptic technique		
5. Changes connector at appropriate frequency		

(Continued on next page)

Appendix 9. Peripherally Inserted Central Catheter, Tunneled, and Apheresis (Long-Term) Venous Device Competency Documentation *(Continued)*		
Skill	**Met**	**Not Met**
F. Caring for the Exit Site		
1. Washes hands		
2. Prepares appropriate equipment		
3. Applies gloves		
4. Carefully removes old dressing		
5. Inspects exit site		
6. Removes gloves		
7. Applies new gloves		
8. Cleanses exit site		
9. Applies appropriate dressing		
G. Assessing and Intervening in Catheter Malfunction		
1. Differentiates between infusion complications, fibrin sheath formation, catheter kinkage, and catheter migration		
2. Is aware of signs and symptoms of infection		
3. Obtains an order for necessary flush medications, as required (e.g., tissue plasminogen activator)		
4. Reassures the patient and prepares for diagnostic procedures, as indicated		
H. Documenting Findings and Patient Education		
1. Documents all assessment findings and procedures		
2. Evaluates the patient's and caregiver's education and response to teaching, including return demonstration of technical tasks and signs and symptoms of potential complications		

Appendix 10. Implanted Port Device Competency Documentation		
Skill	**Met**	**Not Met**
A. Preparing the Patient		
1. Explains the procedure to the patient and caregiver		
2. Performs preplacement assessment of the patient		
3. Ensures that informed consent is obtained		
4. Confirms catheter placement prior to use		
B. Accessing the Implanted Port		
1. Explains the procedure to the patient		
2. Washes hands and obtains necessary equipment		
3. Chooses appropriate size and length of noncoring needle for therapy planned		
4. Applies gloves		
5. Removes dressing, if appropriate		
6. Palpates port and locates center of septum to be accessed		
7. Observes site for edema; erythema; tenderness; condition of the port pocket; or swelling of ipsilateral chest, neck veins, or extremity		
8. Discards used gloves and reapplies new gloves; applies topical anesthetic, if ordered		
9. Cleanses the area over the septum		
10. Grasps the edges of the portal body firmly through the skin to stabilize, pushing the noncoring needle firmly through the skin and diaphragm, and stopping when the bottom of the reservoir is reached		
11. Flushes saline into the port and checks for blood return		
12. Applies appropriate dressing		
13. Attaches IV tubing to the catheter hub if continuous infusion		
14. Attaches needleless connector if intermittent infusion is planned		
15. If continuous infusion, evaluates need to change noncoring needle every 7–10 days or when access is compromised		
C. Flushing an Implanted Port		
1. Explains the procedure to the patient		
2. Washes hands and assembles necessary equipment		
3. If port is not accessed, accesses per procedure		
4. Vigorously flushes catheter using pulsatile technique with 10–20 ml 0.9% normal saline for valved catheters and heparin lock flush for open-ended catheters		
5. If port does not need to be used, deaccesses per procedure		
6. Accesses and flushes port every four to eight weeks when not in use		
D. Deaccessing an Implanted Port		
1. Explains the procedure to the patient		
2. Washes hands and assembles necessary equipment		

(Continued on next page)

Appendix 10. Implanted Port Device Competency Documentation *(Continued)*		
Skill	**Met**	**Not Met**
3. Applies gloves and removes dressing		
4. Discards used gloves and reapplies new gloves		
5. Stabilizes port through skin with one hand, grasps noncoring needle wings or hub with the other hand, and administers flush		
6. While instilling the final 1 ml of flushing solution, simultaneously pulls the needle from the port septum, pushing down on the port edges to prevent tugging the port upward		
7. Applies pressure over the needle exit site, and then applies appropriate dressing, if needed		
E. Blood Sampling From an Implanted Port		
1. Explains the procedure to the patient		
2. Washes hands and assembles necessary equipment		
3. Accesses port per procedure if not accessed		
4. Removes at least 3–5 ml of blood and discards		
5. Removes necessary blood for testing		
6. Flushes the catheter per procedure and either continues infusion, replaces connector, or deaccesses per procedure		
F. Assessing and Intervening in Catheter Malfunction		
1. Differentiates between infusion complications, fibrin sheath formation, catheter kinkage, and catheter migration		
2. Is aware of signs and symptoms of infection		
3. Obtains an order for necessary flush medications, as required (e.g., tissue plasminogen activator)		
4. Reassures the patient and prepares for diagnostic procedures, as indicated		
G. Documenting Findings and Patient Education		
1. Documents all assessment findings and procedures		
2. Evaluates the patient's and caregiver's education and response to teaching, including return demonstration of technical tasks and signs and symptoms of potential complications		

Appendix 11. Hepatic Arterial Infusion Pump Device Competency Documentation		
Skill	**Met**	**Not Met**
A. Preparing the Patient		
1. Assesses the patient's knowledge regarding pump; explains the procedure to the patient and caregiver		
2. Reviews pertinent laboratory values		
3. Provides the patient privacy		
4. Washes hands		
5. Assesses the patient for signs and symptoms of infection over pump location		
6. Palpates pump location, including estimate of refill chamber septum location		
7. Assesses for signs and symptoms of pump complications, such as hematoma, pump pocket infection, flipped pump, malpositioned catheter (e.g., indigestion, abdominal pain)		
B. Refilling Procedure		
1. Washes hands		
2. Maintains maximum sterile barrier precautions, establishes sterile field, applies sterile gloves and mask, assembles supplies, and then verifies that needle is correct for refill procedure		
3. Connects the needle to the extension tubing in kit, attaches extension tubing to stopcock, and then attaches stopcock to empty sterile syringe provided in kit		
4. Cleanses site with an antiseptic, allows to air-dry, and then removes gloves		
5. Applies a new pair of sterile gloves		
6. Repalpates pump and locates refill chamber septum		
7. Inserts noncoring needle perpendicular into the port septum		
8. Advances needle until it comes into contact with the needlestop		
9. Allows the pump to empty into the syringe and does not aspirate		
10. Closes stopcock		
11. Notes amount in syringe		
12. Leaves needle in place and disconnects syringe		
13. Connects new syringe with medication		
14. Opens stopcock		
15. Confirms that needle is still in place by injecting 5 ml of medication in the syringe, releasing pressure on the syringe, and then allowing the 5 ml of fluid to return in the syringe		
16. Keeps downward pressure on the needle and syringe and injects medication into the pump, checking placement every 5 ml until the syringe is empty		
17. Closes stopcock and removes needle		
18. Applies appropriate dressing		
19. Discards syringe and any other contaminated supplies into appropriate waste containers		

(Continued on next page)

Appendix 11. Hepatic Arterial Infusion Pump Device Competency Documentation *(Continued)*		
Skill	**Met**	**Not Met**
C. Assessing and Intervening in Pump Malfunction		
1. Differentiates between inflow and outflow problems, fibrin sheath formation, catheter kinkage, and catheter migration		
2. Is aware of signs and symptoms of chemical versus bacterial infection		
3. Reassures the patient and prepares for diagnostic procedures, as indicated		
D. Documenting Findings and Patient Education		
1. Documents all assessment findings and procedures		
2. Evaluates the patient's and caregiver's education and response to teaching, including return demonstration of technical tasks and signs and symptoms of potential complications		

Appendix 12. Specialty Devices

Procedure	Arterial	Intraventricular	Epidural and Intrathecal	Implanted Intraperitoneal Port	Intraperitoneal: External/Tunneled	Pleural
Short or long term	Arterial ports: Similar to venous ports. Hepatic artery infusion pumps: For longer-term treatment. Percutaneous catheter: For short-term therapy	Also known as an Ommaya® reservoir. Long-term use	External, percutaneous or short-tunneled (short term): For hours to days; exit site in lower back. External, percutaneous or short-tunneled (long term): Exit site in abdomen. Implanted port: Similar to venous ports; contain filters; for long-term therapy. Implanted pump with attached epidural or intrathecal catheter: Long-term therapy	Semipermanent for repeated access	Onetime access (paracentesis) or semipermanent for repeated access (tunneled)	Short term (chest tubes) or long term (indwelling). Include large-bore, "pigtail" nontunneled (chest tubes), and tunneled valved (indwelling) catheters
Insertion and replacement or removal considerations	Placed by trained provider • Short term: interventional radiology (IR) • Port: IR or operating room (OR) • Pump: In IR or OR. Maximum sterile barrier precautions. Short-term catheters can be removed at the bedside or in IR by trained and credentialed individuals.	Placed by trained provider; performed in OR. Reservoir implanted subcutaneously under scalp; catheter threaded through burr hole into ventricle. Maximum sterile barrier precautions. Rarely removed unless malfunction or infection occurs	Placed by trained provider; performed in IR, OR if tunneled, implanted port, or implanted pump; may be placed at bedside if percutaneous. Maximum sterile barrier precautions for all procedures. Temporary catheters can be removed directly using sterile technique at bedside. Ports and pumps are removed in the OR.	Placed by trained physicians; performed in IR or OR. Maximum sterile barrier precautions. Typically removed in IR or OR	Placed by trained provider; performed in IR or OR. Maximum sterile barrier precautions. Not routinely changed unless obstruction or infection occurs. External tunneled catheters can be removed in IR, OR, or bedside under local anesthesia.	Placed by trained provider; performed in IR, OR, or bedside if short term. Maximum sterile barrier precautions. Not routinely changed unless obstruction or infection occurs; short-term chest tubes typically removed within one week; indwelling (tunneled) catheters can remain indefinitely.

(Continued on next page)

Appendix 12. Specialty Devices (Continued)

Procedure	Arterial	Intraventricular	Epidural and Intrathecal	Implanted Intraperitoneal Port	Intraperitoneal: External/Tunneled	Pleural
Aseptic versus sterile access	Requires specialized training and credentialing to access Maximum sterile barrier precautions	Requires specialized training and credentialing to access Maximum sterile barrier precautions No definitive recommendation regarding time interval between placement and first access (reported first day of surgery or delayed up to several days following surgery)	Requires specialized training and credentialing to access Maximum sterile barrier precautions Alcohol cleansing contraindicated; use chlorhexidine and air-dry completely. Povidone-iodine can be used.	May require specialized training and credentialing to access Maximum sterile barrier precautions	May require specialized training and credentialing to access Maximum sterile barrier precautions	May require specialized training and credentialing to access Maximum sterile barrier precautions Pleural fluid typically drained every one to two days
Flush	Short and long term: • No definitive recommendation can be made regarding the frequency or volume of flushing. • During periods where chemotherapy is not infusing, heparinized solution may be ordered as a continuous infusion to maintain patency. • Volume, concentration, and frequency varies; no evidence to support a particular volume or concentration. • Literature reports use of heparin solution 1,000–5,000 IU/ml, 1–3 ml every 8 hours daily to maintain patency. • Port: Heparinized saline (100–1,000 IU/ml), 2–5 ml every week • Pump: Glycerin or 0.9% normal saline (NS) or heparinized saline; volume dependent on pump type	Maintenance flushing not required	Catheter: 1–2 ml preservative-free NS after use Port: 3 ml preservative-free NS after use Routine flushing not needed for ports or catheters Pump: Maintenance flushing not required	20 ml NS pre- and postadministration; use of heparinized solution flush after NS remains controversial.	20 ml NS pre- and postadministration; use of heparinized solution flush after NS remains controversial.	Small-bore tunneled catheters (to dislodge clots or debris): Use 30 ml NS every 6–8 hours.

(Continued on next page)

Appendix 12. Specialty Devices (Continued)

Procedure	Arterial	Intraventricular	Epidural and Intrathecal	Implanted Intraperitoneal Port	Intraperitoneal: External/Tunneled	Pleural
Dressing and securement device change	Change dressing 24 hours after insertion. Sterile occlusive dressing, as indicated. Use securement device and tension loop to prevent needle dislodgment, as indicated.	Occlusive sterile dressing for at least 24 hours, then gauze and tape for several days. No dressing required when healed. Sterile dressing applied following access and administration of medications	Occlusive sterile dressing with securement device or tension loop if external catheter. Use of chlorhexidine-impregnated dressing or sponge recommended	Occlusive sterile dressing with securement device or tension loop; keep in place postoperatively 24 hours, unless soiled. Apply sterile occlusive pressure dressing after the access needle is removed. Dressing not required if not in use	Occlusive sterile dressing with securement device or tension loop; keep in place postoperatively 24 hours, unless soiled. Change three times a week, or up to 7 days. Apply sterile occlusive dressing after the access needle is removed.	Occlusive with securement device or tension loop; observe sterile technique. Change dressing if wet, soiled, or nonocclusive. Use split 4 × 4 sterile gauze around exit site; apply a second sterile occlusive dressing over split 4 × 4. Change gauze-only dressings every 48 hours; change sterile occlusive dressing at least weekly.
Needleless connector	Change after each use, or weekly if not in continuous use.	N/A	Change after each use, or weekly if not in continuous use.	N/A	Change after each use, or weekly if not in continuous use.	Indwelling: Change after each use, or weekly if not in continuous use.
Unique care	Avoid blood pressure monitoring in the ipsilateral limb. Ensure proper labeling of the line on the tubing near the hub. Blood sampling (short term): No definitive recommendation can be made regarding blood sampling from short-term percutaneous arterial catheters. Blood sampling (long term) and ports: Avoid routine blood sampling through a long-term catheter.	Inspect the reservoir for signs of infection prior to access. Keep the patient semirecumbent for at least 30 minutes after medication administration.	Inspect through intact dressing for drainage, erythema, and edema at least daily. Ensure proper labeling of line "epidural" or "intrathecal" on the tubing near the hub. Use a 0.2 micron filter with all epidural and intrathecal infusions, unless the drug is filtered prior to administration or if the port or pump body contains a filter. Change the filter if damaged, leaking, and when tubing is changed. Use specialized tubing to prevent medication administration errors.	Inspect port location for signs of infection prior to access. Ensure proper labeling of the line on the tubing near the hub.	For palliative management of ascites, after first 14 days using sterile technique, the patient and caregiver can be taught to use an aseptic no-touch technique to drain. Ensure proper labeling of line on the tubing near the hub.	Inspect through intact dressing for tenderness, crepitus, or subcutaneous empyema at least daily. Do not strip tubes due to creation of high negative intraluminal pressure. "Milk" tubes gently to dislodge debris or clots, if needed. Do not use petroleum gauze. Ensure proper labeling of line on the tubing near the hub.

Appendix 13. Intraperitoneal Device Competency Documentation		
Skill	**Met**	**Not Met**
A. Preparing the Patient		
1. Explains procedure with the patient and caregiver		
2. Performs preplacement assessment of the patient		
3. Ensures inform consent is obtained		
4. Requests that the patient void before starting procedure		
B. Assisting With Device Placement		
1. Reviews procedure with the patient and caregiver, if present		
2. Performs preoperative assessment and checklist prior to placement; ensures performance of time out in compliance with universal protocol to verify correct patient, site, and procedure		
3. Performs postoperative assessment of the patient, catheter, and surrounding skin		
4. Initiates and reviews patient education (home care)		
5. Confirms proper catheter placement prior to use		
C. Accessing the Intraperitoneal Port		
1. Washes hands and assembles supplies		
2. Locates port site and applies topical anesthetic cream, if ordered		
3. Maintains maximum sterile barrier precautions, establishes sterile field, applies sterile gloves and mask, and assembles supplies (see Appendix 10 for port access)		
4. Is aware that a blood return is not expected as the catheter is not in a vein		
5. Attempts to withdraw peritoneal fluid, if ordered; if unable to obtain fluid, flushes catheter with 0.9% normal saline (NS)		
6. If flush is successful, attaches infusion tubing or connector		
7. If resistance is felt with flushing or if swelling or pain occurs, discontinues procedure and reaccesses using new sterile equipment; if resistance is felt again and it is certain that needle is in right place, discontinues procedure and notifies the provider		
8. Uses securement device or tension loop to minimize tension on the needle		
9. Encourages the patient to stay in bed during infusion, dwell, and drain time to minimize potential for needle dislodgment		
D. Accessing the External Peritoneal Catheter		
1. Washes hands, maintains maximum sterile barrier precautions, establishes sterile field, applies sterile gloves and mask, and assembles supplies		
2. Explains procedure to the patient and ensures privacy		
3. Primes intraperitoneal tubing with NS		
4. Opens supplies onto sterile field; dons sterile mask		
5. Puts on one sterile glove, usually on dominant hand		
6. Picks up sterile syringe in gloved hand and saline in nongloved hand, drawing up 20 ml NS		
7. Drops syringe onto sterile field and puts on second sterile glove		

(Continued on next page)

Appendix 13. Intraperitoneal Device Competency Documentation *(Continued)*		
Skill	**Met**	**Not Met**
8. Cleans catheter and connector with chlorhexidine swab and allows to air-dry		
9. Maintains aseptic technique when disconnecting connector, attaches NS syringe, and flushes system to ensure patency		
10. Withdraws peritoneal fluid for sample, if ordered		
11. Attaches infusion tubing and applies dressing if infusion is ordered		
12. Uses securement device or tension loop to minimize tension on the needle		
13. For palliative drainage of ascites, aseptically attaches drainage bag and allows fluid to drain, controlling rate with roller clamp to prevent the patient from experiencing adverse effects		
14. Assesses the patient's tolerance of the procedure		
15. Clamps catheter per device, detaches drainage bag and tubing, places new connector aseptically on catheter, and disposes of fluid and tubing properly		
16. Ensures that dressing is changed three times a week and catheter cap and clamp are changed once a week		
17. Documents procedure, assessment of site, size of needle, appearance and amount of peritoneal fluid, and the patient's response pre-, peri-, and post-treatment		
E. Dressing the Peritoneal Catheter (External or Implanted)		
1. Changes dressing 24 hours postoperatively or with excess soiling; changes dressings three times a week for an external catheter; is aware that implanted port does not require dressing changes when not in use		
2. Assembles necessary supplies and washes hands; maintains maximum sterile barrier precautions		
3. Explains the procedure to the patient and ensures privacy		
4. Dons nonsterile gloves and removes old dressing, being careful not to touch exit site or needle		
5. Assesses the site for infection or leakage		
6. Opens all supplies and puts on sterile gloves		
7. Cleans around catheter with chlorhexidine swab, working in a circular motion from the catheter outward and being careful not to go over the same area twice; repeats procedure three times		
8. Allows antiseptic to air-dry		
9. Applies sterile occlusive dressing		
10. Disposes of waste in a hazardous waste container		
F. Discontinuing Intraperitoneal Therapy		
1. Allows intraperitoneal treatment to dwell for the amount of time specified by the provider order		
2. Drains fluid into sterile peritoneal drainage bag by opening clamp, or allows fluid to be absorbed, as ordered		
3. Washes hands, maintains maximum sterile barrier precautions, establishes sterile field, applies sterile gloves and mask, and assembles supplies		
4. Removes old dressing, discards properly, and assesses exit site		
5. For implantable port, removes the needle; cleanses exit-site area as described for accessing the device; applies pressure to exit site with sterile 2 × 2 gauze to prevent leakage; and applies sterile occlusive dressing		

(Continued on next page)

Appendix 13. Intraperitoneal Device Competency Documentation *(Continued)*		
Skill	**Met**	**Not Met**
6. For external catheter, removes old dressing and cleanses exit site, catheter, and connector as described for accessing device		
7. Applies sterile occlusive dressing to exit site		
8. Is aware that the external catheter dressing should be changed three times a week or more often if soiled		
9. Documents the patient's response to the treatment and procedure		
10. Disposes of all tubing and supplies into appropriate hazardous waste container		
G. Assessing and Intervening in Catheter Malfunction		
1. Differentiates between inflow and outflow problem, fibrin sheath formation, catheter kinking, and catheter migration		
2. Is aware of signs and symptoms of chemical versus bacterial peritonitis and exit-site versus tunnel-site infection		
3. Obtains orders for necessary flush medications, if appropriate		
4. Reassures the patient and prepares for the diagnostic procedure to determine the cause of the problem, if applicable		
H. Documenting Findings and Patient Education		
1. Documents all assessment findings and procedures		
2. Evaluates the patient's and caregiver's education and response to teaching, including return demonstration of technical tasks and signs and symptoms of potential complications		
3. Refers to an outside agency if the patient and family need additional assistance or education		

Appendix 14. Pleural Device Competency Documentation		
Skill	**Met**	**Not Met**
A. Preparing the Patient		
1. Explains the procedure to the patient and caregiver		
2. Performs a preplacement assessment of the patient		
3. Ensures informed consent is obtained		
B. Assisting With Device Placement		
1. Administers analgesic premedications, as ordered		
2. Obtains necessary equipment and prepares medications and treatment, as ordered		
3. Washes hands, maintains maximum sterile barrier precautions, establishes sterile field, applies sterile gloves and mask, and assembles supplies		
4. Ensures performance of time out in compliance with universal protocol to verify correct patient, correct site, and correct procedure		
5. Assists the provider in placing the catheter as requested, maintaining sterile technique; supports and reassures the patient		
6. Confirms proper catheter placement prior to use		
7. Evaluates the patient for postinsertion complications		
C. Assisting With Intrapleural Drug Administration		
1. Washes hands		
2. Obtains necessary equipment and prepares medications and treatment, as ordered		
3. Maintains maximum sterile barrier precautions, establishes sterile field, applies sterile gloves and mask, and assembles supplies		
4. Assists the provider with removing pleural catheter dressing and drainage of pleural cavity, as appropriate		
5. Ensures that the pleural catheter tube is clamped		
6. Assists the provider with preparing and disinfecting catheter access site		
7. After instillation of medication or treatment, ensures that the tubing or catheter is clamped to allow ordered dwell time		
8. Following ordered dwell time, unclamps the catheter or tubing and allows fluid to drain by gravity		
9. After drainage, disconnects the tubing and discards all equipment appropriately		
10. Washes hands		
11. Documents appropriately in the patient's medical record		
D. Changing the Dressing and Caring for the Insertion Site		
1. Washes hands		
2. Prepares appropriate equipment		
3. Applies clean, nonsterile gloves		
4. Removes old dressing carefully and discards dressing and gloves		

(Continued on next page)

Appendix 14. Pleural Device Competency Documentation *(Continued)*		
Skill	**Met**	**Not Met**
5. Washes hands; maintains maximum sterile barrier precautions		
6. Applies new sterile gloves		
7. Cleanses exit site and allows to dry		
8. Applies appropriate occlusive dressing; includes securement device and tension loop		
9. Discards all equipment appropriately		
10. Washes hands		
11. Labels dressing with date, time, and initials		
12. Documents appropriately in the patient's medical record		
E. Assessing and Intervening in Catheter Malfunction		
1. Differentiates between inflow and outflow problem, fibrin sheath formation, catheter kinking, and catheter migration		
2. Is aware of signs and symptoms of chemical versus bacterial and exit-site versus tunnel-site infection		
3. Obtains orders for necessary flush medications, if appropriate		
4. Reassures the patient and prepares for diagnostic procedure to determine cause of problem, if applicable		
F. Documenting Findings and Patient Education		
1. Documents all assessment findings and procedures		
2. Evaluates the patient's and caregiver's education and response to teaching, including return demonstration of technical tasks and signs and symptoms of potential complications		

Index

The letter f after a page number indicates that relevant content appears in a figure; the letter t, in a table.